Praise for *Beyond th…*

"There is no better guide to 'the dilemma… than Jens Brockmeier. This carefully craf… spirit of Mnemosyne, the goddess of mem… once philosophical, artistic and scientific, bringing together the likes of Marcel Proust, Ansel Kiefer, and Isaac Newton, as well as the most recent neurological research on the human brain. Long after finishing the last page, ideas linger and certain passages beckon the reader back into this exciting world of a universe with an 'infinite multitude of clocks'. *Beyond the Archive* is a true gift for anyone interested in this most fundamental question about the role of memory in human lives."

Molly Andrews, *Professor of Political Psychology and Co-director, Centre for Narrative Research, University of East London*

"In *Beyond the Archive*, Jens Brockmeier masterfully evaluates the limits of traditional approaches to the study of memory. He furthers his argument by insightfully probing the ways in which narrative approaches can enhance our understanding of people's efforts to make sense of the past and thereby ground both their individual and collective identity. Covering a daunting range of literature, from the humanities through the social sciences to the cognitive and neurosciences, Brockmeier's book provides a strong foundation on which to build new approaches to the study of memory."

William Hirst, *Malcolm B. Smith Professor of Psychology, New School for Social Research*

"A large-minded re-envisaging of memory built on an unrivalled depth of learning in cognitive neuroscience, history of ideas and narrative studies… A superb interdisciplinary synthesis that reconceptualises autobiographical meaning as acts of remembering and self-interpretation in the context of cultural memory."

Brian Hurwitz, *Professor of Medicine and the Arts, Director of the Centre for the Humanities and Health, King's College London*

"In this profoundly learned and beautifully written book, Brockmeier draws on Vygotsky and Wittgenstein to debunk the idea that memories are somehow stored in the brain's archive. His skilful and extended argument for seeing remembering instead as a narrative practice embedded in contexts of everyday social life is both exciting and persuasive."

Hilde Lindemann, *Professor of Philosophy, Michigan State University*

"Jens Brockmeier has invented a new field of inquiry. Transcending memory studies, autobiographical theory, neurocognitive science, and narratology, *Beyond the Archive* creates the possibility to imagine and then perceive the real. Memory becomes a living thing almost as human as those who exercise it, while narrative releases those who experience and then remember or forget from the meaninglessness of untold lives. This is a book, above all, about freedom. It is a necessary book."

Rita Charon, *Director of the Program in Narrative Medicine,*
Columbia University

"Distilling decades of work on some of the most foundational questions in the field, *Beyond the Archive* uses a range of resonant case studies to demonstrate the advantages of moving from models of memory based on concepts of storage and retrieval to narrative-oriented models. Even as it draws on state-of-the-art research to develop its argument, this elegantly written book invites the widest possible readership to take part in ongoing discussions about the nature of memory and how best to investigate it."

David Herman, *Professor, Department of English Studies,*
Durham University

"Brockmeier's case for understanding autobiographical remembering—or the 'autobiographical process'—in terms of narrative is based on both an impressively wide-ranging reading of research in psychology and neuroscience, the social sciences, and the humanities and on a close reading of a number of key works of literature, and researchers interested in the concept of memory stand to profit by engaging with it, regardless of their disciplinary homes."

Kourken Michaelian, *Memory Studies 9 (3)*

"Brockmeier's elegantly written new book represents an important and much needed contribution to the interdisciplinary field of memory studies. It is significant because it does not just bring together research from the neurosciences, social sciences, and humanities, but also constitutes one of the first attempts at genuine integration—something that has rarely been done before."

Lucas M. Bietti, *Forum Qualitative Social Research 17(3)*

BEYOND THE ARCHIVE

*Memory, Narrative, and the
Autobiographical Process*

Jens Brockmeier

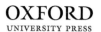

OXFORD
UNIVERSITY PRESS

Oxford University Press is a department of the University of Oxford. It furthers
the University's objective of excellence in research, scholarship, and education
by publishing worldwide. Oxford is a registered trade mark of Oxford University
Press in the UK and certain other countries.

Published in the United States of America by Oxford University Press
198 Madison Avenue, New York, NY 10016, United States of America.

Library of Congress Cataloging-in-Publication Data
Brockmeier, Jens.
Beyond the archive : memory, narrative, and the autobiographical process / Jens Brockmeier.
pages cm. — (Explorations in narrative psychology)
Includes bibliographical references and index.
ISBN 978–0–19–986156–9 (hardcover); 978–0–19–091362–5 (paperback)
1. Memory.   2. Autobiography.   3. Identity (Psychology)   4. Narration
(Rhetoric)   I. Title.
BF371.B747 2015
153.1′2—dc23
2015003217

CONTENTS

PREFACE

We are what we remember about ourselves. We are our memory. It is our memory that makes us human. Everybody knows these claims—commonplaces that pass by easily. More difficult, however, is to give a similarly succinct answer to the question: what *is* our memory? This book argues that it has never been so difficult to answer this question as in the present time. It makes the case that our longstanding view of memory and remembering, the concise and straightforward answer that countless earlier generations would have come up with without much pondering is in the midst of a profound transformation. This transformation does not just affect our concept of memory or a particular idea of how we remember and forget. It is a wider cultural transformation, and in order to understand it we need to step back and observe from a historical perspective what is meant when we say "memory." To offer such a perspective is one of my main concerns because it will help undergird what I suggest: to radically rethink our very idea of memory, to challenge the notion of remembering and forgetting that we have come to take for granted.

Because remembering takes place in many different environments—involving a variety of senses, mental capacities, activities, artifacts, media, and cultural practices—it is a subject of study and reflection in many disciplines. More than this, it is a subject and sometimes even a method of literature and the arts. Do all of them mean the same thing by "memory"? Not surprisingly, they do not. The book, therefore, begins with a cross-disciplinary survey of the arguably most important areas of present memory studies. I distinguish four fields of research and knowledge on remembering, and examine developments in each of them. What are these four fields? One is that of psychology and the neurosciences, the second is concerned with social and cultural memory studies, the third is closely connected with new memory technologies that have emerged in the wake and as part of the digital revolution. The fourth field is made up of literary, artistic, and, specifically, narrative explorations of human remembering and forgetting; that is to say, it centers on autobiographical remembering and its interplay with culture and what is called narrative identity. The complex and contradictory gestalt of narrative identity will also take center stage in the novel vision of the autobiographical process that I present, drawing on the developments in these four fields.

Before getting there, I take a closer look at the new insights and perspectives that have emerged in these various fields over the last decades. Thereby, an overarching trend becomes visible. This trend has taken on the dynamic of a fully fleshed cultural paradigm shift in that it calls into question the venerable notion of memory as a storehouse, an archive of the past. The power of this notion and its lasting presence in our lives cannot be overestimated. Sedimented in Western philosophy, literature, art, and everyday life, indeed even in the sciences, it has shaped the idea of memory for centuries and millennia. The conviction that memory is a kind of archive of past experiences and knowledge goes hand in hand with the assumption that there is a distinctive naturally and, that is, biologically given human capacity or faculty that enables us to remember. This faculty empowers us to encode, store, and retrieve (or recall) the past, to use the technical vocabulary of modern scientific memory research.

This, however, is only one part of the story of how our idea of memory is transforming. The other is about the emergent space for novel ways of imagining, conceptualizing, and studying memory that the decline of the explanatory force of the archival model has opened up. This is where the real action is, where the new happens, where the focus of this book is.

With the traditional notion losing its hold on the cultural imaginary, a number of alternatives have emerged. And more are in the offing. Many of the new conceptions lay out scenarios of remembering and forgetting that are indeed different; they envision them as constructive and reconstructive events, as ongoing, open, and creative processes that have as much to do with the present and the future as with the past. In this light, remembering appears as part and parcel of social activities, as a cultural form of life. This is in stark contrast to the dominant view of earlier times, still widespread today, that confines memory to one individual and, even more, to one of his or hers biological organs, the brain, and, even further, to some specific parts or neuronal operations of it.

I outline several of these alternative models and metaphors of remembering, tracing their imaginative scope. But first and foremost I limit myself to one option, one of the possible alternatives. I call it the narrative option. To explore this approach I concentrate on one area of remembering: autobiographical. Here the narrative approach proves to be especially appropriate because narrative is a human being's most important mode of autobiographical meaning-making. It is the language of our identity. In a number of case studies I show that it is in such meaning constructions where the overarching dynamic of the autobiographical process is unfolded. This dynamic permeates the entire autobiographical process and, in this way, entangles several aspects that traditionally are taken to be separate: the very act of recall, its interpretation, the interplay with an individual's sense of self and identity, and the larger social and cultural context in which all of this takes place. To explain the narrative approach is my second main concern in this book.

Of course, this raises the question as to what is meant by narrative. Synthesizing traditions of research and scholarship in narrative and literary theory, psychology, neuroscience, and philosophy, I put to the test an understanding of narrative that differs from traditional concepts of narration and story. It builds on the fact that not only memory but also narrative is a cross-disciplinary phenomenon, not to mention narrative identity. Narrative, like remembering, involves a variety of senses and mental capacities; it is embodied in a broad range of media and semiotic environments; and it is a socially embedded, cultural practice. In order to resonate and comply with such diversity, my examination of the narrative fabric of the autobiographical process draws on multiple kinds of case studies and other evidentiary materials. Reflecting today's larger media ecology, the spectrum includes interview-based life stories, spontaneous autobiographical narratives in dialogical face-to-face contexts, digital environments, literary narratives, texts that reject the borderline between fictive and factual storytelling (among others, by including documentary photographs as narrative elements), and a sculpture or, perhaps more precisely, an installation.

In all this diversity, what interests me most is how studying the narrative weave of autobiographical processes allows us to understand their fundamentally interpretive, dialogical, and self-reflexive dynamic. What is more, it enables us to comprehend how we localize ourselves—through the autobiographical process—in a cultural world. Such understanding presupposes and advances a postarchival approach to remembering and forgetting, that is, the narrative approach that I set out to explore in this book.

To conclude these remarks, I want to emphasize one more consideration that runs through all the chapters. In elaborating a view of narrative as a particular mode of construing and understanding meaning—I describe this view in terms of a narrative hermeneutics—I want to point out that the study of narrative, the study of mind and memory, and the study of the cultural fabric that weaves them together have a lot in common. They can build on, inform, and enrich one another because they all strive to understand how we bestow meaning to our being in the world. This question is perhaps the most challenging of all.

ACKNOWLEDGMENTS

This project developed out of a number of seminars and talks on auto-biographical memory as a cultural form and practice that I gave in the Columbia University Seminar series *Beyond History and Memory*, organized under the auspices of the Carnegie Council on Ethics and International Affairs, and at The New School, New York, in 2004 and 2005. In 2007, first drafts of some parts were presented in a series of lectures delivered in the United Kingdom at the University of Sheffield, where I was the Marie Curie Senior Research Fellow of the EU-sponsored Research Programme *Memory/Memoir*, and at the Centre for Narrative Research of the University of East London, where I was a Visiting Senior Fellow from 2006 to 2014. A research stay as Visiting Professor at the Center for Dementia Research, Linköping University, Sweden, in 2012, supported by the Social Sciences and Medical Research Foundation of the Bank of Sweden Tercentenary Foundation, allowed me to explore some of the clinical aspects of remembering and forgetting discussed in this book; as did a grant from The Social Sciences and Humanities Research Council of Canada.

I am grateful to some extremely generous colleagues and friends who read earlier versions of the manuscript or parts of it and provided valuable, often extended in-depth comments and feedback: Molly Andrews, Jerome Bruner, Alessandra Fasulo, Michel Ferrari, Lars-Christer Hydén, Hilde Lindemann, Jarmila Mildorf, David Olson, Rom Harré, Hank Stam, Robert Stern, Karoline Tschuggnall, Jaan Valsiner, and James Wertsch.

Mark Freeman has been a most appreciated discussion partner on many of the issues treated in this book—from its beginning, in the early 1990s, when we met at the International Research Center for Cultural Studies in Vienna, Austria, both of us fascinated by the riddles of human identity, memory, and narrative. In numerous meetings and exchanges since then, he has challenged, encouraged, and supported me, and I am particularly grateful that he invited me to publish the results I have come up with, up to this point in time, in a book series with Oxford University Press, of which he is the series editor.

A special thank you also goes to David Herman whose meticulous commentary on the entire draft manuscript provided me not only with a long list of open questions and actual and potential problems—which I tried to tackle as well as I could—but also with an abundance of new ideas demonstrating that a cross-disciplinary mind like David's not only highlights links among diverse disciplines, where none were seen before, but also offers profound and original thoughts within highly specialized disciplines themselves.

Many other people also supported my work on this book with additional comments and helpful suggestions, as well as with offering opportunities to discuss problems or by inviting me to give talks or seminars on critical questions. In particular, I would like to thank Karin Aronsson, Sven Barnow, Jacob Belzen, Mario Carretero and Karina Solcoff, Rita Charon, Carolin Demuth, Andreas Draghun, Paul John Eakin, Gerald Echternach, Peter Frommelt, Arthur W. Frank, Roger Frie, Alexandra Georgakopoulou, Solveigh Goett, Marina Grishakova, Ilaria Grazzani, Martin Hildebrand-Nilshon, William Hirst, Bruce Homer, Brian Hurwitz, Matti Hyvärinen, Martin Klepper, Gabriele Lucius-Hoene, Matias Martinez, Hanna Meretoja, Kyoko Murakami, Katherine Nelson, Jeffrey Olick, Veronica Ornaghi, Sylvie Patron, Daniela Petrelli, Andreea Ritivoi, Linda Sandino, Brian Schiff, Ernst Schraube, Andrea Smorti, Andrea Sormano, Jürgen Straub, Hans-Ulrich Treichel, Steve Whittaker, and Reinhard Wibmer.

I also would like to thank the external reviewers of the proposal and the final draft for their constructive and encouraging comments, as well as Abby Gross, Molly Balikov, and Suzanne Walker at Oxford University Press, New York, for their help, kindness, and guidance in bringing this project to fruition.

My deepest gratitude, however, goes to my wife and closest colleague in matters of work as of life, Maria Medved, for her ongoing backing and patience during the years it took me to write this book.

Some of the research and thoughts on which I build in this book appeared in earlier versions. Though all of this material has been considerably revised and elaborated, I am grateful to the publishers for permission to extract parts of, and use thoughts from, the following papers and chapter:

"Remembering and forgetting: Narrative as cultural memory." *Culture and Psychology* (2002), 8(1), 15–44.

"Austerlitz's memory." *Partial Answers: Journal of Literature and The History of Ideas* (2008), 6(2), 347–367.

"Stories to remember: Narrative and the time of memory." *Storyworlds: A Journal of Narrative Studies* (2009), 1(1), 99–114.

"After the archive: Remapping memory." *Culture and Psychology* (2010), 16(1), 5–35.

"Fact and fiction: Exploring the narrative mind." In M. Hatavara, L.-C. Hydén, and M. Hyvärinen (Eds.), *The Travelling Metaphor of Narrative* (2013) (pp. 121–140). Amsterdam & Philadelphia, PA: John Benjamins.

Ideas and material elaborated in sections of Chapter 7 draw on an invited contribution to a UNESCO (Paris) project on "Social Memory," published as "Localizing oneself: Autobiographical remembering, cultural memory, and the Asian American experience." *International Social Science Journal* (2011), *62* (203–204), 121–133.

I am most grateful to Ralph Turturro for helping me select a painting from the huge collection of beautiful works that he has created, and for his permission to use it for the book cover. As a painter and visual thinker, Ralph has for long investigated the palimpsestic nature of human memory. *Certain Ambiguity* (2008, 66x48" acryl/on canvas), partly represented on the cover of this book, is the result of one of his explorations. I also thank Chuck Marksberry, the owner of the image, for his kind permission to use it here.

For permission to use a photograph of Anselm Kiefer's *Volkszählung* (Census), Nationalgalerie Berlin, Museum für Gegenwart (Museum for Contemporary Art) im Hamburger Bahnhof (© Bildagentur für Kunst, Kultur und Geschichte, bpk, Berlin), I am grateful to Anselm Kiefer and his interest in my work, as well as to Galerie Thaddaeus Ropac, Salzburg and Paris, and Frau Hella Pohl, the gallery representative.

Beyond the Archive

CHAPTER 1

Introduction

The Memory Crisis

WHY IS MEMORY SO ELUSIVE?

We know a good deal about human memory. Yet, as with memory itself, much of what we know is not for certain, and what's more, we only have a vague idea about memory as a whole. We cannot even say whether there is such a thing as memory—or a memory, or a memory system, or a set of memory systems—at all, and I am afraid that the view of memory that I offer will intensify this doubt. I believe that it is, however, not just a subjective impression that what we call memory has become more and more elusive but an observation that is "evidence based" in a strong sense—scientifically, conceptually, and culturally.

One reason for the increasing elusiveness of memory is that it means very different things to different people, especially if they use the vocabularies of different disciplines. And there are only a few disciplines where memory does not play any role. The meanings of memory meander even more if we consider different epochs, cultures, and languages. Many of them do not have a special word, let alone a concept, that suggests a distinct capacity or entity; instead we find terms that indicate an array of abilities and practices. As, for example, in East Cree, one of the indigenous languages of North America where the word for memory, *mituneyihchikan*, embraces the entire spectrum of mental processes from remembering to thinking, knowing, feeling, and understanding, all of them inextricably intermingled and linked to the mental states and social practices of other individuals (Junker, 2007).

On the other hand, Western common sense both in everyday life and in science assumes that there *is* a specific material, biological, neurological, and spatial reality to memory, something manifest in the world. For many, memory—or a memory—is located in the mind or brain of an individual, an island of the past with a clear coastline in a sea of different mental states, a rock in the surf of oblivion. Like a statement of fact, it has a precise beginning and end like, say, a psychological experiment. For others—not only the Cree, but also many of today's social scientists, historians, and cultural and literary scholars—memories are transindividual or collective phenomena. They are cultural creations, like myths, legends, and other stories, reverberating in the minds of generations. They do not even necessarily have to be mental but also can be material and social artifacts, objectified in all kinds of things and activities such as landscapes, monuments, museums, computers, rituals, anniversaries, and other collective practices. Often such structures of cultural memory are embedded in contexts of explanatory and interpretive discourse; they are surrounded by questions and answers, comments and criticisms, personal memories and associations, like issues debated at a town hall meeting. How such interplay works, how words and objects, stories and material structures of remembrance mingle, is a question I examined in an earlier study (Brockmeier, 2002a).

And then there are those who view a memory as a personal, indeed intimate, part of one's consciousness, as well as one's unconscious; those who take it to be a deeply affective thread of the fabric of one's self that, like a line from a poem, a musical theme, or a narrative bond, links us to a world of dreams, forebodings, and early experiences. "We live with those retrievals from childhood," writes Michael Ondaatje (2007), "that coalesce and echo throughout our lives, the way shattered pieces of glass in a kaleidoscope reappear in new forms and are songlike in their refrains and rhymes . . . We live permanently in the recurrence of our own stories, whatever story we tell" (p. 136). Emotions may indeed be strong indicators of what we conceive of as the objective reality of memories, all the more so because the connection between emotions and memories has been given shape in many cultural forms. Among these, the forms and practices of narrative may be the most influential ones, and Ondaatje might have this in mind when he speaks about the recurrence of our stories that forever permeate our lives.

But the diversification of meanings, concepts, and narratives of memory is only one reason why it has become elusive. At stake is not only the old story about modern science and scholarship: knowing more and more about less and less, until the original subject of research vanishes into thin air. This may be one story, yet in order to also permit the exploration of other stories—and for the sake of not already losing the main character of the play while the curtain opens—let me start with an alternative plot. This plot emphasizes the historical dimension of the issue. It assumes for now that there *is* memory, memory in the old sense as an individual faculty and as the place where the past is stored; what has changed, however, are our views about it, our notions and ideas of what remembering and forgetting is all about. Eventually, however, I hope to show that what we call memory is, like Ondaatje's kaleidoscope, one of those tricky phenomena whose assumed material reality cannot really be separated from our views about it.

Using the term "change" is a rather understated way to make the case that the established Western notion of memory is in the midst of dissolving. That is, what is dissolving is the conception that there is a particular capacity, in fact, an entity (or, in more updated scientific terms, a system or a network of neuronal systems) that enables us to store, maintain, or retain, and again recall experiences and knowledge and, in doing so, constitutes an essential part of our existence. In a sense, this is a reverse development to what Ian Hacking (1995; 1996a) has described as the coming into being of "memory" as a specific epistemological and scientific subject, a process he locates in the 19th century. Although memory, in Hacking's analysis, was already viewed as a criterion of personal identity, it became in the latter part of that century "a scientific key to the soul, so that by investigating memory (to find out its facts) one would conquer the spiritual domain of the soul and replace it by a surrogate, knowledge about memory" (1995, p. 198). In this way, memory got a new existence, a new gravitas. Its status changed from a personal and autobiographical concern, a topic of private conversation and the center of moral and spiritual debates, to a subject at the level of factual knowledge. As an objective entity and facility meant to store the past how an individual had experienced it, memory turned into something substantial, into a natural kind.

Hacking traces the constitution of memory as a scientific subject within the framework of what he calls the emerging memory sciences. These include neurology, which locates various types of memory; experimental psychology, which focuses on recall and retrieval; and the psychodynamics of memory that Hacking describes as "the study of memory in terms of observed and conjectured psychological processes and forces," which is, in short, psychoanalysis (1995, p. 199). To these three sciences of memory, which are creatures of the 19th century, Hacking adds two 20th-century branches of science. These are neurobiology at the cellular level and computer-based memory research. Together, the sciences of memory reinvented remembering and forgetting; they established "new kinds of truths-or-falsehoods, new kinds of facts, new objects of knowledge" (p. 198). In this way they laid out an unprecedented ontology of memory.

Now, little more than a century later, this ontology of memory appears again under construction. The framework within which I explore this construction—or perhaps better, deconstruction—is, however, different from Hacking's historical epistemology. It not only embraces scientific and scholarly developments, but also includes literary, artistic, and other cultural and public discourses. Moreover, it takes into account the emergence of entirely new research fields such as trauma theory, Holocaust studies, and social (or collective or cultural) memory studies. Against this backdrop let me qualify my case: What has been challenged in all of these recent developments is the concept of memory as a form of storage, the idea that human memory is to be imagined as an archive of the past. This idea is and has always been at the center of the Western understanding of memory, far beyond the specific gestalt given to it by the 19th- and 20th-century memory sciences. There are many names for it. Often it is taken to be a metaphor; Kurt Danziger, for one, calls it "the storehouse metaphor," which comes with an array of variations (2008, pp. 25–27). But surely it is far older than modern psychology.

This is not to claim that there has only been the archival view of memory. Concepts with such a strong cultural aura and moral weight as memory never simply represent a subject about which there is a general consensus, let alone the shared assumption of a materially identifiable object. Nonetheless, I find it significant that, since Antiquity, the archive is the metaphor most used to portray memory. From ancient Greek and Roman theorists of memory to modern experimental and neurocognitive psychology, there are countless variants of the archival model—I take a closer look at some of them in Chapter 3. The spectrum of memory containers ranges from the warehouse, palace, museum, birdcage, and cave to materializations of writing, such as the book, the library, and the hard disc, where the metaphorical field of the archive again overlaps with that of the ancient wax tablet. All of these structures are firm and solid. Like the archive itself, they are meant to be permanent—even if recently, under the impact of neurosciences and social memory theories, they have become more malleable and dynamic.

Still, our constructions of memory are meant to keep things, to retain them, hold onto the flux of experience and the transience of human existence, which is a desire that has always been associated with the idea of memory in the Western tradition. When long-stay patients at the neurological rehabilitation unit of London's Homerton University Hospital were asked to create objects or installations that might explore their conditions, some built little boxes covered in bright splotches of color. Structures, artworks of minds and selves, they revealed a fascination with the nuts and bolts of what their builders considered to be their memory: receptacles filled with jewels, corals, birds, babies, paper snippets, a leaping dolphin. Broken memories, or metaphors or symbols of memories, all kept together by more or less solid containers, touching storerooms of the past.[1]

For many generations, the entry to the memory archive, remembering, was the key to wisdom and all knowledge that reaches beyond the here and now. Plato, one of the most influential thinkers in the European history of memory, saw in the process of remembrance, which he called *anamnesis,* the key to the deepest truths. The Platonic confidence in the memory archive and its supreme intellectual and moral distinction accompanies the Western tradition all the way through to the modern memory sciences. When I examine this venerable tradition in some detail, in Chapter 3, wondering how it is possible that it has been so powerful for so long, I conclude that these claims and their metaphorical underpinnings, in fact, still determine much of the contemporary view of memory. And they do so in spite of the emergence of novel arguments and evidence in new and old areas of memory studies. These arguments and evidence call into question nothing less than the very existence of memory as we have known it for so long, as an archival entity based on the assumption of remembering as a more or less unitary individual capacity.

An objection from neuroscience

I have used the qualifier of remembering as a "more or less" unitary individual capacity in order to allow for an argument put forward in one important area of contemporary memory research, neurocognitive psychology. Although the development at stake is multidisciplinary, modern psychology of memory no doubt plays a crucial, albeit contradictory, role in it. Even if Hacking maintains that there have been a number of equally influential memory sciences, psychology has claimed, since its academic institutionalization at the time of Ebbinghaus, to be the home base of the scientific study of memory. And in fact, it has influenced thinking about remembering in many areas within and outside of the academic sphere in an unparalleled way.

I, therefore, want to address this important argument right at the beginning. It ensues from a shift in academic psychology in the 1970s and 1980s. Until then the common view of memory was that of an undifferentiated unitary function or operation of information processing that existed throughout (most of) the animal kingdom. During the shift of those years, this view was replaced by a new and more differentiated vision: the idea of several distinct neurocognitive systems of human memory, the systems approach or systems model. The idea that memory is not a single and unitary faculty is not itself new (Squire, 2004); although it necessarily remained peripheral in times dominated by biological universalism, that is, by the idea that all psychological phenomena are governed by the same underlying biological laws and principles. Over the years, the systems model changed from an approach based on cognitive psychology and its models of information processing to what most neuroscientists today see as a more advanced approach based on the study of neuronal networks and other aspects of the brain (cf., for this transformation, Eichenbaum, 2008; Foster & Jelicic, 1999; Schacter & Tulving, 1994). Also, the by now widespread assumption—both in more traditional cognitive quarters and in neuroscientific quarters—that the brain altogether can be viewed as a system (or network of systems) under permanent construction and recon-struction has influenced the concept of system itself (e.g., Schacter, Addis, Hassabis, Martin, Spreng, & Szpunar, 2012). Throughout all changes, however, there has been consensus that even multiple memory systems are realizations of memory as a "natural kind," as a given biological entity (Michaelian, 2010).

Whereas the rise of the systems model was closely connected to the emergence of brain imaging technologies such as computed tomography (CT) scanning and functional magnetic resonance imaging (fMRIs), it was conceptually anticipated by Endel Tulving's distinction between seman-tic and episodic memory (Tulving, 1972; 1983). This distinction entailed more and more distinctions and more and more systems (Tulving,1985a). Although the systems approach has become the dominant paradigm, this is not to say that there is conceptual agreement within cognitive and neu-rocognitive psychology as to what exactly is being investigated, let alone what memory is, despite various attempts to postulate defining concepts (e.g., Byrne, 2008; Moulin, 2011; Roediger, Dudai, & Fitzpatrick, 2007; Roediger & DeSoto, 2015). Often there is not even consensus within one and the same scientific paper or chapter, where the term "memory" can be found to be used for quite different things—for example, for the place or location where a particular piece of information is supposed to be stored, the process of encoding and/or retrieval (be it in the form of recall or recognition), or the very content of a memory. Now, if we highlight the archival aspects of the various visions just mentioned, we notice that all meanings of memory are equally associated with the idea of a storage, whether at stake is a place or structure, the activities or processes needed to access the storage (either in order to store or encode, to reconsolidate, or retrieve or reconstruct information), or its content, however dynamic, process-related, or shaped by neuronal plasticity it might be conceived.

Despite continuous attempts to avoid such confusion and systematize the technical vocabulary referring to specific aspects of memory, the fragmentation of the subject matter goes on. As a consequence, the composition, functions, and sheer quantity of neurocognitive memory systems have become increasingly disputed. All the more as the number of memory systems being discussed in the literature has constantly grown, a phenomenon that prompted a critical ironic commentary by Tulving (2007) in his paper "Are there 256 different kinds of memory?" Still, the growth continues.

Roughly two decades after Tulving's first categorical distinction had turned into the new template of memory psychology, Daniel Schacter summarized what would become the core hypothesis of neurocognitive research since: "memory is . . . composed of a variety of distinct and dissociable processes and systems. Each system depends on a particular constellation of networks in the brain that involve different neural structures, each of which plays a highly specialized role within the system . . . [demonstrating how] specific parts of the brain contribute to different memory processes" (1996, p. 5).

Brain imaging technologies and the systems approach have arguably altered much of psychological memory research, giving it the shape of today's neurocognitive research. Our view of processes of individual remembering has been especially enriched by new insights into the brain's plasticity and its constructive and reconstructive nature. How deeply the idea of a static, all-encompassing memory container was rooted in the scientific and clinical community we know from sources including but not restricted to the published research literature. Memory researchers Loftus and Loftus (1980) asked psychologists to choose between two theories of remembering and forgetting. One theory claimed that every recorded passing experience is permanently and objectively stored in the form of dormant traces in the brain's nerve cells, with the implication that all details of past experience can eventually be recovered with the right experimental technique or therapy. The second theory shared with the first the same basic assumption of memory as a storeroom but conceded that there are experiences that can be lost from this storeroom and irrecoverably forgotten. The results were unambiguous. Eighty-four percent of psychologists opted for the first version. I think it is fair to suspect that today the same study would show a majority of psychologists voting for the second theory. In light of far-reaching scientific and cultural changes in our understanding of remembering and forgetting—which I review in Chapter 2—it has become indisputable that there have been for some time now serious "problems with the idea that all experiences are kept forever in some dark corner of the brain," to quote Schacter's (1996, p. 77) near clairvoyant insight.

As Schacter illustrated in great detail, modern thinking about memory, be it scientific or common sense, has for long tended to conceive of our memories as a series of family pictures; as if they were snapshots from the past stored in the photo album (or, to be more up to date, the digital photography archive) of our minds, which "if stored properly, could be retrieved in precisely the same condition in which they were put away" (Schacter, 2001, p. 9). The snapshot in the photo album—a modern variation of the mnemonic library of memory artists from earlier epochs—is a further important entry to our collection of memory metaphors. It is particularly appealing because it not only shows once again the longevity of the *imagines agentes* of mnemotechnique, but also demonstrates how easily assumptions about memory can gain coherence and plausibility by being metaphorically linked to everyday experience.

Charles Fernyhough calls the idea that we file away our memories in a kind of internal archive, ready to be retrieved when they are needed, the "possession view of memory" (2012, p. 5). And although Fernyhough may be right in observing that even today "no one would doubt . . . that the question of whether you 'possess' a particular memory makes sense" (p. 5), it is fair to say that most memory scientists today—including Schacter and Fernyhough—would challenge this view. Clearly, there is more awareness in the recent literature that the "possession view" of memory is problematic because remembering is taken to be reconstructive and dynamic, rather than static and monolithic. This also has been noted by commentators of my earlier work (e.g., Carretero & Solcoff, 2012; Echterhoff, 2011; Wertsch, 2011).[2]

There are some things, however, that have not changed, in fact, that have remained amazingly constant in mainstream cognitive and neuroscientific memory psychology, and these are of particular significance in the context of my argument. They include, first, the conviction that the diverse memory systems, whatever their number and nature, are reciprocally interconnected to form one brain, one "natural kind." Second, there is the assumption that these memory systems can be constructed—apparently in an amazingly random fashion—using data exclusively from a neurophysiological level. A third supposition that has not changed is that the key research subject, the ultimate "unit" of memory, is the *individual* brain, the head (or, typically, a tiny part of it) of a person. That said, we have to keep in mind that neurobiological brain research almost exclusively works on the brains of animals, not humans. The Nobel Prize-winning biochemist Hans Krebs once said, as his student Steven Rose reports (2010), that for every biological problem God had chosen an appropriate organism in which to study the problem. The organisms chosen for studies on the molecular processes involved in remembering and forgetting range from sea slugs, fruit flies, yeast, rats, mice to chickens—the last ones have been God's organism for Rose. As a result, neurobiological and neurochemical brain research has only very little to say about the mnemonic complexities of human beings. And this is even more true if humans are alive and endued with intentions, agency, and passions, that is, if they are seen as subjects who are at home in bustling life worlds where they are engaged in manifold intersubjective ways and learn to remember and forget according to cultural conventions.

Because this exclusion of people's cultural life worlds continues even in recent neuroscientific research, both at the cellular level and at the level of neuronal and neurocognitive systems, much of the critique directed at it has not changed either. Consider—to refer to just one, psychological line of criticism—Ulric Neisser's (1967; Neisser & Winograd, 1988) efforts to expose the reductionism of what he called laboratory-based "high-road" cognitive memory psychology and to plead for the "low-road" study of more naturalistic, ecological, and situated practices of remembering. Neisser patterned his critique on Frederic Bartlett's (1932) understanding of memory as "an effort after meaning."

Finally, and perhaps most importantly, what has remained untouched is the basic hypothesis that each memory system works according to the model of a storage, that is, as "encoding," "storing," and "retrieval" (or "recognition") of information. As cognitive and neurocognitive psychology has been shaped for so long by models of information processing, the metaphor of memory as an archive has gained even more plausibility because it regularly has been characterized in analogy to the computational storage model. "The computer disk drive analogy also helps us to understand the distinction between encoding, storage, and retrieval in memory," states a widespread introductory book on memory (Foster, 2009, p. 38). The view of encoded, stored, and retrieved memories is also compatible with the reconstruction view. Of course, the memories filed away in the internal archive can change during their storage; they might corrode or get mixed up; they can be (intentionally or unintentionally) overwritten, blackened out, or lost in some dark corner. When we want to take them out of the archive, we thus have to reconstruct them—all of which goes well with the overall archival model.

The storage orientation even prevails when memory does *not* work properly. And that it often enough does not work as it is supposed to do according to the storage assumption has been shown extensively in recent research. There is, in fact, a detailed literature pointing out that autobiographical memory especially is the subject of many biases and distortions and thus commits all kinds of omissions, mistakes, and other "sins" (Schacter, 2001). A point to be made here, of course, is that such "sins" also can be seen as strengths and advantages in the profane thicket of everyday life (e.g., Randall, 2010). Yet my argument is a different one. Admitting such features as "sins" means once more to acknowledge the commandment, the normative rule, the role model of a memory that is supposed to work as an unfailing archive. It confirms the archival circle of encoding, storing, and retrieving memories—even if in a flawed and defective manner (Medved & Brockmeier, 2015).

The work of Schacter (e.g., 1995; 1996; 2001; Schacter, Guerin, & St. Jacques, 2011) and his colleagues is a telling example. Early on it demonstrated a keen interest in not just measuring memory victories, but also investigating the defeats of the archival model—in and outside of the lab. Schacter identified a wide spectrum of what he called "memory failures," or "sins," from everyday life to pathologies such as psycho- and neurotrauma and Alzheimer's disease. Many of these studies "give a properly rounded account of how it feels to be the owner of a memory, detailing all the frustrations of trying to make it work as specified on the box," as John McCrone (2004, p. 4) puts it. On the other hand, however, Schacter's conceptualization of the flawed and sinful memory has remained all the time wedded to the archival tradition, that is, in McCrone's terms, to what is written on the box. Just that the retrieval of dormant traces now also can be a flawed retrieval, and "accurate" memories are juxtaposed with "distorted memories."

Schacter's work is only one example, even if it is the example of a leading representative of some decades of psychological memory research. Although modern experimental research in psychology is teamwork mostly carried out in laboratory collectives, I single out from time to time influential individual researchers whose work, often over long careers, illustrates changes and continuities of dominant ideas in their discipline more succinctly than less individualized "labs." The results of this review are in synch with an overall finding: research publications, psychological and neuroscientific textbooks, memory assessments in neuropsychology and clinical psychology, and informal (ethnographically registered) lab talk provide countless instances of the vocabulary of encoding, storing, and retrieving and the corresponding archivalist mode of thought.[3]

As already noted, this also is the case if memory is conceived of as creative or inventive, constructive or reconstructive (e.g., Gazzaniga, Ivry, & Mangum 2013; Roediger & DeSoto, 2015).

To be sure, creative, constructive, and reconstructive processes are particularly important in the field of memory research that is commonly identified as autobiographical. Technically speaking, this is the field in which one of the central topics of this book is localized, the autobiographical process. Therefore, at the end of this brief first excursion into psychology—which is one of several disciplinary fields of memory research on which I draw in advancing my argument—a short remark on this field as a whole is in order. Bearing in mind that experimental psychologists see the history of scientific memory research beginning with the publication of Hermann Ebbinghaus's *Über das Gedächtnis* (*On memory*) in 1885, it is amazing that it took almost a hundred years until autobiographical memory became a subject worthy of being examined for its own sake. During that century, memory research was mainly concerned with learning, retaining, and recalling of impersonal information presented by an experimenter in a laboratory setting, the classic example being lists of meaningless syllables.

When autobiographical memory finally became a legitimate subject of inquiry in cognitive psychology a leading role was played by David Rubin, who has remained one of the most-quoted protagonists in the field. From the 1980s, when the first edited book that specifically treated autobiographical memory was published (Rubin, 1986), to collections of studies surveying the psychological research on the topic in 1996 (Rubin, 1996) and 2012 (Berntsen & Rubin, 2012a), Rubin's studies have been closely identified with the establishment of a more or less marked-off field of research on autobiographical memory. As Berntsen and Rubin (2012b) summarize it, this field "broke away from the existing field of memory research" (p. 1), among others, when autobiographical memory researchers resolved "the problem of measuring accuracy" by introducing diary studies in which participants recorded personal events, for which their memory capacity was later tested (p. 3). Since then, the area has undergone several changes and extensions, most remarkable, perhaps, the shift from old-school cognitive frameworks of explanation based on information-processing computer models to neurocognitive frameworks based on brain imagining. But throughout these shifts and changes, Rubin's research, as well as the entire field that he helped shape, has invariably centered on one idea: that of memory as a storehouse of information. Rubin has progressively unfolded this idea in what he has called the "basic systems model of autobiographical memory" (2005; 2006; 2012), a model about how information is stored. Although, as he writes, "most storage is in the relevant neural systems of the basic systems model" (Rubin, 2012, p. 23), the gist of this model is to differentiate and integrate a number of memory storage systems that are meant to design ways of how visual, auditory, spatial, tactile, olfactory, and other memories "are stored in individual systems" (p. 23), before they are recalled by a specific "search-and-retrieval system" (pp. 12–13).

But the unfolding of this archival model and its supportive vocabulary of encoding, storing, and retrieving do not make up the entire story of research on autobiographical memory. Nor is it the entire tale of psychological memory research. The story told in this book has more than one plot and more than one storyline. It also encompasses how the traditional notion of memory has been more and more challenged by new neuroscientific findings and alternative ways to conceive of remembering and forgetting. These new views have not least resulted from novel research technologies like brain imaging originally developed to confirm and expand the archival systems approach. Instead, again, the new means have proved to be richer than the ends they were meant to reach. What they suggest are mnemonic scenarios that go far beyond the idea of the archive. How these new scenarios have emerged I discuss in a moment, in Chapter 2, which spells out the radical implications of this dramatic development for the notion of memory.

FROM BRAINS TO PERSONS: OUTLINING THE PROJECT

Psychology and neurosciences play a crucial role in this process—albeit an ambivalent role, as will become clearer over the next chapters. However, they parcel out just one field of memory research, and viewed from the perspective of the overarching shift in our understanding of memory, it might not even be the pivotal one. Let us thus leave aside for a while the situation in psychology and turn to areas of memory studies where it appears to be more obvious that the view of memory as storage is about to disintegrate. We also can recognize here in a more explicit way how, in the same process of dismantlement, new perspectives take forms that go beyond the archival model. It is, in fact, these perspectives in which I am primarily interested. Despite all their diversity, one feature of these visions stands out: they transcend the isolated human mind or brain as the exclusive site of remembering and forgetting. Instead, they localize these subjects within an extended cultural landscape of social practices and artifacts. And as these practices and artifacts are themselves subject to historical change, a further trajectory of time—history—enters the scene.

Abundant evidence suggests a general trend in this direction, a cultural paradigm shift in memory research. Elsewhere I have described this shift as both postpositivist and postmetaphysical, proposing a perspective on human beings as persons who remember and forget, and who do so in material, cultural, and historical contexts of action and interaction (Brockmeier, 2002b). Building on this idea, this book explores the meaning and implications of the dismantlement of the memory archive—the "memory crisis"—in one specific area of our social and cultural memory practices: the area in which the remembering self and the remembered self play the lead roles and which also is called autobiographical memory. To be sure, there are more domains of memory research in which the traditional notion of memory has likewise become precarious. But the field of autobiographical memory is a particularly intriguing case in point because it uniquely interconnects biological and psychological, individual and cultural, and narrative and imagistic aspects of human remembering. I already mentioned that it also is a field in which the constructive, creative, and inventive aspects of remembering are salient.

A second objective of my project piggybacks on the first one. I previously outlined the prospect of novel and alternative vistas of remembering and forgetting that have already emerged or are in the offing. Offering new ideas beyond the archive, they might replace the old notion of memory in the long run. Although a comprehensive investigation of potential candidates for future conceptions of memory would necessitate several research projects covering the many distinct areas commonly labeled as memory, I concentrate in my search on one domain, the autobiographical. To draw the circle even tighter, within this domain I focus on one option, the option of narrative. By this I mean not simply studying autobiographical narratives or narratives of autobiographical memories but something else: using narrative as a model to describe, examine, and explain what is categorized as autobiographical memory within the established order. In other words, narrative serves as a conceptual and analytical blueprint for an alternative approach to what I call the autobiographical processes.

Why can narrative serve as such a model? This question runs through all following studies and I hope that the answer I offer becomes more plausible as the chapters proceed. At this point any remark cannot be but preliminary and provisional. That said, this is what I propose in a nutshell. Narrative, in my understanding, lends itself to such a privileged role because it is the most comprehensive and subtle of language forms, a form of life evolved and culturally differentiated in intimate interweavement with human actions, emotions, and intentions. A ubiquitous social practice, narrative combines several modes that are involved in the autobiographical process: linguistic, cognitive, and affective. The interplay of these modes allows not only for advanced forms of communication and interaction but also of reflection and understanding, with self-understanding being of particular relevance here. Cognitive, affective, and linguistic modes are often—and in psychology typically—investigated separately, whereas it is constitutive of the autobiographical process that they operate together, as components of one complex synthesis. Creating this synthesis is integral to the process of human meaning-making, and I believe that the autobiographical process is exactly such a hermeneutic process: the ongoing enterprise in which we are engaged to make sense of ourselves in time by using the narrative resources of the many cultural worlds in which we live.

To put the same point another way, narrative is so supremely appropriate a mnemonic model because the dynamic of the autobiographical process is at its heart that of a narrative process. Approaching the autobiographical process as a narrative event also sheds new light on the interplay between autobiographical self-understanding and identity formation. To get a better sense of this interplay I employ the notion of *narrative hermeneutics* (discussed in Chapters 4–6), which taps into hermeneutic philosophy and narrative theory.

There is, finally, a third objective, closely connected to the two just presented. I started this chapter by characterizing memory as one of those odd phenomena whose assumed material reality cannot be separated from our views about it. Part of the difficulty in grasping this phenomenon is that it cannot be dealt with on empirical grounds alone. It is inextricably fused with the concepts and ideas by which we define what we mean by empirical grounds in the first place. And this is the crux, because the reasons why we prefer some concepts of empirical evidence over others are not always empirically grounded; rather, they are intermingled with theoretical, cultural, and historical trajectories that are at work when it comes to taking something to be "empirically evident" in contrast with something else.

Let me explain. The assumption that the individual brain, or at least parts of it, is the empirical site of human memory, perhaps even its very substrate, is the premise of contemporary psychological memory research.[4] Shaping the entire project of cognitive neuroscience, this premise appears to be simultaneously confirmed by the outcomes of the research in which it is grounded. As all research is geared to and departs from it, it continuously operates in full circles. This self-referential movement also explains what is left out. Although there is no "empirical evidence" that would justify the exclusion of social forms of remembering, or the role of language and other cultural sign systems and practices of communication that help us to recollect, or the myriad of material artifacts, media, and cultural memory techniques, the chief presupposition of psychological and neuroscientific memory research has remained unchanged: the individual brain is the exclusive subject of inquiry. Moreover, only its neurophysiological and neurocognitive levels provide "empirical evidence."

In more general terms, this third concern could be formulated as an evidence-based effort to de-substantialize and de-ontologize memory. This effort is part and parcel of my main endeavor: to widen the locus of attention from the operations of an isolated organ, the brain, to the biological–social–cultural lives of human beings, that is, to the actions and interactions of individuals who remember and forget in the midst of a cultural and historical world, a world of symbols, language, and media.

The memory crisis expands

To flesh out this project, I begin by mapping some new developments and findings that have contributed to the present memory crisis. "Memory crisis" is a term originally used to dub the changes in the understanding of remembering that have been discussed since the early 1990s in several domains of the new memory studies.[5] In fact, the memory crisis unfolded in a close interplay with the emergence of these new fields of study. It started with a number of authors from different backgrounds setting out to explore forms and psychological consequences of trauma in individuals and communities that had been affected by the Holocaust, the Vietnam War, and the Gulf War. Many of these explorations were autobiographical in nature, and they were followed by a plethora of trauma narratives by individuals from previously marginalized social groups—women, people of color, refugees—and survivors of sexual abuse, to name a few. These literary, critical, social-scientific, psychological, and psychoanalytical lines of inquiry into violence and oppression converged to make both trauma and the nature of remembrance and forgetting of individual and collective experiences the subject of passionate debates.

At first, it might have been an unintended side effect that many of the phenomena under discussion contradicted the traditional notion of memory. In particular, they challenged the idea of memory's continuity, stability, coherence and—based on them—the moral weight and ethical status of memory as an arbiter of truth and authenticity (Gross, 2000). In other words, they challenged what I have described as part of its Platonic legacy. A case in point was James Young's (1993) comparative inquiries on the memory of the Holocaust. In the 1990s, multidisciplinary Holocaust studies were growing rapidly, in large part driven by the historical and biological fact that toward the end of the 20th century the number of witnesses of events that happened about 60 years prior dwindled drastically. Yet Young did not just examine memories of holocaust survivors and the different ways these memories were handed down in various cultural traditions. He showed that although the very facts of this historically unique crime are documented in great detail and considered to be beyond doubt, there was no such thing as one single event called "the Holocaust." Rather, every nation—and sometimes even different communities within one nation—construed their memories of it according to traditions, values, and political agendas that were dominant at a certain historical moment in time. They also changed and reconstrued their memories when these agendas changed. What found its way into a confirmed set of collective memories was the outcome of negotiations, struggles, and decisions that did not depend on events in the past or on the knowledge of these events but on events in the present, the present of "memory policies."

Memories, even if seemingly objectified in historical monuments and memorials, have a "fundamentally interactive, dialogical quality," Young (2008, p. 364) concluded. This quality is linked to what he conceived of as the unit of the memorial and interpretive activity of memorialization: "For public memory and its meanings depend not just on the forms and figures in these memorials, but on the viewers' responses to them" (p. 364). It is this interactional quality, this unavoidable conflation of past and present, and of private and public remembering in the memorial activity that keeps the meanings of a memory—as well as the meaning of "memory"— open and negotiable, even and specifically when time goes on.

Such reasoning was furthered by debates in history. In the wake of the publication in 1984 of Pierre Nora's influential work on French national sites of memory *Les Lieux de Mémoire* and the English translation of its introduction (Nora, 1989), questions of witnessing, remembrance, and the construction of historical and individual memory took center stage.[6] For Nora, the mnemonic continuity of modernity was based on its "constructed histories" that he saw in contrast with the "organic communities of memory" of previous epochs. Nora localized his work in the tradition of Maurice Halbwachs, whose classic *On Collective Memory* appeared in English in 1992. At about the same time and in a related vein, new research in clinical psychology and psychiatry about the so-called False Memory

Syndrome (FMS) began to question the permanence, truthfulness, and reliability of memories and instead emphasized the malleability and plasticity of human memory (Loftus, 1979, 1980, 1994; Schacter, 1995). These discussions, as well as similar ones in law and the political and social sciences quickly transcended the academic arena and connected to public debates about the nature of personal and collective memories. Let us not forget, this was a time when such debates went alongside various efforts to rewrite the history of states and people after the collapse of the power systems of communism, colonialism, and apartheid, a time when unprecedented institutions such as truth-finding and reconciliation committees publicly delved into the significance of remembering and forgetting.

If we look today at these diverse aspects of the memory crisis and the vehement public and scholarly discussions it entailed, we notice that it was not so much about a crisis in the capacity of humans to remember autobiographically and localize themselves in terms of past, present, and future. Rather, it was about the limits of the archive model to represent them. It is in this sense that I use the term memory crisis. Researchers in several disciplines made the same critical observation: Although sophisticated and emotionally moving memory investigations with victims of the traumas of war and displacement, of the Holocaust and other genocides unearthed complicated narrative ways of mnemonic construction and reconstruction, the traditional model of memory as a storage where the past is retained and from where it can be retrieved proved to be increasingly inadequate, in fact, obsolete.

THE MEMORY BOOM

What exactly has given rise to this crisis, which since those early years has developed far beyond the humanities and social sciences where it first came into academic prominence? What has turned memory and remembering from subjects that we believed we knew well for a long time into something of which in reality we did not know very much at all, as we now learn from a variety of sources?

Before reviewing these sources more closely, some background is helpful. Although the memory crisis has manifested itself in diverse fields of research and scholarship, all these fields have been affected by larger tectonic shifts that have pervaded our cultural landscape over the past decades. With respect to the notion of memory, these shifts culminated in the 1990s. What we see unfolding in those years is an unprecedented memory boom—the flipside of the memory crisis—which has not waned since. The term "memory boom" was originally coined by Richard Terdiman (1993) and Jay Winter (2000; 2006) to refer to a new way of actively taking care of the production and historical transmission of memories in the 20th century, beginning with World War I. The unprecedented wave of war memorials erected after 1918 in all countries involved in the "Great War" is only one element in this picture, though an emblematic one. Unlike the post-World War I memory boom, the memory boom starting in the 1990s is first of all associated with cultural and intellectual developments, with processes of rethinking and rewriting memory, even if these processes cannot be understood without taking into account the larger cultural-historical changes of the time.

Memory *boom* seems indeed to be the proper term here. The ISI Web of Knowledge, which combines citation indexes in the social sciences, the arts, and humanities, yields over 11,800 references to collective/cultural/social/public/popular memory, of which some 9,500 appeared during the decade 1998–2008 alone (cf. Beiner, 2008; Blight, 2009). This remarkable flood of attention has even increased since. Again, this cannot be explained only within an academic matrix but needs to be viewed against the backdrop of far-ranging political, technological, and cultural changes. Fundamental to these changes is what sociologists and economists call the postmodern transformation of Western societies. This transformation has been fueled by several interrelated developments. To name just the most important ones: the cascading technological innovations linked to the digital revolution and the multilayered process of globalization, which relate to the emergence of a new global awareness of the fragile resources of our planetary existence. Finally, as already touched upon, we are talking here about a historical period in which the Cold War ended, which closed an epoch but at the same time brought many new problems.

And there is one more background trajectory we should keep in mind in order to understand the new memory boom. The late- or postmodern transformation of Western societies is only the latest phase of a process that started long ago. Radical and incessant change is a fundamental principle of modern life, and so is its consequence, the desire for a memory that makes up for what gets continuously lost. Permanent modernization, historians tell us, has not been imposed on otherwise stable societies; it is, in contrast with traditional communities, the very essence of capitalist societies. Dissolving all traditions and experiencing the never-ending breakdown of certainties is the very essence of modernity and, even more, of postmodernity.

Since Max Weber, the last half-millennium of Western civilization has often been described in terms of an intrinsic relationship between modernity and "Occidental rationalism." Western rationalism, as Weber saw it, led to a process of "disenchantment" that disintegrated an originally unified religious worldview and a corresponding more or less static view of history, of linear *Heilsgeschichte* or salvific history, which teleologically extended from the past to the future. All that changed once a capitalist dynamic had imposed its rules on societal life. In his *The Philosophical Discourse of Modernity* Jürgen Habermas (1987) pointed out that to the degree that everyday life was affected by this cultural and societal modernization all traditional forms of life were dissolved, ruthlessly and without exception. But there was a price to be paid for that. As a consequence of the all-encompassing "modernization of the lifeworld," traditional resources of authority, knowledge, religion, and, not least, memory also dissolved, leaving modern societies with the need to find new forms not only of political self-legitimization and self-justification, but also of sense and meaning on a more fundamental, existential plane. This is the moment where, for Habermas, the *discourse of modernity* sets in, which is a discourse of the intellectual, cultural, and moral problems and crises of modernity. From this perspective, we recognize both the memory crisis and the memory boom as belated parts of the discourse of modernity.

We can even trace back the recent concern with memory to its pre-crisis and pre-boom past. The elaborated systems of public remembering and commemoration developed by modern Western societies, as described, for example, by Paul Connerton (1989), could draw on preceding premodern systems of collective memory. But while, in a predominantly traditional society, mnemonic facilities like the church year, the ecclesiastical calendar, and the seven-day circle served as a tacit background order (Zerubavel, 2003), the organization of continuity became a pressing concern in modernity. The faster modern life worlds change and traditions of knowledge, religion, ethics, and collective memory lose significance, the more energy flows into public practices, institutions, and the creation of artifacts that are supposed to conjure up "lasting" cultural memories in the face of a permanent loss of stability. In the Middle Ages and in early Modern Times, a visitor who entered the center of a European town could be sure to find the cathedral and the castle. Today, when searching for the center of many modern Western cities, we encounter monuments, memorials, and museums, besides the town hall, the traditional administrative hub and site of the town archive. An odd dialectic seems to be at work. It is as if for every ethnic and cultural community, for every tradition obliterated by Western civilization—be it premised as colonialism, imperialism, or globalization—an ethnological museum, or at the very least an exhibition, has opened.

It does not take much to see both the memory crisis and the memory boom as components of this picture. Nor is it difficult to comprehend why it left theorists of memory puzzled and overwhelmed. For decades and centuries limited to a well-demarcated academic terrain of research, they suddenly found themselves in the midst of the storm. A few impressive documents mirror how they tried to come to grips with this onslaught of novel mnemonic phenomena and questions that had never been raised before, such as this excerpt from the preface to a much discussed selection of essays on memory edited by Paul Antze and Michael Lambeck (1996a) in the turbulent early stage of the memory crisis:

> We live in a time when memory has entered public discourse to an unprecedented degree. Memory is invoked to heal, to blame, to legitimate. It has become a major idiom in the construction of identity, both individual and collective, and a site of struggle as well as identification. Memory has found a prominent place in politics, both as a source of authority and as a means of attack; one need think only of recent controversies over museum exhibits commemorating the bombing of Hiroshima or the legacy of Freud. Indeed, we now have not only a politics but a forensics of memory, in which conflicts over memory become matters for litigation and in which talk about memory is increasingly driven by the jural obsession with matters of fact. These developments raise troubling questions. How is our experience of memory being altered by the new political burdens thrust upon it? . . . [How are we] to understand the new importance that memory has assumed in contemporary culture? (Antze & Lambeck, 1996b, vii).

What has changed since the early 1990s is that the memory crisis has come to manifest itself more clearly as a crisis of the archival notion of memory. Numerous more recent books by memory researchers and scholars reflect this tendency.[7] These books are only the tip of a growing iceberg of literature on memory. The case made in this literature is a strong one. In my reading, it suggests breaking with the idea of memory as storage, the view of memory as a given entity, system, or faculty, and instead conceiving of remembering as an activity, a social, discursive, and cultural practice. The point I want to drive home, building on this literature, is that autobiographical remembering is a cultural practice of narrative meaning construction in which human beings' particular hermeneutic capacity of interpreting the world and themselves plays a pivotal role. In this view, as is obvious already now, there is more at stake than merely an issue of memory and autobiographical remembering, traditionally defined; it is for this reason that I prefer the wider and more precise term autobiographical process.

But before the autobiographical process takes center stage I want to examine (in the next two chapters) the implications of the memory crisis by looking more closely at various areas of research and reflection on memory. Given the broad spectrum of diverse phenomena labeled by the term memory, this is not as easy as it sounds. Moreover, there are various ways to categorize and relate these phenomena. The examples already mentioned comprise processes (of remembering and forgetting), entities (that encompass these processes), faculties (through which they are carried out), biological locations (such as the hippocampus), and places (like the *lieux de memoire*) of commemorations. Is there a common denominator to such a variety, except that they are all memory phenomena? Aleida Assmann (2011), for one, favors a classification of memory according to what she calls "media," which can be as varied as writing, images, bodily practices, places, and monuments. Assmann further distinguishes this classification from a second one that lays out different functions of memory, which are individual, social, or cultural.

In my own work, I have come to organize the field differently, dividing it into four semantic domains. These are domains of human knowledge and experience that give mnemonic phenomena their conceptual outline and perceivable shape. I call these domains semantic because they are meaning-endowing. They constitute what counts as "memory," which differs, as we shall see, from one domain to another. The four domains are

(1) the social and cultural,
(2) the technological,
(3) the literary and the artistic, and
(4) the biological and cognitive.

The next chapter is organized according to these domains. In each domain we can identify distinctive traditions of inquiry and discussion of specific issues of memory. All of them open up to different cultural landscapes of knowledge and learning. In all of them the archival tradition has long provided the dominant frame of imagination, but now has been challenged, even if in different ways. Hence, the chapter is entitled *Imagining memory: The archive disintegrates.*

PLAN OF THE BOOK

The gist of this book is on how narrative, the language of meaning-making, tackles the job that the archive model fails. The first part (Chapters 1–3) develops the argument that the metaphor of memory as storage is about to lose its long-standing cultural dominance. This poses the question as to whether there are alternative metaphors, non- or postarchival models, and visions of remembering and forgetting. There are, and there are plenty of them. Many of these have taken shape only recently, be it in the wake of the digital revolution, new neuroscientific and clinical insights, developments in literature and the arts, or theorizing in social and cultural memory studies and in areas such as life-writing. One of these alternative options moves to the fore at the end of Chapter 3 and then is specifically explored in the second part (Chapters 4–9) of the book: the narrative approach. At the same time the focus on what I have called memory phenomena is narrowed down. Rather than treating the entire gamut of memory phenomena, I concentrate on the autobiographical process or, in traditional terms, on autobiographical remembering.

Chapter 2, *Imagining memory: The archive disintegrates*, investigates the perspectives set free by the memory crisis in the four fields of memory studies just mentioned. After surveying how the traditional storage idea dissolves in these domains, the chapter synthesizes the emerging visions of remembering and forgetting that reach beyond the archive. Although I suggest that the four different domains should rather be viewed as parts of one comprehensive cultural process, a large portion of the chapter consists of a discussion of recent developments in neurocognitive psychology and other neurosciences of memory. The thrust of this discussion is to demonstrate that even here, in the heartland of an archival understanding of memory, a new plot thickens that aligns with what I have described as an overarching cultural shift. It is true, this thickening occurs in psychological and neuroscientific research with a certain delay with respect to social, cultural, technological, and literary memory studies. For this reason the chapter sets out with a review of developments in social, cultural, and technological fields. Furthermore, localizing recent developments in the neurosciences within this broader historical context is meant to widen our view of both levels at stake: of what we call "memory" and what we use as our conceptual lenses through which we investigate and theorize it, giving it its quotation marks, so to speak. How then might these quotation marks look in a possible future of memory theorizing, a time after the archive? This is the question raised at the end of this chapter, which concludes with a look at the possibility of a comprehensive multidisciplinary field of memory studies.

One reason why the paradigm shift in the conceptual architecture of our ideas of remembering and forgetting outlined in the first chapters will not radically change the established view of memory any time soon is that the archival model is deeply moored in Western cultural traditions. Sedimented in science, philosophy, literature, and language there are numerous metaphors and models of memory that for a long time have given shape to our ideas of remembering and forgetting. Chapter 3, *Shaping memory: History, metaphor, and narrative* revolves around the question of how these resources have turned an ancient vision of mind and memory into such an enduring conception—elaborated and authoritatively confirmed from Plato to Ebbinghaus, Proust, Freud, and modern cognitive psychology and neuroscience. I am specifically interested in metaphors of the archive because it is this particular vision of human memory that, as I argue in Chapters 1 and 2, has been sliding into a crisis, the "memory crisis." In Chapter 3, I point out that the archive and its two key components, inscription or writing and storing, are in the midst of a metaphorical and narrative field that, over the course of centuries and millennia, has turned the memory storehouse into a natural kind. This field stretches from everyday discourse, literature, and the arts to philosophy, the other humanities, and the social and natural sciences. I conclude with a review of some recently emerged alternative memory metaphors that, significantly enough, break with the archival tradition. One of these alternative metaphors—narrative—is the central issue in all the following chapters.

In Chapter 4, *Interpreting memory: The narrative alternative,* I outline a narrative approach to autobiographical remembering, an approach that conceives of personal memories as inseparably fused with their interpretation in narrative and larger ideas of self, identity, and culture. This view contrasts the strict distinction between pure memory—memory "per se"—and its (linguistic, social, cultural) interpretation, which is characteristic of traditional cognitive memory research. What I am interested in, however, is the everyday reality of remembering and forgetting, and this reality is not cognitively "pure" but always enmeshed with interpretive acts and social actions. As my approach builds on multidisciplinary strands of research and scholarship, it comes with various reconceptualizations. They include the notion of narrative, informed by the narrative turn in the social sciences and the humanities and recent debates on "post-classical" narrative theory. They also include a reformulation of the notion of experience and, more specifically, of narrative experience. After all, autobiographical memories are a special type of experience, entwining past with present experiences in a way that, as I propose, depends on a *narrative* dynamic. To take a closer look at this dynamic I also draw on literary forms of narrative (as well as analytical instruments from literary and narrative theory), which is another aspect of my "narrative alternative" that breaks with traditional research on autobiographical memory. Explaining this broadening of my "database" by including both everyday and literary narrative, I make the case that literary works offer us a long and rich tradition of thinking about remembering and forgetting, a tradition that not only has explored the narrative fabric of memory phenomena but also actively contributed to its very creation.

Whereas Chapter 4 zooms in on the narrative alternative and unfolds the groundwork of my narrative approach to memory and human experience in general, Chapter 5, *Dissecting memory: Unraveling the autobiographical process*, takes the next step. Concretizing this groundwork, it presents a case study of the autobiographical process, which at this point has become my basic unit of analysis: an ongoing interpretive, self-reflexive, and culturally embedded process of meaning formation. My specific "case" is a mental sequence—William James would have called it a stream of consciousness—recreated by Ian McEwan in his novel *Saturday*. McEwan offers an intricate narrative rendering of the autobiographical struggle of his protagonist, the London surgeon Henry Perowne. My analysis of this sequence becomes the fulcrum for a discussion of influential theories about the nexus of self, autobiographical remembering, and narrative. How would, for instance, a neuroscientist investigate Perowne's autobiographical process? And how would a narrative psychologist? The argument I develop in these discussions is that the combination of psychological and narrative theory affords an indispensable complement to the neuroscientific perspective. It is, I believe, particularly appropriate to explore the dynamic of the autobiographical process because this dynamic is at its heart a narrative one.

After unfolding the notion of the autobiographical process and its narrative dynamic in Chapters 4 and 5, the next chapters single out its most important features. Chapter 6 is dedicated to its interplay with identity formation, Chapter 7 to its cultural fabric, and Chapters 8 and 9 to its temporal dynamic. Obviously, all these aspects are closely interlocked. My analysis thus does not distinguish them in a strict sense but foregrounds them in different contexts. The context for Chapter 6, *Creating a memory of oneself: Narrative identity and the autobiographical process* are debates about narrative identity and why it matters. These debates have been ongoing for some decades and I show why they have elicited so much commitment and, indeed, passion. The stakes are high. Questions of self, identity, and how we are to understand ourselves are anything but purely academic. Investigating the identity–memory nexus from the angle of the autobiographical process and pondering the ways it relates to the narrative form of life that we call our identity is, however, not the whole story. Neither is it the whole story about identity and memory, nor about the autobiographical process. An essential part of the story, often ignored, concerns the limits of both the notion of narrative identity (grounded in language) and autobiographical identity (grounded in one's autobiographical story). How are we to understand what identity means for people who do not have a language or autobiographical memories? Or for those who have them only to a severely limited degree because of illness, injury, disability, or atypical development? Exploring these challenges, which are an existential part of the human condition and cannot be neglected in an inquiry into personal identity, leads me to conclude by proposing a postautobiographical perspective on narrative and identity.

In Chapter 7, *Inhabiting a culture of memory: The autobiographical process as a form of life*, my topic is the autobiographical process as a cultural scenario or, as I want to describe it, a cultural form of life. This chapter centers on the idea of remembering as a practice that is part and parcel of living a life, a practice through which we bind ourselves into a cultural tradition, while binding this tradition into our minds. The question I raise thus broadens the view of remembering. What does it mean to conceive of the autobiographical process as an element of a wider cultural economy of remembering and forgetting? In the first part of the chapter, I frame this question historically, investigating the development of modern European and North American concerns with self and identity, a development we have witnessed with the rise of the autobiographical story, roughly, over the last two centuries. Today, there is much evidence that it was not the successive and progressive scientific discovery of universal mechanisms of cognition or brain functioning that has shaped our ideas of memory but the historical emergence of a specific cultural milieu that has promoted individuality, self-creation, and self-presentation. This is the cultural biotope in which the autobiographical process has thrived and flourished. To mark its cultural-historical particularity, I contrast this picture—in the second half of the chapter—with a perspective from the outside, unfolded in a reading of a Chinese American autobiography, Maxine Hong Kingston's celebrated memoir *The Woman Warrior*.

All remembering is about time. Chapter 8, *Dissolving the time of memory: The autobiographical process as temporal self-localization*, is concerned with what I have described in an earlier work as "autobiographical time." Here, I elaborate on this account of autobiographical time as a way of temporal self-localization. Furthering the book's main line of argument, my account traces the narrative dynamic of this self-localization. Whereas previous chapters concentrated on the narrative structure of autobiographical meaning-making, I now extend the focus to include the temporal dimension of the process. The emerging picture is one of the autobiographical process as unfolding a narrative weave of temporality whose primary function is not to localize us in a given, chronological framework of clock and calendar time; rather, it is to create a web of meaning that binds us into a cultural world—and in this process temporal self-localization may or may not play a role. Challenging the Newtonian idea of objective time as a fixed background of all human affairs including remembering and forgetting is not new. It was pivotal to the modernist revolution in the early 20th century, an intellectual and cultural movement that serves in this chapter as a backdrop against which polychronic forms of autobiographical time are played through. To this end, I take a closer look at autobiographical narratives by two key modernist memory writers, Marcel Proust and Walter Benjamin.

Chapter 9, *Beyond time: The autobiographical process as an existential search movement*, continues to explore the relationship between remembering and time, tracing it into a zone of narrative experimentation. Although it builds on the modernist tradition of memory and time narration, this experimentation goes beyond the modernist imagination. The chapter is dedicated to one single work, W. G. Sebald's *Austerlitz*. Sebald's is an unusual work that defies borderlines between historical report, auto/biographical account, psychological case study, Holocaust document, philosophical essay, and literary fiction. Many commentators have pointed out that Sebald—Susan Sontag described him as the Einstein of narrative memory—created a new genre of memory writing, drawing together all the genres just mentioned to offer a unique investigation of the autobiographical process. My reading of one of the most sophisticated contemporary visions of human remembering emphasizes two aspects. One is how Sebald gives shape to autobiographical acts—perhaps more accurately, mnemonic search movements—that have broken entirely with the archival idea of memory. The other is how these acts completely bypass the traditional economy of calendar and clock time. In *Austerlitz*, language and narrative have forfeited their role to "represent" and "depict" remembering and time and, instead, appear to be the very construction site of memories and human temporality.

In view of the two crucial models of memory juxtaposed in this volume, in the concluding Chapter 10, *Reframing memory*, I reflect on how our concepts, metaphors, and models not only mirror but also shape the world in which we live. Memory is a particularly interesting subject here because what it is, its ontology, is not independent from the way we conceive of it, and such conceptions are not independent from the cultural economy of remembering and forgetting of which they are a part. Here, I discuss this argument within the larger epistemological picture of memory's "historical ontology." Historical ontology is a concept suggested by Hacking to capture our changing ideas about the reality of entities such as memory. My summarizing picture borrows from Ian Hacking's philosophy of psychology, Richard Rorty's philosophy of language, and Jerome Bruner's narrative psychology. In order to avoid making these concluding reflections too categorical and theoretical an enterprise, parts of them are arranged around the presentation and interpretation of a contemporary work of art: Anselm Kiefer's *Census*, a memory installation in the Berlin Museum for Contemporary Art. Kiefer has created a case study of sorts in the historical ontology of memory. His installation raises exactly the questions I pose at the end of this book. What remains of "memory" after the disintegration of the archive? How can new models, metaphors, and stories become instrumental not only to reframe our understanding of autobiographical remembering and forgetting, but also guide and organize our mnemonic practices and, specifically, reframe the very processes of autobiographical remembering and self-understanding?

CHAPTER 2

Imagining Memory

The Archive Disintegrates

One view holds that the divisions among the various cultures of the sciences, the social sciences, and the humanities have left their mark on our knowledge of human memory in a particularly obstructive fashion. One of my aims is to show that this is not necessarily the case. More importantly, such divisions do not reflect the "nature" of remembering and forgetting but, if anything, represent a historical division of labor. This division of labor is deeply entrenched in our academic institutions. It is shored up and advanced by the administrative logic of disciplinary parochialism and positivist epistemologies. We are looking here at the same epistemologies that, in the wake of the tectonic shifts in our landscape of knowledge pointed out in the last chapter, have for some time now proven to be highly problematic. In an attempt to ignore the tunnel vision of these various disciplines, I want to offer in this chapter a picture of simultaneous and, in part, overlapping developments in several fields of memory research that pertain to all three disciplinary "cultures." Moreover, this portrait shows them as part of an even larger cultural paradigm shift in our understanding of remembering and forgetting.

If, nevertheless, the psychological and neurocognitive view of memory is given center stage, this is for another reason. Neurocognitive research on memory comes with the reputation of a hard science. Irrespective of the question whether there is a epistemologically stringent definition that distinguishes the many different types of "hard science" from the many types of "soft science," this reputation has been endorsed in recent years by popular academic and educational programs such as the "Decade of the Brain." It also plays a role in the growing public concern regarding degenerative memory problems, such as those encountered in Alzheimer's disease. Neuroscience (and we can include here parts of neurobiology, psychiatry, neurology, and neuropsychology) not only claims a special status in the world of health and illness, but also appears to pervade discourses in law courts, novels, films, and the media. It is likewise present in many social and cultural memory studies, where it is often referred to as the ultimate scientific rock bottom of our knowledge regarding "the nature" of remembering and forgetting. Over the last three decades, few signs and symbols indicating cutting edge neuroscientific and biomedical research have been as widespread as fMRI images and other (MRI, PET, and SPECT) representations of human brains.

It is all the more interesting to notice that many evidence-based findings in the field of biological and neurocognitive memory research are not in accord with the archival model. At times the disagreement is quite spectacular, as we will see more fully further below. Sticking with a popular scientific metaphor, one could say that the memory crisis—which started in the humanities and the social sciences and then went on to technology-oriented areas—has finally reached the scientific "rock bottom" level of memory research, only to reveal that the putatively firm and stable foundations of memory storage are about to be dismantled even here.

Following this chronological sequence, my line of argument begins with the social and cultural field of memory studies, then turns to the technological, and then to the literary and artistic, and eventually concentrates on the biological and cognitive.

MEMORY: THE SOCIAL AND CULTURAL FIELD

To put it in the most general terms, in this field we find research, reflection, and experimentation concerned with the social and cultural constitution and organization of memory phenomena. Academically, this is the terrain of the human and social sciences, including history (especially, oral history, cultural history, history of science and medicine, history of everyday life, and history of mentalities). All of these "proceed from the basic insight," as Astrid Erll summarizes, "that the past is not given, but must instead continually be re-constructed and re-presented" (2008, p. 7). A second insight is often associated with the work of Maurice Halbwachs who played a crucial role in expanding the scope of memory research beyond the traditional focus on the individual and personal, paving the way for the extensive study of social and cultural memory phenomena in 20th-century history and social sciences, as Erika Apfelbaum (2010) argues.

I mentioned the turning point in 1989 when the wall that divided Europe and much of the rest of the world came down. One particular aspect of this made it a momentous event for the study of memory. In the wake of events in 1989 something besides a wall came down: restrictions of access to numerous archives eased, making accessible documents and memories that had previously been unavailable, especially in the former Soviet hemisphere. Countries with newly gained independence began reinventing themselves by negotiating controversial pasts in the light of possible novel stories of national identity. It is difficult enough to rewrite the memory of a person, but now we have to rewrite the memory of entire peoples, stated former Czech dissident and then first Czech Republic president, writer Václav Havel, in a speech at Prague's Wenceslas Square.

Many registers of collective memory had to be newly arranged, and not only in Eastern Europe. In some 20 countries, Truth and Reconciliation Commissions were set up—most famously, perhaps, in South Africa, Chile, and Guatemala—giving public center stage to issues of remembering and forgetting. Similarly, German civil rights activists, writers, and artists published secret Stasi files, autobiographical accounts, and memoirs outlawed during Communism; and Spanish historians unearthed mass killings, documents, and personal memories from a time that Franco Fascism had taken great pains to officially forget.

To commemorate particular aspects of the past publicly, to keep alive the memory of people and historic events deemed to be important to a community is, of course, anything but new. What is new is that we now commemorate an amazing plethora of things and, perhaps even more significant for the issue of memory, that we passionately disagree over what should be commemorated and how it should be commemorated. Tony Judt (1998) has observed that until recently the point of a monument, a memorial plaque, a museum, or an anniversary was to remind people of what they already knew or thought they knew; today, however, these things serve a different end. They are there to remind people of things from their past they may not even know, things they have forgotten, or never learned, or do not want to know. In the United States, discussions of such controversial issues have been described as "memory wars," a term which, as Judt remarks, reflects the enormous importance dedicated to what and how to remember. Yet associating memory with the subject of wars is not only a metaphorical act, and it does not only take place in the United States.

Who has the right to design an exhibition, assign meaning to a battlefield, inscribe a plinth or plaque? These are tactical skirmishes in the greater cultural conflicts over identity: national, regional, linguistic, religious, racial, ethnic, sexual. In Germany (or Poland) arguments about how to remember or commemorate the recent past have been distilled into painful, compensatory attention to the extermination of the European Jews—planned in Germany, executed in Poland. Instead of recording and giving form to pride and nostalgia, commemoration in such circumstances rouses (and is intended to rouse) pain and even anger. Once a public device for evoking and encouraging feelings of communal or national unity, public commemoration of the past has become a leading occasion for civic division, as in the ... dispute over whether a Holocaust memorial should be built in Berlin (Judt, 1998, p. 51).

Obviously, there are a variety of cultural strategies to remember history and shape and reshape the relationship between past and present. These strategies include configuring some events as past and over, other events as still present and alive, and again others as stretching into or anticipating the future. And they also include flexibly changing such configurations in the light of new developments in the present. "As the century drew to a close," state Rossington and Whitehead, "there was an increasing concern with how best to remember the traumatic instances that had punctuated its history" (2007, p. 5). This concern was bolstered by a number of new perspectives emerging out of long-suppressed populations and communities, perspectives that transformed into academic approaches such as postcolonialism, indigenous studies, feminism, and lesbian, gay, bisexual, and transgender studies. Again, the aim was (and is) to re-appropriate and renegotiate individual and collective memories of traumatic pasts. Some historical observers have remarked that the 20th century witnessed the most horrific violence of all human history so far, which might have been a major reason why, toward the end of the century, social and individual remembrance reached a scale never before seen. War, genocide, and terror, writes historian David Blight (2009), have

... challenged us with uncounted numbers of victims and witnesses whose stories must be known. In the twentieth century, it was the victims of wars, not merely those who fought, who became the subject along with their testimony. As never before, the witness to or the victim of great violence is the new and most determining engine of memory—legally and morally, whether in war crimes trials, truth commissions, autobiographies, films, or other mediums. (p. 244)

Blight refers to new global policies supporting this view—and, thus, the discussion of meaning and nature of collective memories—such as those developed by the United Nations. In 2001, for the first time a UN conference on racism and retrospective justice took place in Durban, South Africa. Unexpectedly, a second theme emerged and took center stage: the nature of trauma, testimony, and memory. The conference issued a resolution declaring "We are conscious of the fact that the history of humanity is replete with major atrocities as a result of the gross violation of human rights and believe that lessons can be learned through remembering history to avert future tragedies" (quoted from Blight, 2009, p. 248).

I have used the terms re-appropriation and renegotiation of memories of traumatic events to broach forms and practices of remembrance, individual and social, that are carried out in processes of "testimonial production" and, more broadly, intergenerational transmission. Many of the phenomena under discussion are, in fact, multigenerational processes. "Memory is the faculty that enables us to form an awareness of selfhood (identity), both on the personal and on the collective level," writes Assmann (2008) who views the connection between individuals and their multigenerational community as the key to what he calls "cultural memory," the basis of human beings' "diachronic identity" (p. 109). In more traditional (and more static) terms, we are talking here about individuals' and communities' historical consciousness or the consciousness of historical continuity. Modern "mnemohistorians," scholars of "memoralization," and other memory researchers prefer, however, to refer to "historical memory" (Halbwachs, 1992), or historical "collective memories" (Wertsch, 2009). From all these perspectives, intergenerational memories appear as the result of a variety of social practices and artifacts reaching from haunted topographies to strategies of archiving and narrating (Jobst & Lüdke, 2010). These practices are concerned predominantly with the remembrance of memories of others, and this is what distinguishes them from autobiographical memories. These others also comprise the dead.

Of course, there is no clear borderline between the remembrance of others and autobiographical remembering, just as there is no clear borderline between the living and the dead. Take the consciousness, the autobiographical self, of a person who mourns his beloved partner. Trying to understand his life after the death of his wife, British writer Julian Barnes (2013) points out the experience "that someone is dead may mean that they are not alive, but doesn't mean that they do not exist" (p. 102); it is their constantly remembered absence that makes them permanently present.

Often historical and cultural remembrance takes place in spatial connection with what Nora (1989) described as *lieux de mémoire*, sites of memory. On the one hand, sites of memory can be very personal and ephemeral, which has often made them invisible for successive generations. Keith Thomas (2009) has reminded us that most monuments in early modern England, for example, were temporary ones, garlands of ribbons and paper created by the have-nots and hung in churches or strewn in churchyards before being disposed of by the ecclesiastical authorities like withered field flowers. Even the "vulgar," as Thomas observes, wanted to be remembered and commemorate their loved ones—butchers, carpenters, and blacksmiths of whom nothing more is said than that they had a name, lived so many years, and died.

On the other hand, there are those sites of memory that are conditional for a certain type of commemoration instrumental to the historical underpinnings of national identity. Nora and many other historians and social scientists of memory primarily use the concept in this sense, referring to places where groups of individuals engage in public commemorative activity establishing or confirming a sense of unity through a shared past. Yet the notion of *lieux de mémoire* also allows for a slightly different view. If we understand sites of memory not only as points of reference for those who survived and personally remember historic events, but also for those born long after them, the word "memory" takes on a new meaning; it becomes, as Jay Winter notes, a "metaphor for the fashioning of narratives about the past when those with direct experience of events die off. Sites of memory inevitably become sites of second-order memory" (2008, p. 62), places where people remember the memories of others and in this way re-appropriate a particular tradition.

A turning point in the history of memory studies

It might have been the single most momentous event in the modern history of the study of memory that, in the closing decade of the 20th century, this new multidisciplinary field of social (or collective, or cultural) memory studies came into existence. And it might have been the single most momentous challenge in this field to break with the longstanding notion of memory as an individual archive of the past. However, as we will see, this break was anything but free from contradictions and conflicts. On a theoretical plane, poststructuralist arguments in the wake of Jacques Derrida and Michel Foucault and intertextualist arguments in the wake of Mikhail Bakhtin further fanned the flames. According to these arguments, memories (and associated phenomena like identity formation and life stories) are meaning constructions. Thus, they are in principle unstable. They do not relate to essences past or present but are first of all events in language and other semiotic systems. Interlaced with broader "cultural texts" and situated within "symbolic spaces," they are always incomplete in isolation. And because they are discursively negotiated instead of just given or "retrieved," they clearly appear as subject to orders of power and struggle.

Influenced by these arguments, propelled by historical developments, and underscored by the emergence of new political genres of memory narratives (Andrews, 2007), the surge of vital interests in how the past gets rewritten in the present resulted in the emergence of a new understanding of remembering and forgetting. Across a multitude of academic discourses and disciplines the view became dominant that, whatever it is we call memory, it is the product of social practices, that is, it is shaped by political interests and along cultural trajectories. Conceptually, many authors thus have preferred to use the verbal noun "remembering" to underline the ongoing dynamic of construction and continuous reconstruction and to replace the traditional idea of memory with one of being in a state of constant flux.[1] We also could say that they have shifted the focus from memory as an entity to a process, a liquid and ever changing reality. Obviously this dynamic view of memory is situated in a much wider world, and a much more complicated world. Understanding it, as Lambeck and Antze put it, involves examining "the symbols, codes, artifacts, rites, and sites in which memory is embodied and objectified; the coherence or fragmentation of the narratives, rituals, geographies, or even epistemologies it relies upon; and the way their authority changes over time" (1996, p. xvii).

MEMORY: THE FIELD OF MEDIA AND TECHNOLOGY

A second field of memory studies revolves around the technology and the media, old and new, that shape individual and collective remembering. The hub of this field is the digital revolution, which is, in essence, a global revolution of human memory and communication technologies. Yet the field comprises much more. It extends to the many efforts of conceiving this revolution, its cascading consequences—the permanent production of new technologies and social practices of digital and virtual memory—and their psycho–socio–cultural implications. This interest is a driving force in disciplines such as information studies, communication studies, media and cultural studies, and social studies of technology, some of which have come into being only recently. The question that drives me is: How does this field contribute to a new understanding of human remembering?

Philosophers of mind, information scientists, and cultural theorists have all emphasized the material and technological dimension not only of our processes of remembrance, but also of our notion of memory. Many of them see this notion transforming under the impact of the digital revolution, opening up to new ideas of malleability, mutability, and constructivity. Now, since Bartlett, we cannot say it is a new discovery that memories are mediated and negotiated in social and conversational contexts (cf., for more recent studies, e.g., Hirst & Echterhoff, 2008, 2012; Manier, 2004; Middleton & Brown, 2005; Wagoner, 2012), and that they are grounded, in a Vygotskian sense, in "mediated actions" (Wertsch, 1998). Valsiner (2007) speaks of "cultural systems of semiotic regulation." Nor is it new that their content is shaped through the media in which they exist (photographs, films, narratives, artworks, performances, mementos, other artifacts, and combinations thereof) or that individual memories are often confounded with these media (Ernst, 2013; Kittler, 1999; McQuire, 1998); psychologists would say they are "distorted" by them. But the extensive digitalization of memories surely has drawn sharper attention to these phenomena, and that is, as José van Dijck has it, to the "inextricable interconnections between acts of remembrance and the specific mediated objects through which these acts materialize" (2007, p. 16). Van Dijck, a finely tuned analyst of these interconnections, argues that digital technologies deeply affect the very nature of our remembering processes. Her conclusion is that our view of memory has to be fundamentally reconceptualized to take into account this new type of material mediation. So what in particular, then, is new about it?

There are a number of specific qualities of "digital memory machines," as modern computers are called in the literature of this field, that impact on the cognitive functions and cultural practices of remembering of their users—that is, of us. To begin with, computers are advanced multimedia and multimodal facilities. In combining text, graphic, image, film, and audio media and modalities, they bring about unprecedented "morphing" capacities, to use van Dijck's expression. Likewise, as N. Katherine Hayles (2012) argues, Internet technologies have generated new forms of digital literacy, such as scanning, skimming, linking, "hyper reading," and shifting within hybrid media environments, which are as important forms of reading as close reading once was. At the level of 21st century digitalization these multimedial and multimodal capacities and skills are not just properties of machines but need to be viewed as "mental-technical-cultural processes" (Dijck, 2007; 2013), bound to affect the cultural practices involved in creating and handling memory constructs and, in this way, our understanding of ourselves and others.

In order to see how these processes impact on our ideas of self and constructions of identity we need to bring to mind that digitalized memory media, like older memory media such as photographs or diaries, are not usually understood as exact or complete recordings of past experiences. Rather, they fulfill complex psychological functions, serving as what van Dijck calls "evocative frames" or "building blocks" that we mold in a continuously dynamic process of remembering (2007, p. 24). People use computers (from industrial or scientific mega computers to desktops, tablets, and smartphones) as personal memory machines because they have specific needs, interests, and desires—such as a desire for a sensory experience that, in turn, triggers particular feelings.

> For instance, a song may help invoke a specific mood, whereas a diary is more suitable to inscribe and recall reflexive thoughts. The recording medium once dictated the choice for a particular sensory inscription, but multimedia computers and digital recording devices expand the choices now that digital cameras combined with software packages promote their multiple usage as recorders of sound, text, still pictures, and moving images (Dijck, 2007, pp. 164–165).

But do we not have to suspect that these choices bring "digital memory management" close to acts of distortion, falsification, and forgery? Van Dijck's analyses make clear that these categories do not match the phenomena under examination. She argues that human beings do not engage in autobiographical remembering in order to produce exact, complete, and unchangeable memories of their past. This is not to say that they are not able to remember in an exact and complete fashion. They are, in fact, and it is amazingly often that they do so. But autobiographical reminiscing typically serves more complex functions, as becomes strikingly apparent in digitally mediated acts of remembering. People might, for example, create movies of themselves as future memories, with the explicit intention to look back upon them at an undetermined point in time, or to invite others to do so. This is an involute construction on its own. They also might retouch images, revise texts, and edit films and sounds recorded in the past to attune them to current views of themselves and of others. And they may narratively crossfade "factual" life documents with "fictive" material from various sources. They do this, perhaps, because they want to create comedy-like versions of themselves or others, or tell jokes disguised as "real" memory documents to be shared with friends in a social network or with the virtual global community. It is no coincidence that "remixing" has become one of the buzzwords of *Netspeak*.

Remixing past, present, and future

Let us raise the question again: Is this creative remixing of memories of the past, experiences in the present, and expectations of the future really a new and specific quality of the digital age? Do we not have to acknowledge that our autobiographical memories have always been the subject of narrative interpretation, the stuff of conscious and unconscious elaboration and re-configuration, with or without digital memory machines? For van Dijck there is no doubt that it is the nature of human remembering to be "constantly prone to revision just as memory objects are constantly amenable to alteration" (2007, p. 173). This resonates with a general quality of the relationship between human subjects and fine-tuned technologies like digital tools and "memory machines," which are, of course, not facing one another unmediatedly. From the very beginning, Ernst Schraube notes, technologies have been part of the "sociomaterial world" created by humans; as a consequence, they "go through the subject, showing themselves in . . . the subject's experiences, consciousness, and actions" (2013, p. 29). Schraube backs his view up with studies by the historian of technology David Nye, who claims that "technologies are not foreign to 'human nature' but inseparable from it" (2007, p. 2). In fact, as Nye goes on to say, they "have been part of human society from as far back as archaeology can take us into the past" (p. 7).

There is, however, a specific quality to the new "mental-technical-cultural processes" that have emerged with global digitalization: They are interlaced with novel types of intersubjective networks. These networks interconnect individuals and their memories with others. Blurring established borderlines between the "inner" and the "outer," they redefine the relationship between the private and the public sphere. For Anthony Hoskins, Internet-based social networks dissolve the dichotomy between personal and collective memory-making, creating new "media-memoryscapes" (2009a, p. 29; cf. also Hoskin, 2013a). Transforming a technical term into a social category, van Dijck speaks of an emerging culture of connectivity, "a culture where perspectives, expressions, experiences and productions are increasingly mediated by social media sites" (2011, p. 402).

Social-interactive digital platforms like Facebook, YouTube, MySpace, Twitter, Wikipedia, and Flickr—the subjects of van Dijck's (2013) studies—have become crucial to how many users practice sociality and how they understand friendship, intimacy, trust, and community. This alone profoundly changes traditional conventions for autobiographical remembering, for example, by undermining the idea of memory as a predominantly inward and cerebral property of humans. Rather than being self-confined machines for automated recording, storage, and retrieval of individuals, multimedia Internet technology installations are constitutively "networked." They provide public arenas for shared life constructions and their interpretations, in this way creating a new type of "connective memory." In their analysis of these phenomena, theorists of connective memory like Hoskins (2009b; 2013b) and van Dijck (2011) repudiate the traditional idea of collective memory, which assumes that individual and collective memory are separate entities associated *through* social institutions, practices, and technologies, an idea they attribute to Halbwachs (1992), among others. Instead, they propose that processes of remembering and forgetting are increasingly carried out *by* digital networks, transforming "memory" into an Internet-based social institution, an open forum, a hybrid that is both electronic and human.

This potential becomes particularly manifest in the development of technologies that allow users to operate on autobiographical memory documents by "mixing" and "remixing" them. Consider memory technologies such as multimedia lifelogs or lifeblogs that people use to keep track of their changing lives and those of connected persons. There are, for example, software applications to manipulate digital photographs, interlock them with interpreting texts and sound frames, and link them to other documents, personal and public; mix-and-burn programs that allow one to "customize" existing sounds to particular moods; and digitalized home movies that make it possible to easily reframe a family's contrived past and blend it with historically authentic documents, possibly linked to materials from, say, recognized research institutes. We are looking at digitalized chains of mementos that can deeply affect people's present, or even later, remembrance of things past. They not only impact how and what to remember, over time they may turn themselves into oftentimes confirmed memories that gain more and more "documented" authenticity.

What essentially contributes to such digital-psychological reshaping and consolidation of memories is its social and discursive dimension. Personal collections of electronic memory documents are often embedded in networks or platforms in which users/rememberers share their memories and mutually influence their practices and ideas of creative ("connective") reminiscing. Of course, an important factor is that the 21st-century Internet, in contrast with earlier systems, is not only social, interactive, multimodal, and multimedia, but also truly global. It is ubiquitous—and cheap.[2] As a consequence, cultural techniques and styles of remembrance continuously transform themselves and the results quickly disperse in an uncontrolled and uncontrollable fashion. Occasionally, however, particular genres of remembrance appear to solidify, despite their fluid mode of being, even if only for a brief time. There are, for instance, "global memory places" with a certain continuity, such as Wikipedia and its "floating" wikis (cf. Pentzold, 2009), and digital "memorial landscapes" for the dead (cf. Veale, 2004). Many theorists of digital memory see in the emergence of such new genres interactively connecting personal memories to memories and reflections of others and to public resources the truly groundbreaking qualities of "digital memory machines."[3]

For several authors, the innovative potential of the digital revolution is particularly tangible in new storytelling technologies that break open and radically alter established narrative genres (cf. Hoffmann, 2010; Grishakova & Ryan, 2010; Page & Thomas, 2011). One example is narrative sequentiality or seriality, which has an immediate impact on processes of remembering. The new digital-based forms of seriality that Ruth Page has examined include "reverse-order archiving," the sequenced deletion (rather than addition) of material, and new ways of nonteleological storytelling (Page, 2013). Another example regards new forms of integration of user action within the storyworld. This may entail that in remembering the elements of a story in a certain manner the user/rememberer changes the course of the story and gives it a new turn. Take the Holodeck narrative machine. This interactive storytelling software incorporates every action of the visitor in a way that affects the life of his or her fictional persona, with every different choice leading to a different storyline. "It would be impossible," concludes Ryan in her analysis of this narrative game, which creates stories in real time during the run of the program, "to store in advance all the consequences of all the decisions that can be made by the player" (2009, p. 51).

Traditionally, narrative, whether oral or written, has been considered humanity's most advanced means of contextualizing, whether with respect to propositions, ideas, memories, or ourselves. What has emerged with the advent of multimedial and networked computers is not merely a new device but, according to Roy Harris, "the most powerful contextualization device" ever known; indeed, the capacity for creating and developing new interactive contexts, visual and verbal, "far outstrips that of the human mind" (2002, p. 49). For Harris, this is a much more important fact about computing "than its superhuman capacity for information storage" (p. 49). Drawing on neuroscientific findings about the "morphing nature" of episodic memory, van Dijck (2007; 2013) takes this line of thinking one step further and suggests that multimedial and multimodal computers may enhance this essential quality of episodic memory, that is, its inherent mutability, more than any previous technology. Considering research from neurobiology and neurocognitive psychology, she concludes that we "have to accept human memory as an amalgamation of creative projection, factual retrieval, and narrative recollection of past events" (2007, p. 163). It is exactly this morphing and transformative nature of autobiographical remembering that is supported and enhanced by digital technologies, by "mental-cultural-technical processes" that are not only mnemonic aids but truly creative instruments of reminiscing.

This is all the more evident in the digital creation of fictional and nonfictional autobiographical narratives. Such a creation is amazingly uncomplicated. With the help of appropriate design technologies we easily enter an endless realm of storyworlds that are autobiographically utilizable, seamlessly unfolded in writing, graphic novels, film and television, paintings, photography, graphic and music software. All these various semiotic environments can be employed as imaginative resources for digitally composing one's life story. Viewed in this light, it becomes obvious why the digital revolution plays such a crucial role for the cultural paradigm shift in our understanding of memory. The Internet-connected computer is quite the opposite of a warehouse of the mind that stores memories and other information; it turns out to be an epistemological and narrative model that lends itself to a reconceptualization of memory far beyond the semantic and metaphorical realm of the archive.

Investigating the digital mediation of memories also sheds new light on the fact that our life worlds, in a more general sense, are swamped with mnemonic artifacts and semiotic environments that we readily have come to use as memory resources. This alone challenges the traditional notion of memory as something individual, cerebral, and inward. I already mentioned Nora's concept of memory sites. There is an endless variety of such mnemonic environments, including landscapes and geographies (Halbwachs 1992), cities and urban spaces (Boyer, 1996, Huyssen, 2003), nations (Etkind, 2013; Olick, 2003), places of commemoration (Assmann, A., 2011), memorials (Young, 1993), sculptures and art installations (Brockmeier, 2001a), and all kinds of personal sites and mementos—physical and digital—from the ringlet and the grave in the cemetery to lifeblogs and screenshots (Petrelli, Whittaker, & Brockmeier, 2008). And there is a further mnemonic environment relevant here: language. Even if many of our memories and acts of remembrance are spatially and materially situated, this does not exclude that they are intermingled with language, the oxygen of our social life. Language comes in manifold forms: oral, written, and performative; and it is technically mediated in many ways. It, therefore, is not surprising that the digital revolution and, in its wake, the establishment of a global system of digital literacy has had an important impact on our understanding of language (and writing in particular) as specific forms and practices of memory.[4]

Likewise, the development of new technologies of publicly shared memories has prompted research in the social sciences and cultural studies on another momentous outcome of the digital revolution: the transformation of the traditional archive. Many libraries, museums, collections of documents and other artifacts of the past are undergoing profound changes. Being electronically "rewritten" and "redistributed" changes their reclusive mnemonic status. From a unique and shielded three-dimensional storage space they turn into a virtual surface present and interactively accessible at any time and in any place (Hedstrom, 2002).

MEMORY: THE LITERARY AND ARTISTIC FIELD

The third field with a particular concern for memory is the literary and artistic field. It often has been emphasized that art and literature constitute "a record of human consciousness, the richest and most comprehensive we have," as David Lodge (2002, p. 10) put it. Writers and artists work at the edge of what's understood, and often go even beyond. Many a time the thought experiments executed in the literary laboratory of the mind are more elaborate, reaching further into uncharted territory than scientific thought experiments, Catherine Elgin (2007) has argued. Indeed, often it is literature rather than science or medicine that is responsible for introducing new models and visions of mind, consciousness, and psychological states. The recent history of the sciences of the mind and brain especially provide many examples of this. Historians of ideas suggest, to use Hacking's words, "that the whole language of many selves had been hammered out by generations of romantic poets and novelists great and small, and also in innumerable broadsheets and feuilletons too ephemeral for general knowledge today" (1995, p. 232). Our modern understandings of hysteria, possession, and non-normative forms of personality are, as Hacking has shown, the direct "consequence of how the literary imagination has formed the language in which we speak of people be they real or imagined" (p. 233).

All of these claims hold particularly true for the dimension of human consciousness and mind that is at the heart of this book: remembering and forgetting. It is hardly overstating the point to say that literature represents the longest and most venerable tradition of thinking about memory, with its Western history reaching back to the beginnings of ancient Greece, Israel, and Egypt (Assmann, J., 2011). Literary works from Homer to Proust have provided extensive material for the study of remembering and forgetting, offering what Suzanne Nalbantian (2003) has described as a large variety of fictional test cases of memory phenomena. They also meticulously have portrayed, and indeed examined, the narrative fabric of memory phenomena at work. More than that, literary works even have contributed to the very formation of this fabric and its differentiations and transformations in various epochs and cultures.

In many respects we can recognize close interrelations between the development of autobiographical understanding and the emergence of mind-representing and mind-creating resources of narrative; this nexus is pivotal to the evolution of the modern idea of the self (Freeman & Brockmeier, 2001; Herman, 2011a; Olney, 1998). Autobiographical self-exploration is, after all, a narrative genre. With the rise of modernity it has continuously gained significance. We might even call it an investigative genre, based on the idea that we have to explore what we are in order to establish our autobiographical identity "because," as Charles Taylor has remarked, "the assumption behind modern self-exploration is that we don't already know who we are" (1989, p. 178).

Even if many authors have seen this concern first taking shape in the works of writers from the eighteenth century, such as Rousseau, the sixteenth century, such as Montaigne, or even the fourth century, such as Augustine of Hippo, autobiographical remembering and self-exploration surely reached a new quality in 19th- and 20th-century literature and arts. In fact, as Max Saunders argues, since the beginning of the 20th century, concerns with self and autobiography have been at the heart of the literary discourse. Consider the "surprising number of major works of European modernism and postmodernism"—by Rilke, Joyce, Proust, Pound, Woolf, Mann, Svevo, Stein, Sartre, Musil, Nabokov, and others—that "engage in very profound and central ways with questions about life-writing" (2010, p. 12). This literature has fueled an extensive amount of scholarship and reflection in criticism, literary and art theory, and philosophy. Again, the last decades have witnessed an extraordinary increase in the study of autobiographical and biographical writing or "life writing," to employ the more comprehensive term commonly used today (Jolly, 2001; Saunders, 2008; Smith & Watson, 2010). In light of this critical and theoretical scholarship, a large portion of Western literature appears as an experimental laboratory of human self-examination.[5] And in the center of this examination, we find the question of autobiographical remembering and its manifold interconnections with identity formation.

This interest in the nexus of memory, identity, and life writing can be viewed from two perspectives. One highlights its close connection to the emergence of the individual self as a prominent theme and self-exploratory practice in modern life and literature; the other frames the creation of a rich repertoire of mind-creating and mind-representing narrative forms and techniques, especially since the late 19th century. This repertoire has not only afforded writers an opportunity to develop a particular sensitivity for our manifold practices of remembering. Often this heightened awareness is related to intricate new forms of narrative self-observation and self-investigation, as in many works of the writers just mentioned. In such texts we can explore in great detail how new narrative techniques have advanced significantly the general mnemonic and reflexive potential of modernist writing (cf. Herman, 2011c). That the analytical and reflexive attention paid to memory is not subordinate to the literary and artistic claim was a special concern, for example, of Vladimir Nabokov. Nabokov considered himself a memory artist in so far as he was a memory analyst. And a memory analyst he was indeed, drawing on a profound familiarity with the entire range of contemporary European memory theories from Freud and academic psychology to Bergson and Proust (cf. Foster, 1993).

Beckett's memory

Following the tradition of narrative exploration of memory and self until the present, we notice that many life-writers have taken a critical stance toward the idea that experiences can be stored and preserved over time and finally recalled, whether in voluntary or involuntary fashion. In Chapters 4–9, I use texts from 20th- and 21st-century literary memory-writing to offer what psychologists and psychiatrists would call "case studies" of the autobiographical process. Vis-à-vis this material, it appears that the critical stance I have been taking toward the archival model of memory is not a recent phenomenon. Autobiographers, writers, artists, and diarists have long been aware of the ambivalent and contradictory status of what one takes to be one's personal memories. Samuel Beckett is an emblematic example. James Olney (1998) has pointed out that much of Beckett's work can be read as an effort to think through the insight that one's personal identity construction can never be grounded in autobiographical memory because, as the Irish writer observed, memories of one's past are themselves part and parcel of that very construction.

Few authors articulate as drastically as Beckett the break of the modernist sense of autobiographical identity with the traditional view of self and memory. What then was the traditional view of self and memory for Beckett? It probably was captured best in Augustine's *Confessions* (1991), which famously stated that memory is the present of things past. Now, Beckett asks, does this tell us how we, the rememberers, are situated? Does this say anything about who we are? How can we ever be sure about this, as Olney summarizes Beckett's reasoning,

> . . . if memory is so uncertain or unstable, both epistemologically and ontologically, that we do not even know if a given set of memories is ours or someone else's? To think of autobiography's referentiality as pertaining not to events of the past but to memories of those events solves a lot of problems arising in a good many texts, but Beckett, like other writers of our time, has altered the terms and raised the stakes of the wager by calling into doubt, in the most radical way, memory's capacity to establish a relationship to our past and hence a relationship to ourselves grown out of the past (1989, pp. 7–8).

In Beckett's view, all of the following are formed independently from a physical or otherwise reliably given substrate: what we call our memories of the past, the very idea of past, present, and future, and the order of their succession. Instead of just accepting them as givens, we have to understand them as the outcome of our own creative meaning constructions. Olney maintains that Beckett is acutely aware that endowing autobiographical meanings is inextricably tied to the resources of language. At stake are the "twin acts of memory and narrative in the present" (p. 9). Interestingly, in this respect there are striking parallels between the autobiographical narrations of Augustine and Beckett. Both authors write narratives about the act of remembering as well as about the act of narrating. In Olney's words, "Augustine, like Beckett, tells the story of himself telling the story of himself telling the story of his life" (p. 8). Still, this should not make us forget that more than a thousand years separate Beckett's memory from Augustine's, distinguishing the late-ancient bishop's steadfast trust in the well-ordered stability of our inner memory palaces from the complete loss of such a trust in the modern writer.

When I hence examine in the following chapters examples of literary autobiographical narrative, then this is in line with my main undertaking to explore narrative as an alternative to the archive model of memory. In contrast with other authors I do, perhaps, put less emphasis on the differences between the genres or discourse types of literary and everyday autobiographical narrative because I think that the differences matter less than the common ground, that is the narrative dynamic of the auto-biographical process (I have explained my reasons for this elsewhere, see Brockmeier, 2013a). Furthermore, we should not forget that it was long before psychological and neuroscientific research on memory that litera-ture and the arts first began to scrutinize critically the traditional picture of memory and to evoke alternative scenarios never seen before. Since then, many literary works and other artworks have continued to do so, establishing themselves as an advanced probe of how we situate ourselves in past, present, and future.

The rejection of the naïve notion of the past being preserved in a mental or material (including neuronal) storage, which started in the domain of literary narrative, has been gaining more and more ground in the other fields of memory studies sketched above. We even can discover a compa-rable trend in the fourth field of memory studies, the biological and neu-rocognitive, to which I turn now.

MEMORY: THE BIOLOGICAL AND NEUROCOGNITIVE FIELD

When I was younger I could remember anything, whether it happened or not; but I am getting old, and soon I shall remember only the latter.

Mark Twain

This field is marked by a biological, medical, and psychological focus on the individual and his or her capacities—or inability—to remember and to forget. Here we look at research by neurobiologists, neurologists, psychia-trists, psychologists (mainly in neurocognitive research contexts but also with interests in cultural, discursive, and narrative psychology), clinical researchers, psychotherapists and -analysts (concerned with trauma and Holocaust studies, dementia studies, narrative medicine, and health stud-ies, among others). Several crucial events have influenced the field since the 1990s, although their significance is assessed differently in various academic quarters. While neurobiologists would refer to new research on cellular and molecular levels, neurocognitive psychologists would high-light the systematic use of neuroimaging technologies. At the same time, neurologists, psychiatrists, and gerontologists have been concerned with more medically, socially, and psychologically applied issues, due to, for example, a dramatically growing portion of the population suffering from memory diseases like Alzheimer's. Furthermore, clinical researchers and psychotherapists would emphasize the debates about the False Memory Syndrome and the "memory wars," whereas narrative, discursive, and cultural psychologists would outline novel research on the importance of contexts of interaction, intersubjective and embodied practices, fictional imagination, and cultural models of storytelling for people's narratives about themselves and their autobiographical memories in particular.

I have argued that there is an overarching tendency in these various domains of memory research that challenges the idea of memory as a storeroom of the past. This tendency can also be observed in the fourth field. A caveat is necessary, however, because the general cultural paradigm shift only to a very limited degree has affected the *conceptual* shape of memory phenomena in this domain, where processes of remembering and forgetting typically are still conceived of in terms of archival models. If we consult any standard psychological and neuroscientific textbooks and reference works on memory and learning, as already pointed out in the first chapter, we will find widespread use of a vocabulary that focuses on brain "mechanisms" of remembering and forgetting, with the unchallenged assumption that these mechanisms are to be conceptualized in terms of encoding, storing, and retrieval of information.

This is all the more astonishing because there are many spectacular new findings and observations that contradict and, in fact, are about to erode the traditional idea of memory, even in this field. Although results of neuroscientific research receive wide media attention and become the subject of discourses far beyond the scientific community, their connections with findings and debates in other areas of memory studies are rarely addressed. Even more rarely we encounter discussions about the implications of such findings for our theoretical models of memory, for our ideas of what "memory" is supposed to be. If at all, it is not neuroscientific research we find, but rather the experiences of clinicians and healthcare practitioners working, for instance, with individuals suffering from dementia who have questioned the traditional approach to autobiographical memory (as manifested in neuropsychological tests), especially in respect to its significance for personhood and identity (cf. Brockmeier, 2014). That the established archival models need, however, to be fundamentally reconsidered—and this even and particularly in view of recent neuroscientific developments—becomes obvious when we review some of the findings in this field.

Let me begin with a few new insights of brain research into the long-established distinction between *remembering* and *perceiving* that are of great significance for our understanding of the basics of remembering and forgetting.[6] Storing and recalling past experience is, as pointed out earlier, the common denominator of what the entire tradition conceives of as the essence of memory. One of the most surprising new neurocognitive and neurobiological findings is, however, that there is no evident difference between brain processes operative in remembering and in perceiving. That is, there is no biological correlate that allows us to distinguish between what we traditionally call acts of remembering the past from acts of perceiving the present—whether in a visual, acoustical, and tactile mode; or whether in view of the activation of the brain's sensory areas, emotional (limbic) areas, and executive areas. What is more, there are no neurocognitive indicators that separate the content of a perception in the here and now from the content of a perception we had at some point in the past. As far as the neuronal circuits involved, there is nothing that would discriminate between perceiving, say, a face here and now and having perceived this face a few days or years ago.

If not from a neurobiological configuration, where then does the distinction between the present of a perception and the past of a memory come from? Well, we attribute it afterward, in an act of interpretation and temporal localization—that is, in an act of creation, not just of representation or mirroring. To use a neuroscientifically more established term, this act of interpretation or attribution corresponds to what Tulving (1985b; Tulving & Kim, 2009) calls "autonoetic consciousness." What distinguishes, however, interpretation from Tulving's autonoetic consciousness is that it is predicated not only on the brain and the mind, but also on the social and cultural world of which both the mind and the brain are a part. It is not a brain mechanism that interprets whether the face I have on my mind is a memory, a perception, or an imagination, rather it is I, a person, who interprets it.

That there is no distinction between remembering and perceiving on a neurological level also holds true for the distinction between *perceiving* and *imagining*, as we have learned from other studies. In fact, an entirely new multidisciplinary research field has emerged investigating how the brain "generates" predictions and anticipations, a capacity or a set of capacities described as a "universal principle in the operation of the human brain" (Bar, 2011b, p. v). This means, for example, that the difference between a present perception or thought and an imagined future perception or thought is unverifiable on neurophysiological grounds. Both are constructed scenes, and in this respect they are like a memory. Whether I see a face in this very moment or just imagine it in an act of "episodic simulation"—be it a face that I want, hope, or am afraid to see in the future—the activated neurological functions are the same. Neuroscientists have shown that the brain capacities involved when I recall a scene at my last birthday party (that is, an "episodic memory") and when I imagine this scene to happen at a future birthday party are indistinguishable—whether these capacities are called "prediction," "episodic future thought," "foresight," "future-oriented thinking," "prospection," or "future simulation" (Bar, 2011a; Szpunar, 2010; Szpunar & Tulving, 2011); there is even a slightly poetical variant, "memories of the future" (Ingvar, 1984; Szpunar, Addis, McLelland, & Schacter, 2013). This also applies when we later remember these simulations of future events ("future memories"), a recall that makes use of the same neural substrates as the recall of memories of past events. What matters, it seems, is the content, not the temporal status (past or future), of the remembered episode; and the episodic content—the particular scene at the birthday party—is in both cases the same.

Of course, what also matters is the emotional charge of an episode. Strong and positive emotional experiences are often remembered better and longer; but this is not the main issue here. I like the more careful formulation that what can be demonstrated in experiments using functional brain imaging is "a high level of similarity in the neural substrates of autobiographical remembering and episodic future thinking" (McDermott, Szpunar, & Arnold, 2011, p. 83).[7] This is also confirmed by findings from patients with amnesia. The difficulties these individuals confront in remembering correspond to their problems in imagining new experiences and, especially, in conjuring up holistic scenarios of the future (Hassabis, Kumaran, Vann, & Maguire, 2007; Klein, Loftus, & Kihlstrom, 2002).

A similar picture shapes up if we consider *experienced emotions* and *imagined emotions*. Studies within the same experimental field have demonstrated that feelings associated with perceptions make use of the same neuronal processes as feelings associated with imaginings. There is no way to distinguish the neuronal activities involved in my emotions when I see a face in the present, the emotions that are part of the memory of that face (be it mental or represented by a photograph), or the anticipated emotions—sometimes called "premotions" (e.g., Gilbert & Wilson, 2011)—associated with an imagined future situation in which I see that face. Nor is there a way neurocognitively to distinguish these activities from my desire to see this face, a phenomenon that has been called "desire-like imaginings" (Currie & Ravenscroft, 2002). To put this point another way, the same imaginative capacities and emotional states are in operation when people have certain thoughts, beliefs, or desires, or imagine having these thoughts, beliefs, or desires. This also applies when they envision others having certain thoughts, beliefs, or desires (a kind of imagination that, in a different context, is called "theory of mind" or "mindreading"), be it in the present, the past, or the future. Apparently, there is no such thing as a neurobiological borderline between what we consider and "feel" to be present (what we perceive or experience in the here and now), future (what we anticipate in our imagination), and past (what we usually call memory).

Again, the question arises, what then defines a memory? We already know that it is not a clearly identifiable and reliable psychological mode, or sensation, or feeling. There is no inner special tag that tells me, this is a memory, a memory of a real face I saw in the past, and not, say, the memory of a shot or film sequence of this face that I saw who knows where. Nor is there any psychological indicator that signals, this is a face I imagined after someone else told me about it, or a face I dreamt of, hallucinated, or otherwise made up and then mistook as a real one. All this we knew already. Yet now we also learn that a memory is not characterized through the activation of a specific neurophysiological substrate, a mechanism in the brain that allows me to answer all these questions. In other words, we come to know that there is neither a reliable subjective nor objective neurological answer to this question. The answer, rather, refers to our continuous meaning-making activities, to our interpretive "effort after meaning."[8]

Could time be a further factor in this interpretive effort after meaning? Are memories not temporally "marked" as past events? Indeed, there is a view, especially in philosophical quarters, that memories are defined by their temporal status. To understand this view a little philosophical digression is helpful.

Time and temporalization

Memories are defined by their temporal status, as experiences that occurred in the past. How then, we might ask, do we identify this temporal status, the mnemonic past? Considering that our constructions of memory and time are entangled in multiple ways, there is no easy answer. Localizing experiences in time means, in a basic sense, to envision them as something that happens presently or belongs to the past or the future. Obviously, when we interpret them as past, we take them as memories. Furthermore, we envisage them as something that happens simultaneously, earlier, or later in relation to other experiences. According to a much discussed distinction by John McTaggart (1908), these are the two basic ways in which we temporalize events and arrange them "in time." McTaggart called them the "A series" (which corresponds to the common sequence of past, present, and future) and the "B series" (which orders events in terms of earlier and later). I, for one, find McTaggart's argument convincing that these forms of temporalization do not necessarily reflect a given material structure, an ontological property of the world in which we live (although I could imagine a different rationale for this argument than that put forward by the Cambridge idealist McTaggart when he spoke about the "unreality of time"). Likewise, neither can this or any other notion of time claim to unfold along a neurobiological or physical time trajectory, a trajectory that preexists our concepts of it—as if it were independent of the meaning constructions by which we strive to situate our experiences and ourselves along the "A series" and the "B series." Indeed, McTaggart did not maintain this but rather suggested ways in which we—speakers of English or other Standard Average European languages—make sense of events in temporal terms. To put the same point another way, McTaggart's argument shifted the attention from the question of how we localize ourselves *in time* to how we localize ourselves *by using temporal constructions*.

Yet the ways of the A and B series are not our only ways. If we understand chronological time in the wake of Einstein as a model by which we think and organize our experiences, not as a given condition under which we live, then it is patent that there are many other strategies of temporalization. After all, we use many strategies to give meaning to our experiences. Endowing experiences with meaning is a basic mode of consciousness that is of a higher complexity than exclusively realized on the neuronal level or on the level of Tulving's "autonoetic consciousness," which is not to say that this is not complex enough already. But, as already elucidated, the complexity at stake also spans the dialogical and societal dimension of human consciousness, and thus it also comprises consciousness' interlacement with cultural sign and symbol systems such as language and, especially, the language of narrative. These are the frameworks for specifically human experiences of time. Their meanings are intermingled with the lived contexts and projects of our lives—of work, family, friendship, passions, and desires.

Hermeneutic and phenomenological philosophers, therefore, have suggested understanding our concepts of time and temporality as ultimately emerging out of our practical concerns and life projects. *Sorge*, which is both care and concern, is the term Martin Heidegger (1962) uses to explain the existential root of our sense of time; *préoccupation* is Paul Ricoeur's (1980) concept. One important form in which we engage with these concerns, activities, and events is narrative, the language of existential meaning-making. It is through stories and otherwise performed acts of meaning that we temporalize our experiences, that we give them the shape of dramas, comedies, and enigmas, and in this way situate them in a social world. The argument I put forth is that narrative works as a unique cultural practice of temporal self-localization. Again, on grounds of such narrative hermeneutics, autobiographical remembering is a case in point, for its narrative dynamic provides "the structural glue that ties together the who, what, where, when, and why," as Katherine Nelson (2007b, p. 327) puts it.

But it is not only narrative that affords us such glue. Cultures have developed a broad repertoire of conventional forms and practices that tie these elements together, shaping visions of time, autobiographical memory, and of the interconnected way in which we imagine them. These visions comprise more figures and practices of time than outlined by the A and B series. Besides stories, they include concepts, theories, metaphors, imagery, and other symbolic figurations and social practices. They are comingled with the preoccupations and routines of daily existence (for an anthropological take see Munn, 1992), yet also with the most complex intellectual and artistic creations of philosophy and literature (cf. Currie, 2006; Heise, 1997). Using a concept by Iuri Lotman (1990) we could say that models and visions of time are interlaced with the entire "semiosphere" of a cultural world, the whole of the interconnected sign systems that make up human being in the world—including human time.

Not surprisingly, thus, these visions of memory and time are culturally very diverse. They tend to be, for instance, more contextualist in countries like Japan (and languages like Japanese) where cyclical and spiral gestalts of temporality are widespread in individuals' view of their life course and lifetime, emphasizing a strong sense of intergenerational continuity and connectedness to larger social frameworks and ecological cycles of nature (cf. Minami, 2000; Yamada & Kato, 2006a, 2006b). In contrast, in Western countries and languages models of autobiographical time are likely to resonate with more individualist conventions and self-centered sociocultural imperatives (Brockmeier, 2000b; 2008a).

Against this backdrop it is interesting to account for further findings from neuroscientific research, neuropathological studies, and other clinical observations that underscore a direct link between the *imaginative* trajectories of memory and time. As we cannot on neuronal grounds distinguish the perception of a face from the imagination of this face—whether we set the imagined face in the past or future—we cannot separate "real" acts of remembering from acts of "imagined" or "simulated" remembering. Even if memories are not "real" or "true," but invented, implanted, misattributed, and confused with other ones (including memories of others), this "may not alter the sense of actual lived experience or reality that such memories have," as Oliver Sacks (2013, p. 21) writes. What characterizes the mental simulation of both factual or hypothetical scenarios—past, present, and future—is that they both draw on "richly imagining fictitious experience" (Hassabis & Maguire, 2007, p. 299), and that this experience is reliant on the same brain activities. Other scientists call what happens in these processes "mental scene construction," "self-projection," or refer to the creative navigating of a "prospective brain."[9]

Suppose we are asked what we had for dinner at a party last weekend or asked to name our best friend at school. Taken off guard by the question, we probably will trick our brains into imagining what it would be like if we were about to sit at the same dinner table or school desk again. Where, then, would one draw a line between imagination and recollection? Between semantic reconstruction (which is based on general knowledge), episodic recall (based on the one particular event), and episodic simulation (based on both)? Just as it has always been questionable to draw such lines on psychological grounds, so now we know that it is impossible on neurobiological grounds. As Edelman remarks poignantly, "the very complexity of the brain's repertoires [means that] every act of perception is to some degree an act of creation, and every act of memory is to same degree an act of imagination" (2006, p. 100).

Even if what is created in such joined acts of recollection and imagination are fictive or fantastic scenarios that would not pass the truth exam of old-day cognitive psychology and analytic philosophy, these acts are still carried out by "real" neurophysiological activities. And as not only readers of literature know well, the fictitious is often more likely and plausible than the real; not to mention that it often is also more emotionally engaging. In fact, it is interwoven with all aspects of our everyday life; as Molly Andrews writes, "it guides us from our waking hour to when we go to bed at night. It is with us always, sitting side by side with our reason and perception" (2014, p. 11). Last but not least, it is this imaginative capacity of the human mind that permits us to "time travel" and envision ourselves in other times.

Imagination "is the faculty that enables us to combine objects into possible states of affairs," in Colin McGinn's (2004, p. 145) words. And there are quite a number of different times and temporally distinct "possible states of affairs" we routinely imagine and combine—earlier or future times of our life course, times of possible lives, scenarios of afterlife (Brockmeier, 2002e). In the neuroscientific research field particularly concerned with our capacity to imagine future scenarios there is strong support for the argument that cognitive processes and brain functions did not evolve to remember the past, or even understand the present, but to enable us to anticipate the future (e.g., Bar 2011a; Suddendorf & Corballis, 2007). Foresight and prediction of things yet to happen is seen as a basic, general function of the brain. This view changes the traditional idea of memory not entirely, since it is still compatible with the idea of memory as storing and recalling the past *in as far as* it allows us to predict the future. But it surely de-emphasizes it, shifting from the supposed archival function to its imaginative and creative potentials.

Because they are sometimes still conceptually framed by the traditional notion of memory, the new neuroscientific findings about the astonishing significance of imagination cause worries, understandably. Just consider the issue of distorted, invented, and false memories. One of the few certain outcomes in this highly contested area is that even if we may not be able to testify on a neurobiological basis that memories are "right" or "wrong," we certainly can prove that they are "real." That is, in either case, they come with a solid neuronal correlate. Again, what remains unclear is what exactly is meant when we use the word "memory" (or "memories").

The 21st-century brain

The findings and observations reviewed thus far refer to the temporal status of experiences or memories (that is, of past experiences); more exactly, they refer to the difficulties of identifying this status independently from our interpretation. I want to mention a second area of recent research affecting our understanding of memory because it challenges established ideas of memories' putative permanence or continuity. The keyword here is neuroplasticity, which is central for the new neurobiological picture of the brain, sometimes called the "21st-century brain" (Rose, 2006). Although previous generations of researchers assumed that the structures of the brain were immutable after childhood, this picture has been replaced by one that shows a brain that is anything but completed and stable. Irrespective of age, it changes all the time, continuously adapting to new circumstances. This new emphasis on neuroplasticity and malleability breaks radically with the idea of a permanent memory, which has piggybacked on the "20th century brain," let alone earlier concepts of brain and memory.

A well-studied phenomenon of the new brain is, for example, that every act of remembering mingles elements of experience from the past with elements of experience from the present. To use the terms just explained: its very operation is based on the fusion of elements of realistic imagination with elements of fictitious imagination, elements of "experienced memories" with elements of "imagined memories." Within the "source monitoring" paradigm of memory research this phenomenon is called "source error." I can, for example, imagine that birthday party so intensely—using, among others, my memories from earlier parties in the same house—furnish it with many details such as the flower bouquet on the table, the taste of the cake, the sound of the laughter, that my vivid images and my strong feeling that this was the way it was makes me unshakably believe that this constructed scene is the faithful memory of an authentic scene. "Imagination inflation" is one of the terms used by experimental psychologists to explain the ubiquitous presence of "source errors." Again, although labeling this process in terms of memory "errors" suggests an awareness of the complexity of remembering and forgetting, it also reflects the continued effect of the underlying archival model, because if our memory would work as it is meant to do according to this model, as a warehouse from which items are retrieved in the more or less same unaltered state in which they were reclined and stored, there would be no "errors," "sins," and other rule breaches.

Yet some neuroscientific views, to which I turn now, ignore this conceptual tradition. Here the starting point is that all new experiences (that is new neuronal input) encounter neuronal networks that have already been shaped by previous encounters with the world. This preexisting "neuronal knowledge" powerfully influences the way new experiences are integrated, shaping the content, texture, and emotional quality of what we "recall" of the moment. If we use in this context a term such as "memories" in order to describe these neuronal activities, we must, however, be conscious of the fact that there is no physical correlate to this term; as there is no physical correlate to the entire 20th-century vocabulary of encoding, storing, retrieving, long-term storage, and short-term storage. Nor are there any "mechanisms." As my neurobiology teacher once said: young man, this is about organisms, liquids, and proteins. If you want to deal with mechanisms you have to go to the 18th century or become a plumber.

What might count as a neuronal correlate to processes of remembering is the very opposite of anything resembling an archive: a highly fluctuating excitation pattern, an organismic pattern of activities formed by continuously changing connections of nerve cells in an unending neuron forest, a fickle and unreplicable circuit that in manifold ways is interlaced with other circuits that also are in constant flux. Could there be a permanent memory trace in such environment? "Discrete, fine-grained mnemonic traces," writes Yadin Dudai, "assumed to be formed in encoding, are likely to be ephemeral. What persists is their increasingly diluted contribution to memory palimpsests that keep metamorphosing so long as the brain endures" (2011, p. 38).

Nowhere and at no moment in time can we identify a spot—that is, some cellular or molecular processes, engram, or any other neuroanatomical substrate—where something could be stored, preserved, and kept over time. The closest we get to anything like a spot where the physiological substrate of memories could be located is a place that is hot and almost fluid: the energetic flurry of a cell's interior where proteins and fats are falling apart as soon as they are made. Wolf Singer (2007) remarks about the trajectory of this excitation pattern, that is, the trail of its movement, that it "depends on the entirety of all internal and external factors that have an impact on the system" (p. 17), thereby referring to the entire cerebral cortex as "the system." "During its progression through this multidimensional state space," Singer goes on to say, "the architecture is constantly altered by the experience it gains along the way. Therefore it can never return to the same location" (pp. 17–18).

Edelman (2005) thus calls not only the system of the cerebral cortex but every single event within this system dynamic and context-sensitive: "It yields a repetition of a mental or physical act that is similar but not identical to previous acts" (p. 52). For Edelman, such an act is "recategorical" because "it does not replicate an original experience exactly"; he, therefore, concludes that we cannot assume that such a "memory" is "representational in the sense that it stores a static registered code for some act" (p. 52). What happens in the multidimensional network of neuronal groups is "a non-identical 'reliving' of a set of prior acts and events," irrespective of the fact that there often is "the illusion that one is recalling an event exactly as it happened" (p. 52).

For this reason, neuroscientists emphasize not just the constructive and "recategorical" but the overall creative nature of neuronal activities. For quite a while it has been established knowledge among neurobiologists that, as noted before, remembering is structurally like perception, a generative event occurring in the present, rather than the re-activation of an image or piece of information fixed and encoded in the past and somehow mysteriously retrieved to the present (e.g., Bontempi & Frankland, 2009; Edelman & Tononi, 2000). Each time the "memory" of a face is activated, a creative process of reconstruction, reinterpretation, and reevaluation is carried out, during which the face gains a new meaning, even though it might only be minimally altered. Still, each time the memory is changed.

Especially over the last decades, paradigms of information processing have strongly impacted theories of recall. Accordingly, memories are often conceived of as stored computer files, and remembering would seem to be an act of reloading them from the deep storage of the brain and reopening them; I quoted an example in the previous chapter. "But this mechanical model won't do," Steven Rose (2010, p. 207) contends. And Rose is not the only researcher of the molecular foundations of remembering who describes mechanical memory models as reductionist (cf. also Rose, 2006). Is there a special reason why this skepticism is more common among neurobiologists than, say, among memory psychologists? Could it be that the scientific socialization of biologists gives more space to the idea of an organic brain, which does not go along well with the focus in traditional memory research on brain mechanisms? This is what neurophysiologist Andreas Draguhn (2012) suspects. He also points to some further implications: organs (including brains) are parts of organisms, and human organisms are people—all of which pushes mechanical configurations even farther away. If the basic assumption for neurobiologists like Rose and Draguhn is that "Human beings are not machines, and the brain is no mechanical device (importantly, it is also no computer—it is a brain)" (Draguhn & Both, 2009, p. 5297), then it seems comprehensible why postmechanistic views of the complexities of remembering might likely emerge in these quarters; more likely, at least, than in quarters of traditional memory psychology where conceptual models and vocabularies have always been predicated on the search for memory's "underlying mechanisms"—from Ebbinghaus to cognitive models of computational information processing and neurocognitive memory systems.

However, in light of the new neuroscientific evidence that I have reviewed, support for any mechanical theory of recall dwindles. Memories are not documents that are stored on hard discs or in neuronal engrams and, in the act of recall, reactivated. On the contrary, each act of remembering an experience is itself a new experience which, in the very act, subtly transforms the memory of the "old" experience. In this way, we might add new emotional values, new beliefs, and even new knowledge to our memory of that face, fusing all of it with what we all the same consider an authentic and original memory.

That these findings are reminiscent of Frederic Bartlett's (1932) concept of remembering is no coincidence. The British scholar was one of the few established memory researchers in 20th-century psychology who assumed that human memory was not primarily designed to provide accurate and true representations of past events and experiences but to fulfill a social function. Bartlett pointed out that persons do not remember in an isolated and individualist way but deploy recollections within social interaction and in this way structure their "memories" along with intersubjective intentions within discursive contexts of action. He demonstrated this in his famous experiments of collective storytelling in which people in turn re-narrated their memories of stories they heard from other people. These experiments have led more recent authors to view Bartlett as the first academic psychologist studying the rhetorical (Bruner, 1990a), discursive

(Middleton & Brown, 2005; Middleton & Edwards, 1990b; 1990c), constructive (Wagoner, 2012), and narrative (Straub, 2008) dimension of remembering. Indeed, for Bartlett there was no doubt that everyday life remembering must be understood as a socially and linguistically—that is, culturally—mediated process, and not just as an act of context-free truth finding:

> The actions and reproduction of everyday life come largely by the way, and are incidental to our main preoccupations. We discuss with other people what we have seen, in order that we may value or criticize, or compare our impressions with theirs. There is ordinarily no directed and laborious effort to secure accuracy. We mingle interpretation with description, interpolate things not originally present, transform without effort and without knowledge (1932, p. 96).

It is fair to say that recent neuroscientific research on the generative, constructive, and creative nature of remembering has strikingly confirmed Bartlett's point. What we nearly always envision, when we, as adults, recall an autobiographical childhood memory, is the end product of many processes of transformation and editing, of telling what we believe is the same story in many different ways. We are proactively involved in these processes. They do not just happen because our memory is unreliable or tends toward distortions and other failures, irrespective of how strongly we are convinced that the last memory we bring to mind mirrors an original and authentic event in the manner of a photographic snapshot (a "flashbulb memory") that has been "engraved" or "inscribed" on, or "burnt" into, our brain as though it were written on a hard disc or, for that matter, a wax tablet.

The more the Bartlettian view has become common neuroscientific currency, the more it has become difficult to postulate, let alone localize and differentially identify, a distinctive place or faculty (or a number of faculties or systems) that corresponds to the 20th-century memory vocabulary of encoding, storing, retrieving, and short- and long-term storage of information. This difficulty also haunts efforts to localize, that is, fix mnemonic processes by projecting them onto neuroanatomic structures or regions of the brain as modeled by neuroimaging techniques. "Yes, we can talk about memory systems and memory processes, and we can name them," as Tulving comments on several decades of research, "but we have little idea how 'real' these systems and processes are" (2002a, p. 323).[10]

Against the backdrop of these new findings and discussions, I see the argument affirmed that the archival notion of memory, even in the traditional neuroscientific heartland, is about to lose its long taken-for-granted ontological gravity. That is to say, the idea of memory as a rectified entity, which like the lung or the heart has a safe and sound place in the world or, at least, in the human brain, is dismantling. With its unparalleled rise over the last decades, the neuroscience of memory is about to lose its original subject the more it scrutinizes it.

REMEMBERING AFTER THE ARCHIVE

The cultural paradigm shift in the conceptual architecture of our ideas of remembering and forgetting, which I have traced in four fields of memory studies, will need some time to be digested. This is understandable, we might say, considering the long period when it was taken to be self-evident what memory was and why it mattered—which is basically the Western history of culture. But not only is the old being dismantled, the new is also shaping up. So let me get back to the question of whether there is a novel notion of memory in the offing.

Although there are various efforts to unify the new multidisciplinary memory studies conceptually and institutionally, be it under the leadership of neurosciences or cultural or collective memory studies, my sense is that a great deal speaks against the likelihood that there will be one new conception of memory. Likewise, I do not think there will be one new disciplinary format, let alone one new coherent methodology for the study of memory. The new enterprise of multi- or cross-disciplinary memory studies, that some view as a future disciplinary haven for memory research, only loosely connects a multitude of different subject matters, perspectives, and disciplinary agendas.

This is reflected by a plethora of diverse vocabularies, methodologies, and research protocols, for which "attempting to find a holistic, interdisciplinary model of how the past is remembered by integrating them all, is a difficult and lofty endeavor" (Bietti, Stone, & Hirst, 2014, p. 270). Jeffrey Olick describes the field as "non-paradigmatic, transdisciplinary, and centerless" (2008a, p. 25), which, as he points out—and I agree—corresponds to the status and scope of many of its concepts. If we want to imagine the future of what once was called the study of memory, we must conceive of it as an array of irreversibly poly-centered enterprises that defy organized disciplinary regulation. Envisioning the disciplinary matrix of the human sciences in the 21st century, Clifford Geertz remarked foresightedly that we will continue to have "a more and more differentiated field of semi-independent, semi-interactive disciplines, or disciplinary matrices (and of research communities, sustaining, celebrating, critiquing, and extending them), devoted to one or another approach to the study of how we think and what we think with" (2000, pp. 206–207). Geertz went on to say that, under these conditions, "within such a field, dispersed, disparate, and continuously changing," we have no choice but to simply ignore putatively well-established disciplinary possessions (p. 207).

Geertz's reflections, presented in his essay "Culture, Mind, Brain/ Brain, Mind, Culture," capture precisely the multidisciplinary and non-paradigmatic state of the new memory studies at stake. Yet this, as Olick (2008b) explains—and again, I am in agreement—is anything but a negative assessment. It rather has to do with an altered idea of what concepts are all about. Most concepts in the field of social, collective, and cultural memory do not claim to reflect ontologically the true nature or essence of memory, to say nothing of a physical (or biological) entity, a "natural kind" called memory, but serve as useful instruments meant to sensitize us to important mnemonic aspects or implications of cultural practices and products.

We may call this epistemological nominalism. According to this view, concepts or *nomina* are tools of knowledge, reflection, and communication, rather than representations of things and other *realia*. This orientation links to the assumption, shared by many social and cultural memory researchers, that remembering is a multifarious business, which escapes the traditional realist picture of things and processes on this side and concepts and thoughts on the other side of the equation. "The requisite pluralism of our approaches to remembering is demanded by the world, not imposed by theorists' whim," writes cognitive scientist John Sutton (2009, p. 300), echoing the view of social scientist Olick. Sutton himself proposes an approach to "distributed memory" or "extended memory" (Sutton, Harris, Keil, & Barnier, 2010), drawing on a tradition of studies in cognitive anthropology on "distributed cognition" (e.g., Hutchinson, 1995) and in philosophy on the "extended mind" (Clark, 2011; Menary, 2010).

In spite of this increasing pluralism of approaches to remembering—which alone marks an unprecedented shift in scientific memory research—there are some general tendencies that permit us to remap the remains of "memory" onto the new 21st-century landscapes of knowledge and epistemology. I have already highlighted a few of these tendencies. In conclusion, let me summarize and align them in light of a comprehensive perspective. In all four fields we find emerging vistas of remembering and forgetting as social and cultural practices, which come in tandem with the idea of memories as social and cultural processes and products. Rather than being isolated operations of minds or brains (or of isolated molecular, cellular, or neurocognitive components of these brains), these practices are carried out by people. They are realized by human subjects with agency, intentionality, and the brain states that entail and enable such agency and intentionality.

Another way to think about these matters is to understand practices of remembering as embedded or embodied (sometimes also entangled and entrapped) in environments, Umwelts, eco-niches, media ecologies, meaning contexts of everyday life, and historical *Lebenswelten* (lifeworlds) of action and interaction. More than just brain operations, the making of memories can be understood only if they are grasped as real-world activities, which is an argument that has equally been put forth on social, political, and psychological grounds (e.g., by Dietti, 2014). Ultimately, this involves conceiving of remembering and forgetting as cultural forms of life that are subject to continuous historical alteration (a characterization already pointed out previously and more fully developed in Chapter 7).

A further important element of this cultural approach is mnemonic artifacts. Besides things like mementos, places, and other physical memory objects, which in autobiographical contexts typically are charged with personal meaning, we have to think of media, communication technologies, and semiotic environments (be they oral, written, imagistic, and acoustic) that have always been intertwined with human remembering. It is true, however, that mnemonic artifacts have only recently moved to the center of study and reflection, as mentioned above.

Finally, there is another constituent of the cultural economy of remembering that has become more conspicuous: sign and symbol systems. In part, they overlap and mingle with one another and with other mnemonic artifacts, media, and semiotic environments; this is why I mentioned them there as well. Consider, for example, the sign and symbol systems that underlie social rituals of remembrance or regulate the interplay between present and remembered past in literature, film, television, or digital memory platforms. In all of these settings, acts of remembering and forgetting are not autonomous events but are framed and mediated through semiotic conventions.

Despite the diversity of these conventions, most of them involve two things: images and words. But the word, in this cultural approach to remembering and forgetting, is more than just one element among others. In fact, if we were to single out one of the many mnemonic sign systems as pivotal, it is language, the hub of humans' semiotic universe and the most complex and comprehensive dimension of their cultural semiosphere, to borrow again Lotman's (1990) term. Emphasizing the mnemonic role of language, I want to conclude these reflections on the indispensable elements of a new approach to remembering—to how we can possibly imagine the conceptual outline of remembering beyond the archive—with an important qualification. Language is understood here in Wittgenstein's (2009) sense as a discursive and cultural practice. The reasons why Wittgenstein's philosophy of language is essential for this approach will become even more obvious in the case studies on the relationship between autobiographical remembering and narrative presented in the next chapters. At this point, I only want to stress one advantage of the Wittgensteinian view for this project: it defies exclusive oppositions between the verbal and the nonverbal. To overcome this dichotomy is not only a proposition of the narrative notion of the autobiographical process that I elaborate later on in this book; it also is at the heart of my exploration of memory metaphors in the next chapter.

CHAPTER 3
Shaping Memory

History, Metaphor, and Narrative

Although, as we saw in the previous chapter, conceptions of remembering and forgetting have changed, it is unlikely that the emerging new vistas will radically alter the way we talk and think about memory, which is an inescapable part of ordinary discourse. Furthermore, the languages of literature, philosophy, science, and folk-psychology have given a robust life to the idea that memory is a substantial and physical capacity or structure, and that it is an entity given to us by nature, if not by the creator himself. There are countless invocations of Memory that place it at the heart of the human existence—such as this particularly captivating one by Jane Austen's heroine Fanny Price in *Mansfield Park*:

> If any one faculty of our nature may be called more wonderful than the rest, I do think it is memory. There seems something more speakingly incomprehensible in the powers, the failures, the inequalities of memory, than in any other of our intelligences. The memory is sometimes so retentive, so serviceable, so obedient—at others so bewildering and so weak—and at others again, so tyrannic, so beyond control!—We are to be sure a miracle in every way—but our powers of recollecting and forgetting, do seem peculiarly past finding out.
>
> (Austen, 1992, p. 149)

As emphasized at the end of the last chapter, the linguistic practices of people in various cultural worlds and historical times have given distinct meanings to memory; if we assume for a moment that there is a clear-cut idea of memory in every cultural world. As anthropologists tell us, this is all but certain. In fact, there have been many cultural worlds without the idea of a substantialized memory—the North American Cree mentioned before are only one example.

My question in this chapter is not, however, where and why have there been nonsubstantialist conceptions and discourses of remembering and forgetting in other cultural and linguistic contexts. This is a question Nancy Munn (1995), for one, has tackled when examining the cultural economy of remembering and forgetting of the Oceanian Kaluli. Rather, my question is why has there been such a strong and enduring readiness in Western traditions to objectify such a plethora of practices and objects, processes and products of remembering and forgetting into one entity or capacity? This question is related to another one. Why, among all conceivable ideas and metaphors of memory, have archival metaphors of memory been so crucial in the process?

The chapter revolves around these two questions. Neither can be answered without taking into account the pivotal role of language for our understanding of remembering and forgetting. In the following chapters, I then limit the scope to one particular type of linguistic discourse—namely narrative—and examine how it is suffused with one particular type of remembering, autobiographical remembering.

I approach my two main questions—why have we substantialized memory, and why has the metaphor of storage been so instrumental in the process?—by adopting a historical perspective. Given that the scientific study of memory and remembering tends to ignore this perspective, my first task is to show how a historical perspective can illuminate the way memory is conceptualized and researched. In the second and third parts of the chapter, I again engage with the question of what has made the tradition of archival metaphors so pervasive and compelling. Finally, if metaphors and the narratives that surround them play such an important role in giving shape to the idea of memory, are there alternatives to the archival model? Indeed, there are, and I outline a few such alternative metaphors charting new terrain in the concluding part of this chapter.

THE MANY HISTORIES OF MEMORY

Two of the great values of the historical approach: the explication of the "otherness" of the past and the demonstration of the impermanence of human constructions.

Danziger (2008, p. 15)

In his momentous work *Marking the mind: A history of memory*, Kurt Danziger (2008) argues that we will neither understand the meaning of our memory categories nor what they refer to if we do not view them as historical realities. As rich in insights as Danziger's book is, its most outstanding achievement might be that it radically historicizes memory, as I have pointed out elsewhere (Brockmeier, 2012b). From this historical perspective it also adds weight to the case that memory is one of those peculiar entities whose assumed material reality cannot be distinguished from our views and thoughts about it. Because such a historical picture is in sharp contrast with the typical stance of the scientific community toward history—as something that has no bearing on present research—Danziger, a theoretical and historical psychologist with an acute interest in the philosophy of science, has been labeled as *only* a historian of mind and memory. But everyone who has read Danziger's books knows better. Building on his studies, and thus in contrast with a superficial understanding of the history of science and thought as simply concerning things past and gone, I start by distinguishing four historical frameworks that give shape and significance to our ideas of memory.

The first framework derives from an evolutionary approach, conceiving of remembering as one of humans' "higher psychological processes," as Lev Vygotsky (1978) described them. On this account, the specific human practices of remembering emerged, together with thinking and speaking, through biological adaptation—but only up to a certain point. Like language and other practices of human communication, they are profoundly sign-mediated, that is, mediated through sociocultural forms of life. Their development can only be explained as part of a process of biological-cultural coevolution. Human brains emerged in an evolutionary process in which they specifically adapted for life within a cultural world. In this process of cultural evolution, the social dynamic of fine-tuned communicative and cooperative interaction became more and more dominant—which is a hypothesis recently reformulated on the basis of new evidence by Michael Tomasello (1999; 2008; 2014). In a Vygotskian genetic, that is developmental, view the turning point in this process is marked when communication and cooperation are structurally mediated by social sign systems, which in the process operate as more and more powerful tools of mind (Wertsch, 2007). The universal mediation of cooperation and communication through material tools, signs, and various media has often been seen as the key feature of the specific human mode of existence, practically and psychologically (Deacon, 1997; Donald, 1991; Hayles, 2012). In other words, it is here where the history of specific human practices of remembering sets off (Nelson, 2007b). This makes it all the more amazing, as Danziger notes, that "very little attention has been directed at the huge cognitive changes, particularly in human memory, that took place after the advent of permanent settlement and literacy" (2008, p. 3; cf. also p. 78).

What makes this history especially interesting is that it is a history of practices and technologies of remembering that also is a history of models and metaphors of memory. And given that human remembering, like all other higher psychological functions, has always been mediated by signs and technologies, it is little surprise that there is a large number of different models and metaphors of memory based on signs and, especially, technologies. "Our views of the operations of memory," writes Douwe Draaisma (2000), "are fuelled by the procedures and techniques we have invented for the preservation and reproduction of information" (p. 3). Although Draaisma brings to his studies a view of memory that is grounded in the information processing paradigm of traditional cognitive psychology and draws on an astonishingly narrow empiricist concept of metaphor as "a filter" that we place "in front of our perception of memory" (p. 230), he lays out a broad spectrum of memory metaphors that are influenced by storage technologies. The spectrum ranges from Greek Antiquity to computational and neural memory research. How strong this influence is becomes evident, for example, in Draaisma's review of 19th-century theories on visual memory that exactly reflect the succession of new optical technologies: in 1839 the daguerreotype and the talbotype, followed by stereoscopy, the ambrotype, and color photography; and in 1878 compound photography and shortly afterwards cinematography (p. 3). "The history of memory," Draaisma concludes, "is a little like a tour of the depositories of a technology museum" (p. 3).

Writing and remembering

That the specific human practices of autobiographical remembering are mediated by signs, media, and technologies is an argument that runs through this entire book. In the previous chapter I addressed the impact that technologies of communication and storage have on both the actual process of remembering and our understanding and conceptualization of it. I paid particular attention to digital network technologies. At this point, I want to introduce a second historical framework of memory, a framework linked to the one just outlined. The practice and technology of sign mediation that plays a prominent role in this framework is *writing*. The emergence of writing as a cultural practice of remembering and forgetting has had a lasting influence both on our ways of remembering and our ideas of memory. Specific writing skills, social technologies and institutions of literacy and numeracy, and sign-mediated mnemonic practices such as timekeeping and book-keeping developed entirely as cultural, and not biological, achievements. And so did the kinds of cognition they involved and the societal organization they entailed. But literacy and memory are not just linked because they are results of the same cultural development; one of Danziger's (2008) points is that they are intrinsically intertwined.

Writing is a practice of remembering that also works as a practice of forgetting. We deal here, of course, with processes at a societal level. Literacy is deeply implicated in bureaucratic societies. Literate competences, both basic and advanced, are essential to participate in such "cultures of literacy"; they are practices that allow efficiently to remember and to forget, and to establish, manipulate, and end archival traditions and organize core resources of cultural memory (Brockmeier, 2000a; Brockmeier & Olson, 2009; Olson, 2006). Only after the emergence of writing and the establishment of a culture of literacy in ancient Greece, was "memory" named, defined, and perceived as a distinguishable feature, as in the writings of Plato and Aristotle (Danziger, 2008, pp. 29–31). What is more, it took on the shape of an entity on its own; it became pure memory, memory as such.

Before the written objectification of memory, people conceived of the temporal and transient dimension of their reality in terms of remembering activities that were often indistinguishably embedded in their forms of life. What scholars like Eric Havelock (1963) and Bruno Snell (1982) described as the "Homeric state of mind" was the psychology of a dominantly oral society. In early Greece, as Homer and Hesiod reported, mnemonic practices dwelt in the public space: they were part of conversation and interaction, of epic, poetry, song, dance, ritual performance, and artifacts of art and architecture. In one of his fine books on ancient Greek society, historian and anthropologist Jean-Pierre Vernant (2006) has pointed out how the cultural system of myth that regulated public and private life in preliterate Greece worked at the same time as a cultural system of memory, of public and private memory. The first meaning of *mnemosyne* is not "memory" but "remembrance," the exercise of an activity within a community. Yet with its written conceptualization in Plato's dialogues, as Danziger (2008, p. 29) states, a shift occurred: memory activities changed their location and took up their abode in the individual mind. Locked as an internal faculty of the person and reified in the form of a specific object called memory, they were reduced to just one element of a far more complex set of social practices and forms of commemoration. Although early on, remembering meant listening to and understanding a voice, after the introduction of written records it meant looking something up in an inscribed record; this implied evaluating if and how accurately the inscription was read or re-called. In this way, a multitude of cultural practices of remembering and forgetting transformed into an aspect of cognition, of knowledge and—an important implication—its true or false reproduction.

To characterize the role of memory before its internalization through the literacy revolution in ancient Greece, Mary Carruthers summarizes an often quoted mythical and literary topos, that of Mnemosyne, the mother of the Muses and goddess of the arts—which was the main meaning of the term in the pre-literate world:

> That story places memory at the beginning, as the matrix of invention for all human arts, of all human making, including the making of ideas; it memorably encapsulates an assumption that memory and invention—what we now call creativity—if not exactly the same, are the closest thing to it. In order to create, in order to think at all, human beings require some mental tool or machine, and that machine lives in the intricate networks of their own memories. (Carruthers, 2010, pp. 15–16)

What Carruthers calls the "mental tool or machine" organizing the intricate networks of people's memories altered drastically with the advent of writing and its gradual establishment on a societal level, even if literacy never completely supplanted oral traditions. Rather, coexisting throughout Greece's classical period, oral and written traditions of memory interpenetrated each other (cf. Thomas, 1992; 2009). But what soon would become one of the culturally most important public archives was the library, the storage place of collective knowledge and site of written cultural memory. From now on it accompanied the various traditions of oral transmission. The library archive was the place where collections of clay and wax tablets or blocks were kept. These were everyday writing materials, often stored together with papyrus, stone, and later parchment, which was more expensive and less widespread. When Plato set out his views of how humans remember and forget, he extrapolated several topics from oral mythology. The human capacity for remembrance, Plato wrote, is a godly gift given to humans by Mnemosyne, the goddess of memory.

Memory has been called one of the great primordial concepts of psychology. Danziger has reminded us that there is probably no other established psychological subject that can be traced so far back without even a change in name (2008, p. 14). Yet "memory the godly gift" might have been even in the myth-saturated world of classical Greece a bit of an airy concept and Plato resorted in his explanation of its nature to the more down-to-earth sphere of the library archive, an institution everybody knew. He particularly highlighted one figure, the wax tablet, a common material of inscription. In his dialogue *Theaetetus*, Plato has Socrates pronouncing this metaphor:

> We may look upon it [the wax tablet], then, as a gift of memory/Mnemosyne, the mother of the Muses. We make impressions upon this of everything we wish to remember among the things we have seen or heard or thought to ourselves; we hold the wax under our perceptions and thoughts and take a stamp from them, in the way in which we take the imprints of signet rings. Whatever is impressed upon the wax we remember and know so long as the image remains in the wax; whatever is obliterated or cannot be impressed, we forget and do not know. (Plato, 1921, 191d–e)

Plato's metaphorical equation of memory with a well-known object and a common practice gave clarity and visual concision to this godly gift. Storing knowledge and images by impressing or engraving them, like writing or imprints of signet rings, bestowed a gestalt to the abstract, indeed, mythical notion of *mnemosyne*. This is a general characteristic of metaphor: by fusing the abstract and the concrete, the conceptual and the graphic, the verbal and the visual, it combines oppositions. And in fact, is it not exactly these synthesizing operations that characterize memory as the basis of our psychological apparatus? This, for one, was Freud's (1968) conclusion in his "A note upon the *Wunderblock* (mystic writing pad)." Drawing on the heritage of a long tradition of thinking about memory, Freud adapted Plato's wax tablet to his own theory in which the idea of memory as an (unconscious) writing was pivotal. What this idea missed, however, as Derrida (1978) criticized in his analysis of Freud's conception of remembering and forgetting, was the multilayered, fleeting, and meandering dimension of all three: memory, metaphor, and writing—in a word, their qualities as a palimpsest. It appears that Derrida had a point, because it is exactly this palimpsestic quality of remembering and forgetting in which many recent authors, artists, and cultural memory theorists—in fact, even neurobiologists of memory (e.g., Dudai, 2011)—have been interested. This interest is especially distinct in avant-garde writers and film directors who have set out to explore the intersection between individual and cultural traditions of remembering and remembrance in terms of a poetics of writing and overwriting (cf. Silverman, 2013).

But there is still something more to Plato's writing metaphor, something special and powerful that underlies not only the magic of a compelling figure of speech and a poetics of memory that has lasted until today. It comes to the fore if we consider the historical moment in which this metaphor was coined: the moment of the newly discovered potential of alphabetic writing. In essence, what Plato's metaphor suggests and, in a sense, carries out is to turn memory into a structure of its own, a material thing. "To say that memory is somehow like an imprint on a block of wax," observes Danziger, "is also to say that memory is like an object that can be detached from its surroundings and held up for an examination of its own nature" (2008, p. 30). In this way, it plausibly impressed upon those able to write and to read that with writing definitive versions of verbal texts could be brought into existence—mnemonic inscriptions that lasted and could be kept, re-read, and reproduced. This is not only an ancient perception but a general effect inherent to writing, as David Olson (1994) has reasoned.

Yet this was only one of the implications of Plato's metaphor of memory, which itself, as noted, was an interpretation of writing at an early phase of its historical establishment as a technology of inscription and archival practice. Plato studied the impact of the historically new technology of writing on memory and the mind, and although he did not have a high opinion of literacy, his skepticism must have been ambivalent, at least, given that he wrote down his own works—in contrast with his teacher Socrates who seems to have been an unflinching oralist. Plato, however, was without doubt a writer, even if he imitated the oral form of dialogue and conversation. Irrespective of these considerations and Plato's metaphysical rationale behind it, the wax inscription metaphor was the starting point of a tradition of thought that has lasted until today.

As I indicated earlier, this tradition is not merely one of metaphorical thought. Plato's image, as Harald Weinrich writes, sets out to provide the "underlying conceptual model for many later reflections on remembering and forgetting" (2004, p. 20), whether in philosophy, *ars memoria* (the art of memory), science, or literature. Weinrich refers, among others, to later theorists and practitioners of memory—like memory artists and orators—who imaginatively developed specific aspects of remembering, such as its spatial dimension. This led them to explore what was viewed as the places or *loci* of the mind where memories were stored in the form of inscriptions or images. What is interesting about these "mnemotechnical" investigations is that even if they scrutinized peripheral aspects and *loci* of memory, they always took the overall Platonic architecture as a constant (cf. Yates, 1966). As Roman rhetorician and writer Cicero set forth in a text called *Partitiones oratoriae*:

"Memory ... is in a manner the twin sister of written speech and is completely similar to it, [though] in a dissimilar medium. For just as script consists of marks indicating letters and of the material on which those marks are imprinted, so the structure of memory, like a wax tablet, employs places [loci] and in these gathers together images like letters." (Quoted from Carruthers, 1990, p. 16)

In her study of this tradition Carruthers concludes that the "metaphor of memory as a written surface is so ancient and so persistent in all Western cultures that it must . . . be seen as a governing model or 'cognitive archetype'" (1990, p. 16). Among the numerous reflections on this "cognitive archetype" there are three elements addressed by many authors and researchers of memory. One is the component of inscription or engraving; the second is the storage space or archival structure in which the tablet and its inscription is kept and from where it finally is again taken, re-read, and re-used—which gives us the third element, the re-reading or recalling. These three components have later been called the encoding, storing, and retrieving of experiences or knowledge. Just as the wax tablet with the inscription "remembers," so do persons. The written sign on the archived tablet is not just a metaphor for a physical process, the storage of knowledge, but rather a metaphor for a mental process, for what happens in the "mental archive." Whereas in this scenario center stage is given to storing and maintaining, the frame metaphor of the archive embraces all components, in this way giving shape to the idea of a mental archive or *Memory*. This is what I call the archival metaphor or model of memory.[1]

This metaphorical scenario might also explain why so many memory theories have followed the *ars memoria* traditions and elaborated on the spatial dimension. The common perception of an archive is first of all that of a physical place, a building or structure housing a collection of material, whether it be a storeroom, container, warehouse, magazine, or library. Some libraries are particularly interesting incarnations of archives because they were built, in turn, reflecting the imagined blueprint of the archival structure of human memory (cf. Summit, 2008). Another influential vision of the memory archive is the palace. The most famous palace of memory in the Western tradition is probably presented in Book 10 of Augustine's (1991) *Confessions* where we are guided into an imaginary palace or castle. It is described as full of "large and boundless spaces" which seem to comprise all those halls, theaters, chambers, abbeys, and caverns that have been used by ancient, medieval, and modern philosophers and writers as metaphorical spaces and *loci* to store memories, or their images and symbols. Augustine was for many years a teacher of rhetoric and it has been surmised that his theory of memory reflects his own mnemotechnical expertise, as the fields and caves of memory in his *Confessions* portray the landscape around his hometown of Catharge.

Whereas for Plato and Augustine—a Christian Platonist—remembering (*anamnesis*) was so important because it allowed humans to reconnect with their godly origin, Aristotle set out to suggest a different view. In contrast with Plato's metaphysical vision, Aristotle (1971) saw memory and remembering as sense-based empirical phenomena. He was primarily concerned about the function of memory as a psychophysiological operation, put in modern terms. Concentrating on how the mind stores memories and less on the search for metaphysical meaning through memory, Aristotle took the wax tablet inscription as a metaphor for the mind imprinted by perception, and then went on to examine the factors that influence such imprinting. One important factor was stability because perceptual imprints are difficult to make when the mind is distracted or distressed by emotion, just like carving wax tablets under water. Whereas Plato's confidence in the archival power of memory was existential and metaphysical, the Aristotelian confidence was psychological and physiological, or at least that was how both theories of memory were read in the following centuries and millennia (Bloch, 2007). Despite their differences, both the Platonic and the Aristotelian tradition shared the same basic assumption of human memory as a storehouse of experience and knowledge, the archival model. Authorized by the two towering founding fathers of Western philosophy, the archival metaphor indisputably turned into the "governing model" for all subsequent thinking on remembering. It became the "cognitive archetype" of memory.

Archetype, though, is not phenotype. A third historical framework of memory comes into sight when we consider the many phenotypes, the changing variants of this basic model of remembering and forgetting, which have entered the metaphorical discourse over the centuries. There could be an entire history of memory based on these changing versions, so rich is the material for such an enterprise outlined by various intellectual historians of memory.[2] What is highlighted within this framework are the metaphorical and conceptual models of memory that have been formulated against the backdrop of the first, evolutionary and sociocultural framework, and the second framework, which brings into prominence the material and practical conditions constituted, for example, by writing technologies and material archives of knowledge.

Although my account centers on the "governing model" of the store, we should be aware that not all memory metaphors are archival. To envision certain aspects of memory even Plato referred to an aviary in which the birds—individual memories—have a certain degree of unpredictable mobility. Medieval monks, quenching their thirst from the Scriptures and taking nourishment from God's Word, saw memory as a stomach; Rene Descartes described it as a muscle; and Heinrich Heine saw it as sea. Quintilian referred to remembering as hunting and the alchemists understood it as something done by a little homunculus residing in our brain, which is an idea that has enjoyed an astonishing resurgence in recent discussions among cognitive and neuroscientific memory researchers about a "narrator in the brain." Among all memory metaphors reported in the literature—Draaisma (2000) lists a few dozen of them—archival memories are only one category or genre. It is the one, though, I am particularly interested in because it has gained paradigmatic status for the modern understanding of remembering and forgetting. Yet, not only are there more memory metaphors than those of storage and inscription; there also is great variety *within* the archival tradition. Obviously, storage and archive are umbrella terms. They cover all kinds of metaphorical storerooms for all kinds of things: for knowledge, experiences, and information, there are libraries, palaces, boxes, and inscriptions; for goods and materials, there are warehouses, depots, and wine cellars; for animals, there are dovecotes, aviaries, and zoos; and for valuables, there are treasure chests, vaults, and leather purses. Surely this classification is all but complete.

It is less amazing that there are so many different versions of the archival model if we consider that there also have been numerous transformations of technologies of writing and practices of storing knowledge (cf. Danziger, 2008, Chapter 2). With each step in the development of inscription and storing techniques, new metaphors and models of memory have appeared. And there have been many steps linked to the use of materials such as wax, stone, papyrus, parchment, paper, books, libraries, print, photography, film, magnetic tape, digital computers and networks, technologies of brain imaging, experimental molecular biology, and chemistry. In synchrony with these material and practical changes, we can trace the history of changing memory gestalts from Egyptian, Greek, and Roman Antiquity all the way down to figures crucial for the 20th-century memory sciences such as Hermann Ebbinghaus and the members of the Göttingen School of experimental research who, by systematically standardizing Ebbinghaus's methods, have determined the shape of academic memory psychology until today's neuroscientific models. Research on the various stages of this historical memory parcours has provided abundant evidence as to the importance of the experience of writing as a practice of inscribing knowledge. Intertwined with the metaphor of storage space as a container for these inscriptions, the image of remembering as inscribing (encoding), preserving (storing or retaining), and re-reading (decoding or retrieving or recalling) "information" has served for two millennia as model and empirical confirmation of the Western idea of memory: a cognitive archetype, indeed.

This plethora of conceptualizations marks the third level on which memory is historicized.

THE MEMORY EPISTEME

Plato, then, was only the beginning, and it is tempting to think of what I have just sketched in terms of another series of footnotes to the Greek thinker. Philosophers, writers, scholars, and scientists have many a time rewritten and reshaped memory as a subject of human knowledge, reflection, and investigation. But this—the third framework of memory—is not only a matter of conceptual or intellectual history; it is not only about thoughts, theories, and metaphors. The first and second frameworks already outlined some material and practical technologies providing the experiential conditions for the possibility of a certain kind of theorizing about memory. Yet Danziger proposes a further explanatory order that helps us to frame the multifarious metaphorical gestalts of mnemonic inscription and storing. This order—I view it as a fourth framework giving shape to memory—encompasses both material and conceptual factors, in Danziger's words, "memory concepts, technology, mnemonic values, institutional practices and memory performances" (2008, p. 9); moreover, there are social and political forces that contribute to a historical memory constellation or, again in Danziger's terms, to the "historical linking of memory culture, memory technology, and memory theory" (p. 10). I call the subject of this fourth framework a *memory episteme*.

The term episteme is borrowed from Michel Foucault (1970; 1980) who tried to capture the interpenetration of all these factors with a further one, that of power. Power? It is true, for most memory researchers the issue of power has little do with their subject. So why does it surface within the framework of a memory episteme? For Foucault, the basic intellectual and conceptual assumptions of the human sciences are part of an overarching order or discourse that is intermingled with the exercise of power. Now, power is a multilayered concept. It is not necessarily restricted to the political or military regiment of rulers, governments, business corporations, and the like, but also refers to historical formations of knowledge and thought. One of Foucault's most discussed case studies of such a formation is about the rise of the episteme of the modern individual, the "episteme of man."

The historical formation of the modern subject is not only a telling example of an emerging episteme, it also is of interest in our context because it is linked to an array of new archival strategies. These strategies enable, for example, the positioning of individual-centered themes, norms, and values, while they effectuate at the same time the transformation, devaluation, and repression of others. All archives in the public sphere—libraries, museums, schools, universities, media, publishing houses, Internet repositories and encyclopedias, and so on—unavoidably are sites of selection and rejection. Realizing a double operation of conservation and destruction (Weiten & Wolf, 2012), they are places of potential censorship and manipulation. This translates into a dialectic of remembering and forgetting, which has been emphasized from Freud and Halbwachs to Orwell and Borges. One aspect often singled out is that the archive embodies a mode of power that is operative even without violent enforcement and spectacular interventions. The archive is soft power. More often than not this power escapes our attention. But despite the objectivity they postulate, archiving techniques are far from neutral and innocent, a point particularly emphasized by Foucault's colleague Jacques Derrida (1995). The archive, he noted, even if untouched from outside interests, is per se a site of violence. Its acts of assembling, classifying, and storing are acts of distinction, interpretation, and control.

Derrida (1995) begins his essay *Archive fever* with the reminder that the Greek word *arkhe* names at once the *commencement* and the *commandment*. The term coordinates two principles in one: "the principle according to nature or history, *there* where things commence," which Derrida calls the physical, historical, or ontological principle (p. 9). And a second principle, which he names the nomological—*nomos* is the Greek term for law—because it brings in the "law, *there* where men and gods *command*, there where authority, social order are exercised, *in this place* where order is given" (p. 9). Derrida argues that the concept of the archive "shelters in itself ... this memory of the name *arkhe*," that is, its dual meaning; but at the same time "it also shelters itself from this memory ... which comes down to saying also that it forgets it" (p. 9). This is particularly the case with concepts of the archive that mask the fact that it works intrinsically as an institution of power or, perhaps more precisely, as a mode of power executing the "commandments" of an overarching memory episteme—concepts, in other words, that ignore that the physical and the nomological principle are always interlaced.

One reason why this is ignored, Derrida adds, is because the modern term archive stems from the Latin *archivum* whose meaning comes from the Greek *arkeion,* which initially meant a house, a domicile, and an address; what is not present any more in the Latin *archivium* or the modern English *archive* is that it also is the address of the superior magistrates, the *archons*, those who command and rule (p. 9).

To summarize, a memory episteme captures the totality of all factors that make a certain cultural economy of remembering possible. I take a closer look at the *cultural* fabric of this economy in Chapter 7; here I want to call attention to what Foucault referred to as the *historical* a priori of such a cultural economy of remembering, namely, the memory episteme, as I have dubbed it, which binds all ideas, concepts, and metaphors of remembering into a historical framework. This is the fourth framework of meaning that helps us historicize memory. It complements the first framework, that of biological-cultural coevolution; the second, which outlines the history of technologies of sign-mediation in general and writing and inscription in particular; and the third, comprising the history of the various conceptualizations of remembering and forgetting that have articulated the many versions of the archival model.

It is within the fourth framework—that of changing memory epistemes—that I also read Danziger's (2008) studies. They demonstrate that the various theoretical and metaphorical conceptions of memory, with all their pretheoretical presuppositions, hidden imagery, and philosophical assumptions, do not constitute an isolated domain but must be seen in accordance with more basic exigencies and requirements of their time. These epistemic requirements correspond to Foucault's historical a priori. That is, they are anything but merely conceptual, literary, and academic but reach beyond the sphere of thought and imagination into the fields of technology, society, and politics—and these are no doubt fields of material power. To put the same point another way, at issue is the particular historical constellation within which memory concepts, material technologies, institutional and individual practices of remembrances, and memory values are mutually interlinked.

As far as I can see, Danziger's approach is unique in that it situates remembering and forgetting within the context of such a multifaceted sociohistorical episteme. This allows us also to envisage some further elements of a memory episteme introduced earlier: literature and the arts, as well as everyday practices of autobiographical self-resolution and self-writing. All of these have advanced our knowledge of the intricacies of autobiographical remembering and its narrative fabric, perhaps more than anything else. Hence they must not be left out of this epistemic perspective.

These epistemic elements also relate to what Danziger calls memory tasks and mnemonic values, which can be seen as one component of a memory episteme. Individual practices of remembering and forgetting are not only closely linked to historically changing technologies of memory, they also "work in the service of tasks whose parameters are set by changing social demands and conventions" (Danziger, 2008, p. 5). Similarly, mnemonic values are culturally grounded assumptions about what, within a given memory episteme, "ought not to be or need not be remembered, how the shards of memory should fit together, which kinds of tasks memory should be expected to serve" (p. 8). Again, what we face here is Foucault's amalgamation "power/knowledge." For memory values also specify which functions practices of remembrance are expected to serve, which tasks they should solve. It is hard to find a memory concept, a metaphor, a theory, an experiment, a fMRI brain scan, any practice of public commemoration that does not expose or at least echo cultural values. Ancient Greek writers expected memory to offer a contemplative way to the deepest primordial truths; Romans wanted it to be a rhetorical expedient for legal and political debates; the medieval cultivation of monastic memory was meant to foster the virtuous life and valued remembering as an act of emotional and spiritual immersion, as a way to connect with God; the Renaissance practitioners of *ars memoriae* appreciated memory as an intellectual and artistic construct, an object of deliberate invention meant to improve mnemonic and imaginative skills.

Again an entire new set of mnemonic values came about with the European Enlightenment, a period that, in part, overlaps with the Industrial Revolution and the establishment of capitalism. Rather than existential reflection, moral improvement, religious self-reassurance, or aid for intellectual exercises, the epistemic significance of remembering now was to provide accurate, useful, and efficient factual knowledge—facts. Memory was expected to work like a mechanical archive, a copying machine. This idea resonated well with the empiricist view of memory as an inner storeroom for copies of sensory impressions, a tradition reaching from Aristotle to Locke and further to many modern psychological theories. At the same time, it related to new visual and auditory recording devices (such as cameras and phonographs) and other sociomaterial technologies demanded by industrial and commercial expansion. Finally, on the "subjective side," the particular value of this kind of memory work was promoted by new educational institutions and methods, not least by the political program underlying compulsory schooling introduced in the

19th century. It is no coincidence that learning and memory have always been one theme, one problem, one subdiscipline in academic psychology. In fact, since Ebbinghaus, psychology textbooks have treated memory as an aspect of learning (cf., e.g., Byrne, 2008; Schacter & Wagner, 2013).

With Ebbinghaus's experiments we have reached the scientific center of this episteme. Rather than investigating actual experiences of remembering or forgetting, the aim of these experiments was to demonstrate memory's successes and failures in accomplishing very specific memory tasks, typically related to learning. Crucial to all tasks was the correct recall of precisely defined items of knowledge such as isolated syllables. As a consequence, the idea of a reified memory separated from the psychological, material, ecological, social, and cultural contexts in which people remember and forget was to become the hallmark of experimental psychology. "From the start," as Danziger puts it, "the experimental science of memory had been dedicated to demonstrating the importance of experimentally manipulable factors in the memory process while turning a blind eye to other factors" (2008, p. 134).

MEMORY AND METAPHOR

For many psychological memory researchers, the work of Ebbinghaus stands out as a watershed between the past and the present of the discipline. Often there is even a precise date attributed to this turning point, the year 1885, when Ebbinghaus's book *Über das Gedächtnis* was published (in English it appeared in 1913 as *Memory: A Contribution to Experimental Psychology*). One might say that 1885 is a considerable time ago, especially if one takes a closer look at the research settings of today's neuroscience. All the same, for many memory researchers this date is very present. I personally learned this when I worked for some years at the University of Toronto, a school that has a reputation for cutting-edge memory sciences. As Canada's biggest university, it is admittedly quite a labyrinthine institution and I had a hard time getting the lay of the land. Who was dealing with what issues of memory and the mind, and in what places? The kind of research and scholarship I was interested in was lodged in a variety of disciplines, schools, departments, institutes, laboratories, research centers, and writers' studies—a confusing landscape that seemed to me as difficult to navigate as the universe of human practices of remembering. Things were even more complicated because there was a second school in Toronto, York University, where people were said to have "a different approach" to memory altogether. There was, however, one body at the University of

Toronto where it was undisputed what the scientific study of memory meant and where it took place: the Department of Psychology. The department defined itself as an experimental discipline, as the "Ebbinghaus Empire." The "Ebbinghaus Empire" remains an unmistakable label and program. In a number of regular events with names like Ebbinghaus Lectures, Ebbinghaus Meetings, and Ebbinghaus Conferences, the cultural memory of the first experimental scientist of memory is cultivated. This, of course, is not a Toronto specialty; in the tradition of experimental psychology, as well as in many publications on the history of psychology, it is generally acknowledged that with Ebbinghaus's first experimental psychological memory laboratory in Berlin, the age of modern memory science dawned. Many of today's leading psychological memory researchers and cognitive neuroscientists view themselves in an uninterrupted genealogy that started with Ebbinghaus.

Historians of science, however, tell a different story, the outline of which I have already sketched. This story is about how memory and oblivion, remembering and forgetting have been continuous subjects of study and reflection since Antiquity. This continuum was not really altered or interrupted by the "Ebbinghaus event," if viewed in terms of models and metaphors of memory. It is, perhaps, for this reason that some prefer emphasizing that Ebbinghaus invented a new method—controlled memory experimentation—or, at least, the precursors of such a method. Draaisma (2000, p. 4) has observed that the change with which Ebbinghaus is associated on the level of methodology can hardly be found at the level of content and theory; if one brings to mind the long tradition of metaphors and models of memory, one is struck more by the underlying continuity than by a break or sudden start in 1885.

To take this argument one step further, we can see this continuity not just in the scholarly attention dedicated to remembering and, importantly, its improvement; nor is there simply continuity in the metaphorical and theoretical grounding of this tradition; rather, this continuity is first and foremost due to the startling endurance of the archival metaphor. Consider how Ebbinghaus sets out his famous book. The first chapter, titled "Our Knowledge Concerning Memory," poses the basic question of memory research: How can past experiences survive? The answer it offers is well-known.

> Mental states of every kind,—sensations, feelings, ideas,—which were at one time present in consciousness and then have disappeared from it, have not with their disappearance absolutely ceased to exist. Although the inwardly-turned look may no longer be able to find them, nevertheless they have not been

utterly destroyed and annulled, but in a certain manner they continue to exist, stored up, so to speak, in the memory. (Ebbinghaus, 1913, p. 1)

What Ebbinghaus calls the "inner survival" (1913, p. 3) of mental states indicates the royal road that has been taken to explain their "continued existence" over time. These mental states "must have been present somehow and somewhere," and that is, they must have been "stored up" in memory (p. 1). Note that Ebbinghaus signals "stored up" as a figure of speech by adding the expression "so to speak." I already broached a few times the metaphorical existence of memory that we see here again in Ebbinghaus's wording. Now let me tighten up this line of argument. Envisioning memory, in whatever way, one cannot but make use of a discourse that is pervaded by metaphors and—as we will see in more detail further on in this chapter—stories. In this respect everyday language does not differ from scholarly and scientific memory research; both are deeply rooted in metaphors and stories. I believe that one reason for this metaphorical and narrative surplus of memory discourse is exactly because there is no such thing as "memory." I have put forth this argument more fully in Chapter 2, where my research review showed that it is impossible to identify a generally accepted tangible or otherwise delimitable material reality of human memory. Only "so to speak" can memory become a natural kind.

This distinguishes the archive metaphor from many other metaphors. In "man is a wolf"—Thomas Hobbes's famous expression that takes up the Latin *homo homini lupus est* (man is a wolf to his fellow man)—we clearly find two natural kinds on each side of the metaphorical equation. At the same time, both terms belong, according to various "grand narratives," to different kingdoms: that of civilized and compassionate humans and that of cruel and instinct-driven animals. This tension makes this expression work as a metaphorical interaction or, more precisely, has made it work when it was pronounced in the context of those grand narratives that it obviously set out to challenge. Likewise, when William Harvey introduced the metaphor "the heart is a pump" he related two very different but in his time highly comparable natural kinds, the heart and the pump. As Draaisma (2000) expounds, Harvey's metaphor had great heuristic value for theorists and empirical researchers—Harvey himself was a physician—because the pump provided theories on the operation of the heart with missing links such as the *circulation* of the blood. More than this, Draaisma goes on to suggest that "it organized separate empirical findings into a coherent representation and explained experimental results" (for example, on the relation between blood pressure and distance from the pump), which in terms of an earlier metaphor—the movement of blood seen as the movement of the tides—could not be explained (2000, p. 18).

The memory archive, however, is a different type of metaphor. In contrast with the heart, which Harvey and his colleagues were able to take out of the body, at least post mortem, and examine as an isolated muscle, human memory does not have such an existence. It is an abstraction, an idea. Without any distinct and tangible substance, without any rectified entity that has "memory" written over it, its ontology remains elusive. That there is something internally "stored up" is an imaginative visualization, even if one with a long history. In reality, neither Plato nor Augustine, not to mention Ebbinghaus, Tulving, Kandel, or Schacter, have ever seen such a place where memories are stored up. This distinguishes them from Harvey who actually viewed, on the operating table, the blood vessels and valves of the hollow muscular organ he was interested in and that he localized at the center of the circulatory system, which he understood as a mechanical system, by analogy with the most advanced machines of the time. The archival view of memory, however, draws exclusively on the imaginative power of the metaphorical discourse by which Plato and his followers—that is, all of us—have given visual and conceptual shape to this idea. Ultimately then a fictive shape, it has turned into memory's primary reality.[3]

How could this stunning transformation happen? How can we account for such a constructive force of the archival metaphor?

At this point I should make good on something I have avoided so far: to clarify what I mean by metaphor. Metaphor is one of the most important forms and practices of figurative discourse—other figurative or rhetorical figures are metonymies, allegories, parables, personifications, proverbs, and oxymora, to name a few. To avoid unnecessary complication I comply with what has been, since Aristotle's *Poetics*, the standard understanding of metaphor as a type of comparison or analogy that relates two otherwise unrelated phenomena (Aristotle, 2013). Metaphor, on this account, is a figure of speech whose literal meaning originally is bound to a specific context but then has shifted to a different area where it brings a new perspective to bear. That said, most debates on metaphor and its workings today agree that at issue is not just a matter of language but also of thought and mind. It is not just about figures of speech but also about figures of thinking and imagining and, perhaps, of acting.

To be sure, human language in all its various genres and numberless forms of life is shot through with metaphor. Anything but merely illustrative, decorative, or aesthetic add-ons, metaphors provide "nuts and bolts" reasoning and problem solving. They make our imagination streetwise, whether in the market places of everyday life, the venues of fiction and poetry, or the workshops of theoretical and abstract reflection, where metaphors often are the backbone of thought. To believe that any kind of pure thought exists without metaphor is, as Charles S. Peirce put it, to imagine "an onion without peel" (1992, p. 392).

One of metaphor's important functions is to make sense of new or unfamiliar phenomena, which makes it play such a crucial role in so many life worlds, from everyday experience to science. Opening unusual vistas, fresh metaphors break new ground, often operating as heuristic and visionary instruments. Recall what might have been Plato's original idea in comparing the well-known phenomena of inscription and storing with phenomena little known or even mysterious such as "mental states" that must have been "present" somewhere and somehow. As a result of this interplay of two different phenomena, both appear in a new light—which is the effect of a mutual meaning transfer. Aristotle had this effect in mind when he described it using the verb *metapherein*, to transfer. We also could say that metaphors offer an interpretation that creates something, if only a novel way to look at things. It is not just the nuts and bolts of speaking and thinking that metaphor provides; it also "is the dreamwork of language," as Donald Davidson remarked, "and like all dreamwork, its interpretation reflects as much on the interpreter as on the originator" (1978, p. 31).

Following Max Black (1962), metaphors today are mostly viewed in this sense as a form of interaction—to which Davidson has added the variant of an interaction of interpretations—that affects both parts, man and wolf, heart and pump, archive and the idea of memory. Davidson's "dreamwork of language" points to one extreme within a spectrum of interaction possibilities; the extreme to be found at the other end of the spectrum is that metaphors lose their innovative capacities and turn into fossils. How can a metaphor "fossilize"? The archival memory tradition is a case in point. Let us suppose that Plato, one of the finest writers in philosophy whose prose has often been described as bordering on poetry, came up with a compelling new idea—in the form of a metaphor. This metaphor emphasized an aspect of many practices of remembering and forgetting that had become salient with the invention of writing. Let us further suppose that with the cultural diffusion of writing as a system of communication and storage of knowledge this metaphor too became widespread and successful, so successful that its usage slowly but surely transformed into a linguistic and intellectual routine carried out countless times. In this manner it became what metaphor theorists call a dead metaphor. A dead metaphor is an idiomatic and cognitive fossil, both with regard to its inscription element and its storage element. What originally might have been an invitation to ponder certain aspects of remembering took on the semblance of a literal expression. It transformed into a simple representation of what appeared increasingly as the prelinguistic, external reality of memory. Each time an archival metaphor was used, this reality seemed to be confirmed anew.

That many expressions and descriptions that we take as literal representations of an external world have, in fact, a more complicated genesis—that is, that they are the outcome of a linguistic and cognitive construction—has also been emphasized in recent research on metaphor and figurative discourse. One argument is that much of what we normally see as literal language and literal thought is itself constituted by more fundamental processes of figuration (e.g., Gibbs, 1994; Lakoff & Turner, 1989). Although cognitive linguists tend to localize these processes in the individual mind, it is, however, also possible to conceive of them in a pragmatic and historical context. From this perspective, the results of such figurations appear as literal and realist representations only within a certain cultural context. Viewing, for instance, the heart as a mechanical pump was highly plausible and hence was taken to be a literal expression in an epoch in which the world view of mechanical physics was the all-dominating scientific paradigm. Applying such a universally proven paradigm equally to pumps, hearts, and even minds was more than plausible; it was self-evident. This changed with the rise of organismic paradigms and biological models of explanation in the 19th century—even if not for the memory sciences.

Occasionally, a student of memory's "mechanisms" of inscription and storage might have felt some hesitation, noticing, like Ebbinghaus, that he or she uses a figure of speech, "so to speak." But if we reviewed, in a hypothetical ethnographic investigation of this metaphorical field, memory discourses in today's psychological laboratories, journals, textbooks, and at research conferences, we could be pretty sure that the archival and mechanist metaphors employed are as "dead" as it gets. And that means linguistically, they are taken at face value, as literal representations, as depictions of a given and natural reality. Not only have they lost all innovative and creative tension, but their users, too, have lost any awareness that they apply a fictional description of one aspect of a much more complex social and cultural phenomenon.

An ongoing question in this chapter is what has made the archival metaphor so exceptionally capable of shaping our understanding of remembering—irrespective of the many centuries that have passed since its inception in Ancient Greece; that is to say, irrespective of the many different subsequent memory epistemes to which it was integral, the rise of experimental memory research in the wake of Ebbinghaus, and other scientific undertakings up to the emergence of contemporary neuroscience. In seeking an answer to this question I have identified a number of key factors. One is exactly this long and multilayered history that has enhanced the perception of memory as natural-kind storage. Consider that there has been support from numerous epochs and areas of practice and knowledge, plus the most authoritative cultural acceptance, indeed nobilization, an idea can possibly achieve—from Plato and Aristotle until today. Another factor is, linguistically speaking, the early cognitive fossilization of the archive metaphor. To abide by the geological field of metaphor, it appears that the enormous pressure of diverse rock formations from different ages superimposing each other has formed a *pietra dura*, a granite-like hard stone. A further reason that might help explain the taken-for-granted reality associated with archival metaphors is their intertwining with the most efficient technology of communication and storing of knowledge evolved in human history, writing, and its many diversifications in analog and digital media.

To add one more aspect to this far from complete list I turn to the narrative environment in which most metaphors are at home. We should keep in mind that a metaphor, like most human expressions, is rarely a stand-alone entity. Typically, a metaphor is part of a discourse, which extends its interpretive scope. More often than not, it is surrounded by stories; it is embedded in a narrative milieu. In his book on metaphor, Paul Ricoeur (2003) points out—in Chapter 3, *Metaphor and the Semantics of Discourse*—that the focus of traditional metaphor theory on names, words, and expressions falls short of capturing the entire dynamic of metaphorical meaning constitution. He argues, in a first move, that the only appropriate frame of reference is the statement or proposition in which a metaphor unfolds its meaning. In a second move, he shows that the statement opens to discourse, which has a different semantic and rhetorical dynamic, and it is this dynamic that gives rise to the real "contextual milieu within which the [metaphorical] transposition of meaning takes place" (Ricoeur, 2003, p. 74). He calls this a "discursive conception of metaphor" (p. 75). In his metaphor book, Ricoeur still envisions this conception on the grounds of a theory of rhetoric that ultimately "'focusses' on the word" (p. 3), the word that, as a metaphorical act, has "the power to 'redescribe' reality" (p. 5). But then he seems to have come to the conclusion that, within discourse as the larger context of all linguistic and rhetorical meaning constitution, another discursive form and practice might be more fundamental for the study of complex acts of meaning. This is narrative. After finishing his work on metaphor, Ricoeur went on to elaborate his theory of narrative. If in *The Rule of Metaphor* his interest was in poetic discourse as a productive activity, it shifted, as Andreea Ritivoi notes, to discourse as a basic form of human action, with language and, especially, narrative as the realm in which such action—including the action of metaphorical interpretation—is produced (2006, pp. 44–45).

Considering the relation between metaphor and narrative against this backdrop, it appears on the one hand that metaphors are narratively "generative" (Danziger, 1990b). They can bring to bear a "narrative potential," which is even stronger if several metaphors are interconnected to form a "figurative nextwork" (Biebuyck & Martens, 2011). We have seen this in Plato's *Theaetetus*, where multiple plot strands and seemingly disparate elements are drawn together: writing and the wax tablet, the public archive, imprints of signet rings, human remembering, and the mythical goddess Mnemosyne. Clearly, such meandering metaphors are more than mere images. They rather work like those "imaginings" that Theodor Sarbin (1998) has described as narratives. To understand the imagery of these extended metaphorical imaginings, as we could also say, one has to enter a storyworld. Instead of construction, Sarbin also speaks of *poetics* because poetics, in Sarbin's sense, more neatly reflects the making of such metaphor-induced stories while "avoiding the architectural flavor of *constructions*" (p. 19).

On the other hand, there is a counter-tendency to this poetic or narrative potential of figurative discourse: Metaphor needs narrative explanation. Often, it is the function of narrative to elucidate the point of new and unusual tropes. Why is our memory supposed to be a "palace"? Augustine's students might have wondered. The answer was given to them by the story of a guided tour through the many rooms, halls, and chambers where memories could be stored. The meaning of other metaphors might be given through the discursive and political context (as in Derrida's deconstructive reading of the word "archive"), or provided by personal anecdotes (as in my autobiographical presentation of the "Ebbinghaus Empire"), or by references to culturally well-known narrative resources (such as a novel by Jane Austen). Sometimes a metaphor encapsulates these resources in a condensed way. "Man is a wolf," is the metaphorical nutshell of moral, political, anthropological, and religious doctrines that all draw on extended narratives. In order to establish his theory and its central metaphor of the pump-like human heart, Harvey delivered innumerable talks rife with narrative illustrations to convince his audiences, which ranged from his colleagues at the London College of Physicians, to Kings James I and Charles I, Galileo, and the Roman Jesuits.

Likewise, the memory archive is entangled with an array of stories that are presupposed and ensue from it. They flesh out content and form of the rhetorical figure and bind it into the discursive context in which they fulfill a function. When Wittgenstein characterized the meaning of a word as its use within a given context, then this holds all the more true for metaphorical expressions. Narrative, in a sense, *is* the context within which archival memory metaphors operate.

Draaisma refers to the computer as an example of a memory metaphor that is so "all-embracing that it would be better to speak of metaphoric *themes* than metaphors" (2000, p. 20). These themes, he goes on to write, not only furnish metaphorical terms for separate mnemonic functions, they also provide a background against which separate elements have meaning (p. 20). In view of extended memory metaphors like the archive we might want to say that this background is woven out of stories, stories that are entwined with other stories, which would make it even more appropriate to speak of semantic and narrative *fields* that encompass various metaphorical themes. Let me add one more illustration of this vision.

In the dark

It is the narrative environment, as just described, that affords metaphorical interpretation to be fine-tuned to a specific discursive situation. One reason why such fine-tuning can be required is because archival metaphors are composed of several elements and sometimes the proper combination of these elements poses problems. Take Augustine's "large and boundless" palace of memory. Although this palace is built to celebrate humans' mnemonic abilities, it also is a place where it can be particularly difficult to recall. Sometimes it seems hard to find again the spot where a certain memory was stored, precisely because this compound is so large and boundless. "When I am in this storehouse," Augustine writes, and

> I ask that it produces what I want to recall, and immediately certain things
> come out; some require a longer search, and have to be drawn out as it were
> from more recondite receptacles. Some memories pour out to crowd the mind,

and when one is searching and asking for something quite different, leap forward into the center . . . until what I want is freed of mist and emerges from its hiding places. (Augustine, 1991 [10, viii, 12], p. 185)

If everything is safely stored in the palace of memory, how can I have difficulties in remembering some things? Where does the mist come from? This is the question that Augustine's little story seeks to answer. Searching for memories that are hiding in the archive, possibly even in one that is cluttered and poorly lit, can demand a serious search effort. This leads to another question. How can we remember that certain memories are stored in our memory palace at all when we have forgotten where exactly they are located? Does not any memory have a particular spot within the archive? The answer calls for some narrative elaboration. Of course, Augustine writes, all memories in the palace are stored in their particular places, but some are "so remote and pushed into the background, as if in most secret caverns, that unless they were dug out by someone drawing attention to them, perhaps I could not have thought of them" (Augustine, 1991 [10, x, 17], p. 189).

In this way, the narrative field extends to include the theme of light and darkness. From ancient writers and medieval memory artists to today's neuroscientists, the lack of light in the various memory containers is an amazingly ongoing concern. Again, the frame of reference is a common everyday experience: We are searching for something and cannot find it because there is not enough light. In many memory conceptions this problem is even aggravated because they share the assumption, widespread among memory practitioners, theorists, and scientists, that what is stored are mnemonic images. But how can I recognize, catch sight of an image in the dark of a storehouse, a cellar, or a cave? Not to mention closed spaces such as a stomach, a cranium, or the interior of a cell without any daylight at all? Clearly, this is not only a challenge for Augustine and Renaissance memory artists.

On February 9, 2007, the London newspaper *The Guardian* offered its readers a stunning front page. The eye-catcher covering nearly one half of the page was a picture of a transparent human head viewed from the side, the prominent headline stating: *The brain scan that can read people's intention.* The accompanying front-page article stated that "World-leading neuroscientists developed a powerful technique that allows them to look deep inside a person's brain and read their intentions before they have acted on them." The article reported that a team of neuroscientists from the Max-Planck-Institute for Human Cognitive and Brain Sciences, together with colleagues at University College London and Oxford University, used a new high-resolution brain scanning technology to investigate neuronal activities during and before thought and decision processes. The newspaper then engaged in a discussion of what was described as the controversial ethical implications of the research. What makes, however, this report particularly interesting in this context is the language the scientists applied in their own description of their findings: "Using the scanner," the lead researcher, John-Dylan Haynes, is quoted as saying, "we could look into the brain for this information and read out something that from the outside there's no way you could possibly tell is in there. It's like shining a torch around, looking for writing on a wall" (Sample, 2007, p. 1).

These metaphors are, of course, not really exceptional but well known from history; they also are rather common in neuroscientific brain and memory research. That digital technologies "read" information about mental states, which are "hidden" and "inscribed" in normally inaccessible areas of the brain, is part of standard neuroscientific vocabulary. Notably, it is also evident in the academic version of the research covered by *The Guardian* (e.g., Haynes, Sakai, Rees, Gilbert, Frith, & Passingham, 2007). Still, I have chosen *The Guardian's* front-page report because it speaks to something important about this narrative field that extends seamlessly from Antiquity to today's laboratories of brain research, as well as from philosophy, literature, and the arts to the other humanities, social and natural sciences, and everyday discourse. Not many metaphors can boast such a ubiquitous pervasiveness.

Not surprisingly then, this metaphorical and narrative field also comprises scenarios that permit us to come to terms with the problem of darkness in the storerooms of memory and the brain, besides using the torches of Professor Haynes and his colleagues to read the writing on the walls of the cortex. For Proust, one of the most successful rememberers engaged in the search for memories that got lost in the dark, this is the illuminative moment of narrative imagination. His own writing about his memories, he once remarked, works best when it is done at daylight, possibly in the morning. In Proust's *À la recherche du temps perdu*, the autobiographical narrator evokes the fragments of his memories only to elaborate and interpret them in the bright light of the present, which permits him to experience the original events even more richly than when they happened in the first place.

If Proust seemed to create the light he needed to recover the past in the act of autobiographical writing, in the premodern vision of memory the trouble results not least from the nature of the often badly lit store. Thus, the remedies, too, stay within the same premodern horizon. If recalling is seeing or re-reading, there is no retrieval from the dark storage of the past without proper lighting, which means the use of fires, candles, oil lamps, and, indeed, torches. The idea of forgetting as losing something in the dark must have been so threatening that the memory artists of the *ars memoriae* tradition went to great efforts to organize their mnemonic stores and retrieval processes in a way that they were always lit, clear, and transparent. There are manifold "topical" memory landscapes through which the mnemotechnicians walked and mentally picked up the memorable items that they had single-handedly located there beforehand in a well-ordered fashion (cf. Carruthers, 1990). The ever important precept: walk through these landscapes or architectures only during the day.

Darkness, the night, sleep, dreaming in the twilight, buried and being entombed in deep underground strata not accessed yet by the archeological digging of conscious remembering: all these expressions have been applied by researchers and writers on memory to refer to the absence of memory, to repression, and forgetting. Weinrich's (2004) collection of metaphors of forgetting and oblivion from the last 2,500 years can be read as a variation on Pindar's remark that all forgetting is dark, or in the dark: Dante sees the place of forgetting in the dark depth, *il pozzo scuro*, of Hell from where no word nor memory escapes; Friedrich Schiller speaks of *finstere Vergessenheit*, dark and saturnine oblivion; and Victor Hugo pictures *le sombre oubli*, gloomy oblivion. This narrative field also comprehends remote and not easily accessible corners of the memory store, where it is not only dark but downright dangerous, where remembering becomes abysmal and transforms into its contrary. The deeper we climb down into the cellars, caves, slots, and holes of memory, the deeper we move into the sphere of forgetting and of being forgotten. In his *Phenomenology of the Spirit*, Hegel describes this border zone as *den nächtlichen Schacht des Ichs,* the nocturnal pit of the I, through which knowledge falls down into the depth of forgetfulness.

Against the backdrop of this narrative field, which has grown over many epochs and penetrated a broad range of cultural discourses and memory epistemes, we have come to understand our memory metaphors—and, as I have argued, metaphors of the memory archive in particular. Modern psychologists of memory, as Danziger (2008) has shown, are an outstanding example: they inherited an everyday psychological language that already positioned memory in a certain way; and like all users of everyday language and metaphors of memory they "generally took for granted the kind of psychological reality that was presupposed by this use" (p. 13; on psychology's linguistic inheritance, see also Danziger, 1997). I believe that this multiple historical rootedness of the idea of memory's "psychological reality" helps explain its perseverance as a root metaphor, even in the face of evidence to the contrary. Endlessly reiterated, reflected, and corroborated by many cultural discourses, the very nature of memory has come to look like the metaphorical vision on which it was modeled. The various aspects of history, metaphor, and narrative pointed out in this chapter all have to be kept in mind when we tackle the question as to why there has been such a persistent readiness to objectify a great many practices and objects, processes and products of remembering and forgetting, rectifying them into one entity. Surely, without its metaphorical and narrative clothes, the notion of memory is a highly abstract construal, an elusive emperor.

I started this book with some reflections on the elusiveness of memory that seems to have become more manifest the more our basic cultural certainties about its alleged existence as a natural kind have come to be challenged, not least by the "memory crisis." Now, in these pages, I have tried to understand the "rationale" behind the archival model of memory, exploring what has led to these certainties in the first place. I have suggested various historical, metaphorical, and narrative factors that have shaped the idea of the archive and its two key components, writing and storage. Taken together, these factors have bestowed it with a robust ontology that has resonated for so long with the full panoply of Western memory values.

METAPHORS BEYOND THE ARCHIVE: CHARTING NEW TERRAIN

I want to add a coda to these conclusions. In this chapter, I have been seeking answers to why there has been such a willingness to objectify remembering into one entity, and why archival metaphors have been so crucial in the process. The latter question takes on particular importance because there also have been other ideas and metaphors of memory, just as there have been many other experiences and stories of remembering and forgetting that do not match the blueprint of the archival discourse.

What is more, in the wake of the changes in our understanding of remembering and forgetting outlined in the first two chapters, it has become obvious that the figurative and conceptual registers of the archive increasingly fail to capture recent scientific and cultural-historical developments. This was one half of my story. The other half was that these very changes also afford new ways to conceive of human remembering and forgetting, which, again, is linked to the emergence of new, alternative metaphors and models. And one does not need a crystal ball to predict that there are more of them in the offing. Far from offering a satisfying examination of these alternative metaphors, I want, however, to point to a few candidates that have gained a remarkable profile in present discussions. Eventually I single out one: narrative. It is to the alternative metaphor of narrative that the remainder of the book is dedicated.

To view remembering as a process in which the past is creatively constructed, a process that is not restricted to the individual and his or her brain but unfolds through social and materially embodied practices in cultural environments, calls for a design that not only conceptually but also metaphorically and narratively goes beyond what any inscription and storage model would permit. Although the archival model has been, as we have seen, enormously flexible and comprehensive, ultimately it was reductionist, fixating just one element of a larger and more complex whole. What every storage metaphor conceals, as Wagoner remarks, is "the temporal, cultural, contextual, and constructive nature of remembering" (2012, p. 1039). In contrast, the alternative metaphors at which I now take a look try to overcome this constricted focus and emphasize instead aspects of the novel vision of remembering as constructive social practice through which persons—not brains—create cultural scenarios of past and present events, and often also of future events.

The metaphors that I want to highlight fall into three categories. The first category of figurative models is brain-based; the second underlines the discursive and, more generally, social qualities of remembering; and the third has as its frame of reference Internet-related digital technologies and practices.

Much of the figurative language of brain and memory used in neuroscientific communities reflect discoveries such as the extent of the brain's plasticity and malleability (an assumption that, as noted, until recently was firmly ruled out; once the brain had finished its ontogenetic development, its neurophysiological layout was seen as immutable). This discourse thus "interacts" with aspects of the brain's dynamic, constructive, creative, and inventive organization. On a conceptual level, this is the home base of models of complex self-organizing systems (e.g., Singer, 2009), for which there are many suggestive metaphors. I personally like the metaphor—which circulates in several variations—that projects brain and memory as a large and busy restaurant, a place where numerous waiters, cooks, food runners, stewards, and other specialized support staff serve different people with diverse tastes and sometimes complicated individual orders and moods. A frenetic place with a milling crowd. People arrive and leave the restaurant at different times, coming from and going to different locations. This also holds for the restaurant staff, and the food itself that is delivered to the restaurant from various shops and markets. At the same time, the waste is brought away to other places. This scenario often looks like chaos, but most of the time it works amazingly well, making sure that many people not only feel satiated but also enjoy the setting and the company of others. Isn't it a telling coincidence that, in a reverse transfer, the organization of big restaurants is often compared to a "brain business" where hundreds of people keep numerous overlapping networks of production, delivery lines, and subsystems of remembering running as smoothly as possible? This is how, for example, *The New York Times Magazine* describes one of the city's big restaurants, *Balthazar* (Staley, 2013). Even the scene of a minimal accident that might occur in the coordination of the various networks of food, pleasure, and work comes metaphorically close to what we know as an initially minimal cerebrovascular accident, which can end up in a stroke: "This could prove disastrous, the sort of domino effect that a kitchen might not bounce back from: dishes could go out cold and come back for refires, clogging up the line for the rest of the night, creating delays, angry customers, cuss words" (Staley, 2013, p. 48).

There are a few other recent metaphors comparable to the restaurant. Some emphasize the organic—in contrast to the mechanic or technical of many computational metaphors—as in the figurative equation of autobiographical memory to a compost heap (Randall, 2007). A compost heap memory is not only different from the "memory" of a computer, it is not even a thing but a process, involving several organic/mnemonic phases (again, in contrast to the computational encoding, storing, and retrieving): "laying it on, breaking it down, stirring it up, and mixing it in"—completed by a continuous transformation dubbed "letting it be" (Randall, 2007, p. 618). The compost metaphor suggests a permanent process of change that also is emphasized in what neurobiologist Yadin Dudai (2011) calls "a 'phoenix' type of metaphor" to characterize the high plasticity of so-called long-term memory traces. Whereas, as Dudai explains, traditional hypotheses of long-term traces or engrams favor "a 'storehouse' class of metaphors," more recent research has identified "cyclic" trajectories of neuronal activities as reflected by the phoenix metaphor: "Occasionally, items in memory get the opportunity to be reborn again and again" (2011, p. 36).

Other metaphors relate the neurobiological dynamic of human remembering to a jazz performance (Pipa, 2010) or the performance of an orchestra without a conductor (Singer, 2005; 2007). The orchestra fashions a postarchival metaphor that foregrounds the spontaneous and self-emergent aspects of neuronal activities. The idea of memory as an entity or capacity is transformed into the performance of many different players engaged in countless acts of interpretation. These interpretations are twofold: they refer to the score of the music to be interpreted and they carry out the interplays in which the players mutually respond to the interpretations of other players, given that there is no conductor who centrally coordinates and merges the countless musical or mnemonic activities into one coherent sound.

A slightly different aspect is brought into prominence by Edelman's (2005) metaphor of memory as a permanently shifting glacier. In order to emphasize the flickering neurobiological choreography of the brain, the open, fluid, and continuously transforming nature of its neuronal networks, Edelman has suggested what he calls a nonrepresentational concept of memory that he sees resonating with an Alpine glacier. Whereas a representational memory would be like a "coded inscription cut into a rock that is subsequently brought back into view and interpreted," as Edelman (2005, p. 52) puts it, a nonrepresentational memory would be

> ... like changes in a glacier influenced by changes in the weather which are interpreted as signals. In the analogy, the melting and refreezing of the glacier represent changes in the synaptic response, the ensuing different rivulets descending the mountain terrain represent the neural pathways, and the pond into which they feed represents the output. Successive meltings and refreezings due to changes in the weather could lead to a degenerate set of paths of water descending in the rivulets, some of which might join and associate in novel ways. Occasionally, an entire new pond might be created. In no case, however, it is likely that the same dynamic pattern will be repeated exactly, although the general consequences of changes in the pond below—the output state—could be quite similar. In this view, memories are necessarily associative and are never identical. Nevertheless, under various constraints they can be sufficiently effective in yielding the same output. (Edelman, 2005, pp. 52–53)

Interestingly, the brain-glacier analogy also seems to work conversely, for instance, when glaciologists characterize what they see as the life of glaciers in terms of the brain's neuronal activities (Christensen, 2011).

The second category of alternative metaphors brings to the fore the discursive and social qualities of remembering. There is a long tradition of viewing joined or collective practices of remembering and forgetting in terms of interaction, conversation, dialogue, discourse, and narrative. Sometimes these metaphorical vehicles include writing, understood, however, in a sense different from the inscription tradition. It is different because writing is not viewed as objectifying or consolidating, as "cutting into a rock," to use Edelman's phrase, but through the lens of concepts like instable traces, palimpsests, and "permanently moving" meanings. An example is Derrida's notion of *écriture*, which itself is a metaphorical transformation of models from molecular biology (cf. Brockmeier, 2012c). In studies on conversational and discursive remembering, the figurative vision has turned into an investigative strategy, a research approach dealing with the nuts and bolts of discursive practices of remembering; we can trace back this approach to authors like Bartlett and Halbwachs.

Still, there remains a figurative surplus, a dimension of the metaphorical theme of "conversation" that relates to a meaning of shared activity and community, which invites more interpretations. One possible further interpretation of the metaphor of conversation has been put forward by Oliver Sacks. Sacks (2013) has made the case for an intersubjective notion of autobiographical remembering that builds on new neurobiological evidence. In contrast to the Ebbinghaus tradition of memory research, he argues that human remembering is fundamentally subjective. From a neurological point of view, the brain has no binding obligation to veridicality; there is no "mechanism" meant to produce something like objectively true memories. On the contrary, we assimilate what we read and what others say, think, and believe as intensely and richly as if these were our own primary experiences—and we remember them accordingly. Yet Sacks conceives of this not as shortcomings, failures, or "sins," as Schacter (2001) did. Rather, he views it a part and parcel of humans' special intersubjectivity, as element, we might say, of a never-ending dialogue, an ongoing conversation so characteristic of our social being in the world. For the biologically in-built subjectivity of human remembering

> ... allows us to see and hear with other eyes and ears, to enter into other minds, to assimilate the art and science and religion of the whole culture, to enter into and contribute to the common mind, the general commonwealth of knowledge. This sort of sharing and participation, this communion, would not be possible if all our knowledge, our memories, were tagged and identified, seen as private, exclusively ours. Memory is dialogic and arises not only from direct experience but from the intercourse of many minds. (Sacks, 2013, p. 21)

The third category of metaphors charting new ground beyond the archive uses Internet-oriented digital technologies and practices as a domain from which the metaphorical transfer takes place. Even here we can draw on the material reviewed in the last chapter: visions of networks (which already is a fossilized metaphor), of processes of mutual human-computer and human-computer-human interaction, mediated and embodied communication and remembering, and multimodal and multimedia transformation or "morphing" of memories that are paramount for new figurations in this field. There are interesting forerunners; for instance, the ideas of embedded, distributed, and ecological memory, or wild remembering in the wake of the metaphor of "cognition in the wild." Such remembering was studied outside of experimental laboratories in "natural" or "wild" environments that include multiple subjects, their interactions, and the material world (e.g., Hutchins, 1995). Yet with the unparalleled rise of digital technologies over the last two decades, the Internet and the types of "mental-technical-cultural process" (Dijck 2007; 2013) it has produced have turned themselves into most powerful and comprehensive memory metaphors. "Connective memory," "memory network," and "hyper memory" are only a few of many Internet variants within this metaphorical and narrative field (cf., e.g., Hoskins, 2009b; 2013a).

The digital revolution has produced practices and visions of remembering and forgetting that are truly global (cf. Assmann & Conrad, 2010). This indicates one more difference from the archival metaphor tradition that emerged with the literacy revolution in European Antiquity and, in a sense, has always remained linked to it. A case in point is the global reach of a set of digital technologies that have become known as "lifelogging" devices. Lifelogging refers to the process of digitally archiving all possible "live" information about one's life, in as far as it gets in touch with the digital sphere (Whittaker, Kalnikaite, Petrelli, Bergman, Clough, & Brockmeier, 2012). And there is a lot if we include paper and digital documents: e-mail, paper mail, and instant messages; content of telephone conversations; websites visited; and credit card transactions. Further, this comprises information relating to everyday activities and material, nondigital things, documented in still images, video, ambient sound, and location data. These "personal archives" might also be supplemented with environmental measures and even biosensor data (heart rate and galvanic skin-response) reflecting our physical and emotional state and desires (Rose, 2014). If "total recall" is understood in this sense, it appears increasingly feasible, if only technologically, as Whittaker et al. (2012) conclude. Technological feasibility and personal relevance aside, what is interesting here is that lifelogging has become a metaphor that "interacts" with autobiographical narrative, life story, and storied self-presentation and self-exploration: a figurative expression that is increasingly used on the Internet, especially in social networks and what is called the blogosphere.

One reason I have brought up the metaphor of lifelogging at the end of my coda to this chapter is because it paves a way for the shift in focus to *autobiographical* and *narrative* forms and practices of remembering that will take center stage in the next chapters. Within the three categories of alternative metaphors, I have mentioned narrative only in passing. In the remainder of the book, I will mainly concentrate on this metaphor, the idea of autobiographical remembering as a narrative process. This is not meant to downplay the power and cultural scope of the other alternative metaphors; nor does this short list of examples claim to be exhaustive in any sense. Rather, it is important to bear in mind that narrative is only one alternative to the archival model of remembering and forgetting. I see this shift more as an act of zooming in on one metaphor, which permits me to demonstrate in some detail that the "narrative alternative" affords a comprehensive and sophisticated exploration of autobiographical remembering.

And there is more to it. My exploration not only breaks with the archival tradition, it also oversteps the limits of a merely metaphorical discourse altogether. What I outline is a *theory* of the autobiographical process. And, not least, this also expands the disciplinary horizon of memory studies by drawing on literary and artistic forms, practices, and studies of remembering and forgetting.

CHAPTER 4

Interpreting Memory

The Narrative Alternative

"If only I could take my heavy burden off my breast and shoulders, if I could forget my past!" exclaims Madame Ranevskaya in Chekhov's *The Cherry Orchard* after she has returned to her country house. The place is somewhere in the provinces of Russia. She left it with her family many years ago to live in Paris. When the view of the blossoming cherry orchard calls her to the days of childhood it seems that for a moment she might be able to forget at least some of the troubles of her later life. But the moment is short. The estate is heavily in debt and stands in danger of being auctioned. Quick and determined action is needed. But Lubov Andreyevna Ranevskaya and her brother cannot bring themselves to do anything about it. As if paralyzed, they live in a world of reminiscence and nostalgia.

Chekhov's play has been said to be all about remembering and forgetting. Each character struggles with personal memories, acting them out within an emotional spectrum ranging from hope to despair. Ranevskaya, for one, tries to seek refuge in the past from her unhappy life. She wants to revive her earlier life in order to escape the present. Yet in doing so she not only is about to lose her idyllic house of the past to the ruthless present. The estate itself is saturated with memories of her father and ancestors and, more than anything, of the death of her son that begin to haunt her as soon as she arrives. "Can't you see them, all these people? Behind every branch, every leaf, every tree trunk a human being looking at you. Can't you hear their voices? . . . How can we begin to live in the present if we don't come to terms with the past?"[1] Yet while Ranevskaya continues to hope that her innermost wish—If I only could forget my past!—comes true in some miraculous way, the events make strikingly clear that her past neither can be forgotten nor does it have to be remembered because her past *is* her present, a present in which she has already been living for a long time.

Ranevskaya longs for the state of mind that the Greeks associated with Lethe. Lethe is a river in the underworld that conveys forgetfulness on the souls of the dead. In his analysis of the mythological image and image field of Lethe, Weinrich (2004) emphasizes that both memory and forgetting are wholly immersed in the fluid element of the water: "There is a deeper meaning in the symbolism of this magical water. In its soft flowing the hard contours of the remembrance are dissolved and, so to speak *liquidated*" (p. 6). What also resonate with the Greek view is that Ranevskaya appears as a person who yearns for her death, while at the same time being deeply horrified by the idea of dying. Perhaps it is for this reason that Chekhov's main character seems to act—or more precisely, not to act—like a prisoner of her memories, unable to see her actual life as anything but a reminder of time past. She finds herself drawn into a world that at few moments is elegiac, but more often despair has taken over all perception of the here and now.

And so the tale of Madame Ranevskaya's memory ends—and goes on. The visit to the ancestral estate leads to the house being sold, the cherry trees cut down, and she and her entourage once more escape to Paris. They leave the estate as though a long-winded attempt of fleeing the past had come to a bitter close. But soon, we sense, a new wave of memories of the cherry orchard will take over as if a new dream starts and Ranevskaya will again sigh, if I only could forget my past. In lengthy conversations and even longer soliloquies she will continue to conjure her life long ago and we again will be unable to distinguish between what are bittersweet memories and what are eloquent meditations about them, what is remembering and what is interpreting.

But then, can we ever do so? Does it make sense to draw a clear-cut line between a memory "as such" and the language of memory that so compellingly takes center stage in *The Cherry Orchard*? Within the psychology and neuroscience of memory the answer traditionally given is yes, it does, because memories are stored and recalled prior to, and thus independent from, language and interpretation. But then, we wonder, is not Chekhov one of those writers who went to great pains to seek out the intimate interplay between remembering and language? Was he not one of the first authors—the *Cherry Orchard* premiered in 1904, four years after the publication of Freud's *The Interpretation of Dreams* and three years after *The Psychopathology of Everyday Life*—who saw the desire for autobiographical self-reflection as a form of life inherent to the modern condition? Moreover, was he not one of the narrative and dramatic artists who explored what they viewed as the continuum of a river, a stream of consciousness and practices of remembrance in which memories are inseparably fused with their interpretation in language and larger ideas of self and identity? So another question springs to mind. Can we at all envision a memory and bring it to mind as a pure memory without interpreting it? These questions aim at the very nature of the autobiographical process. They are at the heart of this chapter, in which I want to advance the narrative alternative to mind and memory.

NARRATIVE, LITERATURE, AND THE AUTOBIOGRAPHICAL PROCESS

It is hard to overstate the role literature has played in our understanding of memory. In Chapter 2, I described literary works as constituting the longest and richest tradition of thinking about memory available to us, a tradition that not only has unfolded the narrative fabric of memory phenomena, but also essentially contributed to its very cultural formation. Crucial to this formation is that literature does more than merely represent memories and processes of remembering and forgetting; it gives shape and meaning to them. And this is all the more true for more complex autobiographical memories, memories of the kind with which Madame Ranevskaya struggles. This links to the argument that language not only reflects but also creates realities, including the realities of memory; and here I refer to reality in a robust and realist sense. In this chapter, I qualify this claim by making the case that there are autobiographical memories that only come into being *because* of narrative. Without narrative—and without narrative interpretation—they would not exist. I call this the strong narrative thesis.

I also already mentioned another crucial role literature has played for our understanding of remembering and forgetting: the role of a laboratory, a place of investigative experimentation. In its long history, literature has laid bare the interplay between memory and narrative, creating a prime site for probing the constitution of the narrative mind. There are many ways in which exploring practices of narrative worldmaking can inform, and not just be informed by, the sciences of the mind, as Herman (2012; 2013) argues. If I, therefore, use literary texts from fiction and nonfiction as well as from dramatic genres—as in the case of Chekhov who moves from narrative to drama and from drama to narrative (Bowles,

2010)—to make sense of the autobiographical process, this is not just to offer some examples and illustrations but first of all to take advantage of the rich hermeneutic potential of literary narrative. I want to build on narrative where it is at its most sophisticated. Gregory Currie, a philosopher who combines a background in epistemology with expertise in narrative, points out that literature, while it shares many features with other vehicles of thought and communication, is particular in the way it gives shape to human subjectivity. When it comes to understanding character and personality, action and intentionality, Currie concludes, "it is fictional narratives that show the most developed, most imaginative resources" (2010, pp. viii–ix).

Over the last decades, the significance of narrative for human subjectivity has become a subject of discussion and inquiry far beyond the traditional field of literary and linguistic narrative studies. At the same time, things within this field have changed. Roger Sell has argued that a perception has become central, which he sees as closely linked to the area of postmodernity, namely, "that the writing, transmission and reading of literary texts really are human deeds, with a fully interpersonal valency" (2000, p. 22). This is in contrast to the perception that literature is a *representation* of those deeds and, as a consequence, has to be investigated with a focus on formal textual features, which in most of narratology's history were seen as structural or structuralist features. Of course narrative scholars and researchers are still preoccupied with what has been their exclusive subject for centuries, written texts. But they also have become increasingly concerned with different kinds of texts and media, including "texts of the mind," an expression meant to highlight the linguistic and narrative fabric of human consciousness that reaches far beyond the sphere of writing and bookishness (Brockmeier, 2005). This shift beyond the written, primarily literary text to the manifold everyday forms, practices, and semiotic (including digital) environments of narrative also has been called the narrative turn.

Yet there is, of course, more than this to the narrative turn—in the wake of which I also see this book. Matti Hyvärinen (2010) has argued that there has not been one narrative turn but a number of turns. The first turn to narrative took place in literary theory in the 1960s and it was strongly influenced by structuralist theory; before that the field was mainly defined in terms of literary subjects such as the novel. This was followed, second, by historiography and, third, by the social sciences, broadly speaking (ranging from anthropology and sociology to philosophy, education, law, psychology, and certain areas of medicine), where narrative began to play an increasing role from the 1980s onwards. Finally, there has been a turn to narrative in cultural studies and related disciplines, including the arts, film, and architecture. Although Hyvärinen (2010; 2013) recognizes some overarching trends, he shows the concept of narrative did not simply travel from discipline to discipline but was re-created and re-evaluated. In fact, many disciplines reinvented the narrative wheel, as Brian Schiff (2013) puts it, spreading it out as "narrative psychology," "narrative medicine," and "narrative anthropology," to name a few. It is important, though, to be aware that, at the same time, the understanding of narrative also underwent radical changes in its home base of literary theory, linguistics, and narratology.

The relative disconnectedness of these narrative turns and their rootedness in local, disciplinary traditions might explain a certain narrowing in the interests of many social scientists on the subject. This is nowhere more obvious than in the focus on narrative as a method or methodology, which characterizes a large portion of social science publications on the subject. A method is a means to an end. It is, as it were, not the real thing but what gets you to the real thing. Adapting narrative to specific "methodological needs" of the social sciences—that is, its transformation into an instrument in the repertoire of "qualitative research" methods—has come at a price. To a large degree, the appropriation of narrative as an apparently freely "travelling concept" (Hyvärinen, 2008; 2010) has paid no attention to the discussions in literary and linguistic theory on the topic of narrative. Materialized in an immense research literature, these discussions have not just been about narrative and stories but about the workings of a large variety of different types, practices, and techniques of narrative discourse. By ignoring this world of advanced knowledge, the turn to narrative in the social sciences has basically been a turn to a metaphorical discourse, Hyvärinen (2010) maintains. For the most part, "narrative" and "story" have been adopted as metaphors conveying an everyday meaning that seemed to need no further specification. There are countless texts, in fact, entire textbooks, in the social sciences where "narrative" and "story" are used interchangeably with "account," "report," "description," "interview," "testimony," "information," or simply "data."

The promise of narrative and its skeptics

What has drawn social scientists to narrative, albeit if only on a metaphorical level? Hyvärinen believes that the idea of narrative has allowed them to see human action, identity, life, and mind in a new and promising light: as something changing, evolving, and adapting to social circumstances, rather than as a fixed store of intrinsic features. But using narrative as a method or model to capture something else also meant that "the metaphoric discourse was not primarily interested in the study of narratives as such, but rather in their use as . . . models for the study of lives" (Hyvärinen, 2008, p. 262). A case in point is the narratological distinction between "story" and "discourse," where story refers to the presumed sequence of events (for example, the chronology of a life) and discourse to the actual, typically nonchronological, way in which the sequence is presented, say, in a memoir. According to Herman (1999a), this distinction is one of the most important insights social scientists could gain from narratology. However, it is almost nonexistent within the metaphorical discourse of the social sciences, with the implication that narratives and lives have been the more easily understood as "homologous sequences of events" (Hyvärinen, 2008, p. 262), to be recorded, for example, in autobiographical interviews.

Another fallacy of narrative research in the social sciences, especially widespread in the literature on self and identity formation, is to assume, as Jarmila Mildorf (2010) has noted, that the storyteller who shares experiences in the first person with an audience equals the narrator (from whose perspective the story appears to be told) and, moreover, equals the protagonist or character presented in the story. Paying no attention to the "fine-tuned narratological sensors" (Mildorf, 2010, p. 251) that come with these distinctions among various narrative personae or positions ignores important ways of identity formation and negotiation.

Perhaps it is not least because of such limitations that social science approaches to the narrative structure of life and human identity have become the subject of criticism (e.g., Sartwell, 2000; Strawson 2004; Williams, 2009). There is, however, little in this critique that exceeds the narrative-theoretical resources of the metaphorical discourse itself. The critics appear to share with the criticized the same narrow concept of narrative that dates back to 19th-century genre conventions of the realist novel. Privileging sequentially ordered, well-formed, and coherent plots, this idea of narrative can be traced back to Aristotle's *Poetics*. Moreover, the understanding of narrative underlying these criticisms seems also to have been shaped by structuralist narratology with its emphasis on narrative as a rule-regulated, self-referential, and concealed language system. Structuralism dominated academic ideas of language in general, and narrative in particular, for most of the second half of the 20th century.

Viewed in this way, the aim of much contemporary criticism of narrative then is, not surprisingly, to contrast an Aristotelian-structuralist idea of story with the much more complex reality of lived experience.[2] What

I find astonishing about this is that neither the metaphorical discourse nor its critics seem to be aware of the broad spectrum of narrative practices and techniques that have developed since early 20th-century modernism and that radically undercut the traditional view of what narrative is supposed to be. Consider, for example, what Saunders (2010) calls the fields of "modernist auto/biografiction" and "postmodern experiments in meta-auto/biofiction," which includes works by James Joyce, Thomas Mann, Vladimir Nabokov, Fernando Pessoa, and Italo Svevo, to name just a few. Nor do the metaphorical discourse, on the one hand, and its critics, on the other, show any familiarity with or even interest in contemporary research on narrative in general or on any specific subdomains in particular. One could imagine that the detailed discussions concerned with life writing, narrative identity, and the mind-narrative nexus should be of particular interest here. After all, there is, as Eakin (2004) put it, an entire class of literature—life writing—in which people tell life stories where the questions of what is life and what is narrative and how do they mingle are pivotal.

So let me raise a question that for a number of reasons—from disciplinary protocols to a possible reluctance, reminiscent of Madame Ranevskaya, to take cognizance of challenging knowledge—has been skirted in these debates, as well as in the metaphorical discourse. Namely, what gives literature its particular quality of a magnifying lens for exploring the autobiographical process and, more generally, the core qualities of narrative experiences, whether these are present experiences or past experiences, that is, memories. While I defer the first half of this question about the investigative and hermeneutic potential of literature to my discussion of some autobiographical case studies later on, I now embark upon the more far-reaching second half regarding the core qualities of all narrative experiences in life and literature by reformulating it: What *are* the core qualities of narrative experience?

NARRATIVE EXPERIENCE

There has been a remarkable revival of the issue of narrative experience and, more generally, the relationship between narrative and experience in recent narratological discourses. The spectrum ranges from the humanities to the social sciences, psychology, and medicine. In speaking of a revival I allude to an idea of Walter Benjamin, one of the most original 20th-century theorists of experience. In trying to understand the intricacies of the nexus between narrative and the mind, recent discussions can be seen as bringing back to the notion of experience something that Benjamin called the color of our experience, a color that he saw historically lost with the rise of the modern paradigm.[3] The modern paradigm, for Benjamin, was the empiricist paradigm of capitalist rationality and, in philosophical terms, Kantian theory of knowledge. Repudiating the opposition "Grey is every theory, ever green is the tree of life," as posited by Mephistopheles in Goethe's *Faust*, Benjamin had in mind a theory of human experience that gets its color and vitality, its curious detail and nuance by being rooted in the checkered cultural life worlds of people, of body and mind uniting persons.[4] More than Cartesian and Kantian protagonists of reflexive thinking, real people have fantasies and fears; they suffer from anxieties and traumas; they live in the midst of moods and fancies and ever changing bodily states—all of which shape their experience of the world and of themselves and create the humus for their stories. And it is not least their stories that make them feel at home in particular places and at particular times, such as in a cherry orchard in the Russian provinces at the beginning of the 20th century.

Along similar lines, philosophers such as Paul Ricoeur (1981) and David Carr (1986), psychologists such as Jerome Bruner (1990a) and Mark Freeman (1993), narrative scholars such as David Herman (2009a) and Monika Fludernik (1996), and medical scholars and theorists of the experience of illness such as Rita Charon (2006) and Arthur Frank (1995) have all outlined approaches to the weave of human experience that they consider as narrative, albeit if within diverse conceptual frameworks. And there are quite a number of frameworks on offer.

Some strictly distinguish between experience and narrative, others conceive of them as interrelated or even inseparably fused, respectively drawing attention to psychological processes and capacities that give rise to narrative experiences or, conversely, are grounded in such experiences. Most discussions on the relationship between narrative and experience assume that there is a difference between life and experience, on the one hand, and narrative, on the other, a distinction that gives plenty of room to the unfolding of diverse forms of interplay between experience and narrative.[5] Now what are the various relationships that can be allotted to experience and narrative? In the most general terms, we can distinguish three positions. The first one takes experience as being articulated and represented through narrative; the second one views experience as being ordered or otherwise organized or shaped through narrative; and the third one conceives of experience, or at least ways of experience, as created through and in narrative. To my mind each of these positions can be viewed as grounded in some kind of everyday experience. This view obviously assumes that there are various kinds or categories of experience; yet because this distinction is rarely explicitly made, discussions on experience and narrative are often difficult to interconnect as they refer to quite distinct things in using the same terms.

Before taking a closer look at these various categories and their corresponding theoretical frameworks, let me point out one critical property of the nexus of experience and narrative on which, I believe, all authors just mentioned would agree. This is that narrative experience revolves around meaning and processes of meaning-making. In all accounts, the constitution and transformation of meaning appear as central dimensions of both narrative and experience — if we want to separate them out for a moment. "Experience is meaningful," as Donald Polkinghorne concludes, "and human behavior is generated from and informed by this meaningfulness" (1988, p. 1). In this way meaning turns into a pivotal notion for the study of human experience and, what is more, the experience of being in the world. Experience, then, is the key category of what can be described as narrative hermeneutics, a project centrally concerned with meaning-making (Brockmeier, 2013a; Brockmeier & Meretoja, 2014). It resonates with Polkinghorne's view that human experience "is hermeneutically organized according to the figures of linguistic production," with narrative as "the basic figuration process that produces the human experience of one's own life and action and the lives and actions of others" (1988, p. 159).

Although I agree with Polkinghorne's outline of narrative experience—which is shared, as I said, by many narrative theorists—I think it is important to be aware that his claim does not apply to all human experience.[6] Not all experiences are narrative experiences, that is experiences, as I want to qualify them, that cannot be disentangled from narrative practices. First and foremost this applies to conscious and complex experiences that grow out of, and are part of, lived and reflected human reality. Not all experience is conscious, however, and not all conscious experience is reflected. Often we consciously experience something but make sense of it only afterwards, in hindsight, typically by reconfiguring the past experience in light of a new present (Freeman, 2010a). For the sake of clarity, I call complex only those experiences that are consciously reflected on, whether this is in language or in any other cultural sign system. Complex experiences reach beyond forms of pre- and nonconceptual modes of sense-making that comprise "interpersonal attunement" and other habitual and corporeal practices that fall outside the domain of language and narrative (Herman, 2013; cf. also Zahavi, 2007). That is to say, complex experiences tend to be interwoven with language, with language at its most complex level of organization, that is narrative. Only here does it make sense to talk about narrative experience—experience closely entangled with narrative. Whenever things get messy, problematic, and involute, we use narrative, if we can, to make sense of our experiences. Narrative, as Freeman puts the matter, "exists the very moment we try to make sense of living"—which under conditions of Western modernity can surely count as a complex task—"if not the full blown sort [of narrative] we find in memoirs and autobiographies, then the more inchoate sort, the rough draft" (2010b, p. 274). A case in point of complex experiences, of both present and past events, in an ever changing modern world, is the autobiographical narrative of Madam Ranevskaya.

To further explore complex experience, as well as its relation to narrative, I want to take a closer look at what I see as its four essential qualities. These are, first, its entanglement with language and other forms of sign mediation; second, its inherent temporality; third, its capacity to capture the *what's-it-like* quality of experiencing, sometimes called *qualia*; and fourth, its interpretative nature.

Language, signs, symbols

To begin with the first quality, it is helpful to bring to mind an idea by Lev Vygotsky. For the Russian psychologist, both narrative and complex experience would be located at the level of psychological activities that are culturally mediated; that is, they are organized through signs—Vygotsky (1978) called them "psychological tools"—such as language, symbols, and counting systems. He saw language as the most important societal mediator of humans' psychological relations to the world and to fellow humans.

Does this make Vygotsky a narrative theorist? Well, he surely has important things to tell to narrative theorists. We can allocate narrative along the same trajectory within which he understood language and its development. In this way, storytelling emerges and unfolds as humans' most comprehensive language practice, as a form of discourse that is pivotal for the development of our ability to experience the world and ourselves in such a differentiated way.[7] It is true, although Vygotsky set out as a literary scholar in his short academic career—his first book was about Hamlet and the psychology of art—and dedicated a great deal of attention to the relationship between language, including literature, and consciousness, he was not specifically concerned with narrative or narrative experience. Yet if we today examine the interplay of complex experience, interpretation, and narrative we recognize a number of themes that seamlessly continue and extend Vygotsky's ideas about language and thought. One is that language is the "chief instrument of integration and order in human mental life," as Bruner (1987a, p. 15) summarizes a crucial idea of Vygotsky. Bruner goes on to write that for Vygotsky language is not just an instrument but "a powerful system of tools for use—for use initially in talk, but increasingly and once inwardness is achieved, in perception, in memory, in thought and imagination, even in the exercise of will" (Bruner, 1987a, p. 15). A third theme is that complex experiences are interwoven with language and hence with larger cultural meaning systems in whose dynamics they unavoidably partake. To couch this Vygotskian point using a hermeneutic vocabulary we can say that complex experiences are the likes of being that can only be understood in language.[8]

Yet make no mistake, neither the Vygotskian nor the hermeneutic claim—both of which, in my reading, are connected in several ways—is that there are no other experiences that are mediated by sign or symbol systems other than the language of words. Think of sign languages, of mathematical or musical systems, or of the language of quantum physics in which physicists talk about their experiments within the particle zoo. Visiting a museum, some paintings strangely speak to you; and we conceive of a building's facade as being engaged in a dialogue with the architecture of a surrounding square. Moreover, there are practical, ethical, aesthetic, and sensuous experiences where the significance of language may be altogether minor, if there is any at all. At the heart of the experience of riding a bicycle, playing a piano sonata, or suffering from a serious accident or a natural disaster is not a linguistically mediated and reflected act. This is not to say that language is not helpful in teaching or learning how to ride a bicycle, and it may even be essential in interpreting a piano sonata or any other work of art. Still, there no doubt is a nonlinguistic dimension to certain experiences. To name it, or at least one aspect of it, Benjamin (2008) used the term *aura*.

On the other hand, this does not rule out that such concrete, singular, prereflexive, and unarticulated experiences have a generalized meaning. In fact, they typically originate not in an isolated and unique event but in repeated events; they emerge in a series, a pattern, a generalized meaning structure within which something stands out like a figure before a ground. In the realm of human culture—to resort again to the Vygotskian framework—there is no perception without categorization, as perception researchers like Bruner (1973) and Holzkamp (1973) stated drawing on an old philosophical argument. "Perception," Benjamin (1917/1996) wrote, "is reading." In their ways, Bruner's, Holzkamp's, and Benjamin's point was that if we register a sensation, that is, if we perceive, we are about to transform information into experience: making it conscious by giving it a meaning, preliminary and temporary as it may be. We do not do so because of a personal decision or an individual penchant but because we live in a social and cultural world that also comprises perceptions. For this reason, experiences, whether linguistic or not, are to be seen as always occurring within a symbolic space, a space of history and cultural significance. It is this symbolic space that makes them *experience*; without it they remain psycho-physiological processes, bodily sensations, unconscious perceptions.

To put the same point differently, we can say that all experience is generalized, even if not necessarily in a linguistically mediated way. Besides language and, by extension, narrative there are cultural systems of semiotic mediation like sign languages, images, music, dance, and other performative practices—often intertwined among one another—through which experience can be shaped, reflected, and interpreted (Brockmeier & Homer, 2014). These interpretations can be quite different in scope and character. Visual arts and music, for example, may only center on certain moments or figures or feelings in the interminable flow of life. Notwithstanding, here, too, we are talking of complex experience. I thus believe it is overstating the point to assume that narrative is a *necessary* condition for experience, a "basis or context for the having of (an) experience in the first place," as Herman (2009a, pp. 153 and 212) has suggested. I even suspect that it is difficult to claim that "narrative might be viewed as a basis or condition for *conscious* experience itself" (Herman, 2009a, p. 143; emphasis added).[9]

Following the line of thought developed so far, we arrive at a notion of experience that embraces what Benjamin called the dimension of praxis and history. One of Benjamin's main concerns was to anchor his notion of experience in historical forms of life and in doing so distinguish it from the physiology-based concept of perception that has underlain the idea of experience in the empiricist tradition. A few words on these two overarching traditions of understanding experience are helpful, because they also permit us to localize better the concept of narrative experience. Despite Vygotsky, Bruner, Holzkamp, and other psychologists aware of the cultural and historical dimension of this issue, the empiricist tradition has dominated academic psychology and scientific research on perception and experience from the very beginning. In contrast, the notion of experience associated with the concept of narrative experience belongs to a tradition different from empiricism. In this tradition, reaching from Aristotle and Hegel to Benjamin, modern hermeneutics, sociocultural and poststructuralist approaches, experience is not modeled on empirical immediacy, that is, on psychophysical and physiological perception; it rather is conceived of as always already generalized within a larger context of individual and social experiences. The experience of a thing, as Aristotle (2004) points out in his *Metaphysics*, needs some previous understanding of this thing; Aristotle speaks of a memory of this thing without which there cannot be any experience of it (980 b 28). According to this view, experiencing something means experiencing something *as* something or, as I described it earlier, as a figure against a ground, a ground of cultural meanings. In this process, experiencing an object or event is not simply to capture or to represent it, but to create it anew, "to re-create it for us," as Hegel (1977) summarizes the central proposition of this tradition in his account of phenomenology.

The notion of experience in this tradition also has kept an element of real-life or applied knowledge and thus a connection to Benjamin's color of life. Aristotle referred to both practical skills and abilities, *techne*, as well as practical wisdom, *phronesis*, terms that have retained a reference to the knowledge and virtuosity of an experienced practitioner, say, a craftsperson, a physician, an artist, or a trained ancient rhetorician. In this meaning, experience became central to the hermeneutics of Heidegger and Gadamer. Ricoeur, well aware of this tradition, took great pains to argue that narrative, too, is a practical knowledge and skill anchored in the experience of what it means to live a life. Ricoeur even went so far as to see life as a mere biological phenomenon as long as it has not been interpreted in narrative. Narrative self-experience, as he put it, is inherent to humans' specific "living experience of acting and suffering" (Ricoeur, 1991a, p. 28).

Being entangled with language and other sign systems and thus inextricably fused with larger cultural meaning contexts is one important factor that makes experiences complex and, given a certain degree of complexity, seamlessly interweaves them with narrative experiences—experiences that cannot be distinguished from narrative practices.

Temporality

A second quality of complex experience that makes it so intimately entwined with narrative is its inherent temporality. Complex experiences are temporal or, more precisely, they are or at least can be temporally extended. This distinguishes them from the immediacy of the passing moment, the experience in the here and now, and from pure physiological sensations, which are not necessarily extended in time. Clearly, narrative interpretation and reflection presuppose and bring about temporal extension. To understand a memory *as* a memory (and distinguish it as past from a present sensation or imagination) is predicated on an awareness of the past *as* past, which only is possible if there also is an awareness of the present *as* present. It is this awareness that Tulving (1985b; Tulving & Kim, 2009), though in a different conceptual frame, has described as "autonoetic consciousness" and that I discussed in terms of self-interpretative meaning-making in Chapter 2 (and will further qualify in the rest of this chapter). This autonoetic—that is, literally, self-knowing—feature of consciousness also holds true for our awareness of the future: "When I pronounce the word Future,/the first syllable already belongs to the past," writes Wislawa Szymborska in one of her poems (1998, p. 261). There are, however, forms of what is called traumatic experience where this double awareness is challenged. At times, for Chekhov's protagonists the catastrophes of their past are present in a way that makes the past feel as if it were the real here and now, as if it had never passed.

Obviously such forms of time consciousness, whether troubled or not, do not exist in an either-or way but are a matter of degree, like the reflection and interpretation they entail and presuppose. Yet it seems that there are certain forms or gestalts of temporality or temporal experiences, gestalts of complex experience, that are only possible in narrative. In *Time and Narrative*, Ricoeur (1984–1988) expounded the hermeneutic thesis that there is an inner correlation between narrative and human time experience. More than this, he concluded that narrative is constitutive of human time, that human time *is* narrated time. How we can envision this narrative redefinition of time is the central issue of Chapters 7 and 8, which explore the interrelations among time, narrative, and the autobiographical process. In those chapters I return to the question of narrative experience, building on the qualities identified in this section.

What is it like?

The third quality of complex, narrative experience is its capacity to capture or realize not just the experience of something—its aboutness or intentionality, as it is called in phenomenological and analytical philosophy—but also the specific subjective feel of this experience, the sense of *what it is like* to have a particular experience. *Qualia* is another term by which philosophers of mind refer to this property of certain experiences that permits us not only to experience something, but also to experience it in a particular, subjective, personal way.

In certain trauma accounts the felt quality of the traumatic event, the sense of what it is like to have gone through an experience as a lived experience, an *Erlebnis*, often is more prevailing than the very event. It is not the catastrophe, the disaster, the rupture that is at the center of many stories of those who went through such an event but its subjective quality—the sense of being stunned, overwhelmed, helpless, powerless, speechless, humiliated, paralyzed. All these were feelings and emotional states described in accounts of eye witnesses to the events of 9/11 in New York City. In a study on how people remember 9/11, eye witnesses were asked to tell what had happened a few days after the attack.[10] A 53-year-old woman from Brooklyn, for instance, who was walking near the towers when the first plane exploded above her, reported:

> Whenever I hear an airplane, I get tense. I am using the wrong keys for my door.... . Have nightmares and my alpha stage before asleep has very discombobulating thoughts. I am petrified, tired + not myself. I feel like I have been through a twilight zone episode. *Masks Military Police State Troopers Scary*
>
> (quoted from Brockmeier, 2008b, p. 23).

Although the attack on the World Trade Center and its subsequent pulverisation were unique events, many eyewitnesses seem to feel that the ultimately definable and describable extent of the disaster did not match the magnitude of *what it was like* when they experienced it firsthand. Countless reports, films, and pictures caught those scenarios, but what could capture the lived and felt experience, the *Erlebnis*, of falling while running away from the debris, the dust, the deafening noise of the crashing towers?

In accounts like this of the woman from Brooklyn it is not the events as such that are foregrounded but rather that which is unbelievable, mind-boggling, terrifying, or staggering about them. We may call it their subjective and emotional quality. This is not only the case in historical occurrences that are collectively and simultaneously experienced by a great number of people. Rita Charon, reflecting as a clinician and medical scholar on the story a cancer patient told her in the course of their conversations, notes that "like any illness narrative, hers was not simply a report of a particular set of symptoms but, rather, an *exemplification* or *showing forth* of what it might mean for any of us to live with illness" (2012, p. 346).

The focus on subjective meaning and emotional, intensely lived experience is, however, not only a quality of trauma or illness narrative. Emphasizing and interpreting the lived experience of events in order to come to terms with it is the point of all oral storytelling, argues Fludernik

(2009, p. 59), even if, we might add, this applies to different genres or kinds of stories to different degrees. Perhaps it is particularly in trauma and illness narratives where this moment is unfolded to the point that it overpowers the entire story, in fact, the entire narrative event and sometimes even an entire life. But then, there are many who maintain that much of literature is, in principle, exactly about this experience, because "literature not only reports on what happens and on what may happen, it is itself 'a form of lived experience'," to borrow Michael Wood's (2005, p. 9) words. Wood refers to Dorothy Walsh's (1969) remark that "literary art, when functioning successfully as literary art, provides knowledge in the form of realization: the realization of what anything might come to as a form of lived experience" (p. 136).

It is one of the essential properties of narrating, whether as form of art or as everyday activity, to "make present." Schiff (2012) has pointed out the phenomenological significance of *making present* or *giving presence* to. There is a German word for this making present, *vergegenwärtigen*, that figures prominently in Hegel's phenomenology. Here it comes to mind because it simultaneously means giving presence to, bringing into the present, and reflecting. Other nuances of the meaning of *vergegenwärtigen* are showing, taking shape, and giving corporality to something, all of which Schiff (2012, p. 36–37) conceives of as features of narrative. Making present, in this sense, also alludes to socially connecting and entangling with the world and stories of others. And indeed, "when we tell," Schiff writes, "we make experience and interpretations of life present in a social scene of action, using the terms of some particular linguistic, historical and cultural community" (p. 37). He goes on to say that in communicating the feel and texture of our lives, ambiguous and vague experiences, and inchoate thoughts may take form and become, as it were, objectified; they turn into "something other than internal wanderings and become active as they are entered into the here and now of the social world" (p. 37).

There are good reasons to assume that in question is not only the critical property of particular categories of stories (besides trauma or illness narratives we may think of confessional narratives, stories told in therapeutic settings, and the "novel of consciousness") but a quality of all narrative. Herman (2009a; 2011a) considers this "consciousness factor" to be a basic element of narrative. For Fludernik (1996; 2009), as already insinuated, the particular sensitivity of stories to what she calls "human experientiality" is the defining feature of narrativity. As there are experiences that are highly amenable to being understood in narrative terms, there are stories that are "tailor-made for gauging the felt quality of lived experiences," remarks Herman (2009a, p. 139), who sees at the basis of this an "isomorphism" (p. 157) between the structures of experience and narrative.

How can we account for this amazing structural equivalence? Why do stories, in Herman's (2009a, p. 145) words, "orient themselves around the what's-it-like properties of experiencing consciousnesses"?—which is, by the way, what they do both within the narrative worlds they evoke and in respect to their tellers and listeners or readers. One reason may be that narratives, across all media and social contexts, are told and understood because their inherent intersubjective (or interactional or dialogical) resources allow them to fine-tune themselves to the way people—tellers and listeners—experience, feel, and imagine the minds of others and themselves. Stories take place in a discursive environment where they unfold a psychological dynamic. Thanks to this dynamic they are not just *about* something; they do not merely convey information or present a certain content but also, and sometimes in the first place, carry out what it is like for a human mind to experience this content, to make sense of it. More than just representing experience, stories evoke and enact ways of experiencing (Herman, 2009a, p. 157). This makes narrative, as Herman goes on to conclude, "uniquely suited to capturing what the world is like from the situated perspective of an experiencing mind" and thus distinguishes it from other forms of discourse such as descriptions and deductive arguments and from nonlinguistic sign systems such as the periodic table of the elements (p. 157).

Fludernik (1996) offers a similar explanation of the narrative enactment of the experiencing mind, though within a slightly different framework. In her view, what qualifies narrative *as* narrative is not that it represents a sequence of events or construes them as structured plot or "story," but that it precisely acts out the way humans experience something. Her point, if I understand it properly, is that there is something about narrative that "embodies" human concerns and human existence. Fludernik calls it narrative's "experientiality." Stories center on a human experiencer and his or her consciousness, which can be the consciousness of the character within a story, of the narrative voice, or of the narrator or listener/reader. Again, the point of Fludernik's experience-focused reading of narrative is that this is not the property of a particular genre or type of narrative but of narrativity in general, as it makes itself felt in everyday, performative, and pictorial narrative practices, as well as in literary prose.[11] It is interesting to see that Fludernik does not recognize, across the entire spectrum of narrative practices, the existence of two qualitatively different types of narratives, fictional and nonfictional. In her account, narrative is fictional per se because it does not deal with events and facts but with experience and mental states, with consciousness. Narrative, as we could say, is, or perhaps more precisely, includes a mode of experiencing the world that involves the experience of its own interpretation (cf. Brockmeier, 2013a). This brings me to the fourth quality of narrative experience.

Interpretativity

The fourth element that makes complex experiences indissolubly intertwined with narrative is its interpretive nature: narrative experience is experience interpreted. This chapter is entitled *Interpreting memory* for its chief point is that autobiographical memories cannot be understood independently from their interpretation; the chapter's subtitle, *The narrative perspective,* further qualifies this interpretation and refers to the overall approach to autobiographical memory suggested in this book. To put it pointedly, memories and their interpretations are inherently interconnected elements, aspects of the same autobiographical process.

Just to identify certain mental phenomena as memories, or certain mental states as processes of remembering, involves interpretive attention that allows us to distinguish these phenomena or states from others, for example, from imagination, hallucination, or daydreaming. What is it about the sudden appearance of a face that I cannot make sense of? Do I fantasize, make it up? Am I lost in reverie? Is it how I seem to envision the main character of a novel I have been reading in these days? Or am I floating in retrospect and encounter with this face an autobiographical memory, but a memory of whom? Perhaps the face of someone I saw this morning on the subway, or in a photograph I glimpsed for a second in a magazine ad, that for who knows what reason got carried away with my stream of consciousness? Or is it the face of someone I met in my earlier life, and later tried to forget? And then, can I rule out that I have blended two or more of these mental states into one another, creating something new that appears both familiar and strange?

To ask such questions is to *interpret* the status of this "face," with one option identifying it as an autobiographical memory. Let us assume for a moment that I succeed in qualifying it as the face of a person from my past whom I hoped to have forgotten, that is, that my interpretations allowed me to identify or, at least, to narrow down what experimental memory psychologists call the source of a memory. This may evoke further and possibly even more intricate acts of interpretation. Such acts of interpretation—acts of meaning—are at the heart of the autobiographical process. Their intricacy may even increase when these acts occur within discursive and conversational formats; and they indeed often do. Yet whatever their discursive form, the more extended and complex they are, the more they are interwoven with narrative. If I am able to figure out the status of that face, it is because language allows me to ask those questions and consider possible answers. This is not to say that I eventually know what this face is all about. But when we understand anything at all, we understand it by means of language; and the more complex our understanding is, the more it takes the form of narrative.

Viewed in this light, the idea of a pure and autonomous autobiographical memory turns out to be an abstraction, even if it may be artificially construed and materialized in scientific memory experiments. That there is an individual "memory per se" that must and can be studied in isolation from its social and cultural reality appears all the more problematic for social or collective memory researchers who take the primary and most fundamental existence of human beings to be social, as Jeffrey Olick, Vered Vinitzky-Seroussi, and Daniel Levy (2014) elucidate. It may help to clarify this point by looking at it against the backdrop of such memory experiments, which, in fact, have been quite common in psychological and neuroscientific research. For decades, the basic assumption of this research has not changed. The assumption is, as we remember, that memory consists of multiple memory systems operating on the basis of cognition. In earlier days, these operations and their "mechanisms" were understood in terms of computation and in more recent days in terms of neurocognition. But in whatever form cognition is conceived of, in respect to memory it means first of all *pure* cognition, cognition "per se." The pure cognition underlying acts of retrieval is unaffected by any act of interpretation or linguistic reconstruction. If it does so, another severe sin is committed, as Schacter (2001) has maintained in his catalogue of the seven capital sins of memory. Therefore, research of declarative memory (memories that can be articulated or otherwise expressed) is viewed as only dealing with the "postretrieval" nature of such expressions.

Specifying declarative memory systems, Schacter and Tulving state that "the final productions of all these systems can be, and frequently are, contemplated by the individual introspectively, in conscious awareness" (1994, p. 27). However, within neuroscientific memory research, these "final productions" do not have much to do with what are taken to be the very mechanisms of recall; they rather are transformations or conversions of memories. "Any conversion of such a product of memory into overt behavior, even symbolic behavior such as speech or writing, represents an optional postretrieval phenomenon" (Schacter & Tulving, 1994, p. 27). In a nutshell, it is not memory anymore.

The view that I want to advance in this book is in clear contrast with this distinction between experiences or memory and its interpretation, between "pure retrieval" and not so pure "postretrieval" meaning construction. Whereas traditional cognitive and neuroscientific memory research takes great pains to experimentally create conditions that appear to separate "pure retrieval" from "postretrieval" interpretation (sometimes called "expression"), the approach I suggest is only marginally interested in the construct of pure cognitive memory and its universalist claims. Instead it is interested in the everyday reality of remembering and forgetting, and this reality is all but cognitively pure because it is always situated in interpretive communities. "Interpretive communities," a term coined by literary theorist Stanly Fish (1980), can be viewed as specific cultural worlds. These worlds are made up, however, not only by communities that share the same literary or aesthetic canon but also, say, by the community of an experimental laboratory of memory research or, in a wider sense, by the communities of all memory researchers who do experimental research under laboratory conditions. This view, elaborated by many sociologists, historians, and philosophers of science in the wake of Ludwig Fleck (1979/1935) and Bruno Latour and Steve Wolgar (1979), helps me to understand better the interplay between experience and narrative, whether in the context of science, literature, or everyday life.

To drive home the points made so far, we can take experience as a notion that embraces memory or past experience but obviously is broader than it because it also holds for the interpretive dimension of experience. It thus relegates in an existential sense to the interpretive condition under which humans live their lives (cf. also Meretoja, 2014a). To say that certain experiences are complex is another way of saying they are intrinsically interpretive, being the subject and outcome of processes of sense-making. Herman's (2009a) incorporation of the what's-it-like quality of stories into narrative theory draws on Daniel Dennett's (1997) definition of qualia as *the way things seem to us*. In the context of my argument the way things seem to us is, however, not a given that comes with the things themselves, as Dennett suggested, but the result of how we experience and, that is, interpret them. It is the meaning we give to things *re-creating them for us*.

The re-creative constitution of meaning is not necessarily a single act. This does not remain without consequences, because the conditions for repeated interpretation are never exactly the same. The flux of time does not stop; understanding is always different. "It is enough to say," as

Gadamer put it, "that we understand in a *different* way, if we *understand at all*" (1989, p. 296). In this way, the ongoing interpretability of narrative experiences and memories keeps the entire process open-ended, at least in principle. Understanding narrative, be it in contexts of everyday life, literature, or academic investigation, rarely ends with closure, and this is not only because our stories about past experiences do not automatically turn events into memories. "Who was it said," writes Julian Barnes "that memory is what we thought we'd forgotten?" (2011, p. 63) And Barnes goes on to say that "time doesn't act as a fixative, rather as a solvent" (p. 63). It turns every story into a story of interpretation.

Perhaps we can see this interminable quality as intrinsic to narrative form; put differently, we can never be sure that there is a last word, to use Andrews's (2013) expression. Consider the discursive interchange of conversational narratives as it shows, for example, in turn-taking, an activity extensively studied in Conversation Analysis. In a typical Western conversational storytelling setting, an interlocutor may interrupt or otherwise react to the storyteller at any moment, giving the telling a new and unexpected twist, if not initiating a new story (Sacks, 1992). Yet the open-endedness is also evident in more extended and monologic narratives, oral or written, where listeners and readers constantly try to make sense of the story they hear or read. The smallest cue counts.

To make it completely clear: all of this is not external to narrative. It is nothing that has to be added to it after the fact; rather, it is part and parcel of the very enterprise. Narrative is predicated on interpretation in a way that every new interpretation endows it with a new level of meaning (or, at least, a new aspect of meaning) and, in doing so, transforms it, as Kermode (1983) explained. This even holds when the interpretation is tentatively given to a particular sequence while the entire story is yet unfinished.[12] Narrative, as Kermode writes, is a continuous "dialogue" between a story and its interpretation; it emerges "as the product of two intertwined processes, the presentation of a fable and its progressive interpretation (which of course alters it)" (1983, p. 136). In view of these observations, I have suggested that the telling and listening or reading of a story requires and induces a mode of experience that comprises the experience of its own interpretation.

To put the same point more straightforwardly, whatever we experience occurs in the form of its interpretive re-creation. It is in this sense that we can understand Charles Taylor's claim that interpretation is constitutive of human experience (1985a, p. 37). More precisely, Taylor aims at one particular kind of interpretation that he views in the tradition of 20th-century hermeneutics outlined above: self-interpretation.

Accordingly, the human imperative to world- and self-interpretation is not just a matter of knowledge, curiosity, or individual inclination but is inscribed into the human condition, into our existence as what Taylor calls "self-interpreting animals" (1985b). Further developing this idea, Taylor (1989) describes human beings as engaged in continual processes of enquiry and reflection about what makes life worthwhile.

Although Taylor leaves no doubt that language is crucial to these processes, he is not mainly concerned with language, let alone narrative. How a conceptual reframing of this view of interpretation would look in terms of narrative has, however, been the central question in this section. In making the case for a narrative hermeneutics of experiencing and remembering I have suggested complementing the notion of narrative as a "gestalt of experience" (Brockmeier, 1998, p. 279) by a notion of experience as a gestalt of narrative. To do so I have built on the proposition that it is "in narrative we give our experience and imagination the form in which they turn into a subject of consciousness," as I formulated it earlier (Brockmeier, 1998, p. 278). Although I still believe that this assumption stresses an important aspect of the interconnection of experience, consciousness, and narrative, I have emphasized in this section why it is necessary to qualify the experience in question in a more precise manner, namely as a particular, complex experience. This may seem just a minor conceptual nuance. Yet it brings about an essential qualification of the notion of narrative experience that helps us understand what makes this kind of experience—experience that cannot be disentangled from narrative—special.

THE STRONG NARRATIVE THESIS

As we have seen, efforts to understand how linguistic, temporal, and cultural trajectories of human experiences intermingle are all but new. It did not require a narrative turn, let alone a series of narrative turns, to reveal that the complexity of our experiences and their interpretation has a lot to do with the narrative nature of the human mind. Nor have narrative theorists discovered that meanings and processes of meaning-making are essential for what we consider to be our identity, and that these processes are tied up with manifold actions and interactions and situated in a cultural world. What narrative research and scholarship *has* gained is the insight that the more complex these acts of meaning become—that is, the more they become interpretive, constructive, and creative—the more they are inseparably intertwined with complex sign systems. Among these systems, I am particularly concerned with language and, more specifically, with narrative language because, as I argue, it plays a crucial role in the interpretive dynamic of the autobiographical process. Put differently, to understand the complexities of human meaning-making there is no getting around narrative.

To account for this elective affinity, I want to take the argument about narrative's constructive and creative potential one step further. I propose that the intricacies of autobiographical meaning-making are not just represented or expressed by narrative, they only come into being through and in narrative. I call this the strong narrative thesis. The strong narrative thesis applies to a set of phenomena that only exist due to the specific kind of action that is carried out in acts of narrative meaning construction. A case in point, already mentioned, is narrative's capacity to create complex temporal scenarios that are typical for the autobiographical process. Another phenomenon illustrating the strong narrative thesis is the what's-it-like quality of conscious awareness, which I have described as a critical property of narrative experience. Endorsing Herman's (2009a; 2013) view of narrative as enacting and evoking and not just representing ways of experiencing, I have referred to the accounts of trauma survivors as an example. What is foregrounded in many trauma stories is not the traumatic event as such but its felt quality, the emotional impact of what it meant to have gone through it. It is hard to see how this sense of what it is like, which is pivotal for an entire spectrum of experiences, would come into a meaningful existence without its narrative shape.

To better understand the meaning-creating potential of narrative I have examined it as a form and practice of human agency. In my study *Reaching for meaning: Human agency and the narrative imagination*, the starting point was that neither experiences nor stories just come upon us; it is we who make and re-make them (Brockmeier, 2009). Both making experience and telling stories are not external to human subjectivity but always already belong to the very business of living a life. The narratives we tell about ourselves may be influenced by established cultural conventions and traditions, yet we do not simply reproduce them but instead actively engage with them in ways that can go far beyond the common ground.

What is possible

To view narrative as a form and practice of human agency also sheds new light on a phenomenon already well known. Making sense of emerging experiences and giving new meaning to old experiences can constitute in and of itself a new experience, and this experience again invites us to further investigations and interpretations. "There will be no end of interpretations," as Bruner has it, employing a well-established hermeneutic insight, for "the object of understanding human events is to sense the alternativeness of human possibility" (1986, p. 53). Building on the idea of narrative and experience as forms of agency, I have suggested in the 2008 study that narrative imagination enables us to probe the reach and range of our options—in Bruner's words, their alternativeness—both in everyday and literary discourse and thought. I have described this probing in terms of exploring possible actions or action possibilities (Brockmeier, 2009), taking up a concept by Holzkamp (1983; 2013). Now I want to frame it this way: If meanings are *options for acting*, then narrative appears to be the most advanced practice by which we envision, scrutinize, and try out these options, and, in fact, realize an important portion of them.

Exploring possible actions is always a proactive endeavor. One aspect of it, its interpretive nature, has already been examined; but there is more to it. When Bruner says that narrating is "being in the subjunctive mode"— a "trafficking in human possibilities rather than in settled certainties" (1986, p. 25)—he brings into focus a slightly different approach to our action possibilities. Interestingly, we find this approach further detailed in the work of a literary scholar, Wolfgang Iser. Iser (1993) outlined a narrative theory of the *imaginary*, which he sees as a general human faculty, and the *fictive*, which he takes as a way of using this faculty. Iser mainly considers literary narratives, investigating what he calls literature's "limitless patterns of human plasticity" that, in his view, is reflecting and shaping the plasticity of human life itself (1993, p. xiii). Yet obviously the idea of openness and plasticity of human life goes far beyond the scope of literary theory and, in fact, Iser conceives of his project as a "literary anthropology" in which literature figures as a "heuristics for human self-interpretation" (p. xiii). As in many postclassical narrative theories, the fictive here is not confined to literature; it stands for an operational mode of consciousness that makes inroads into existing and nonexisting, possible and impossible versions of the world. In their interplay, the fictive and the imaginary engender narrative's specific sensitivity for the openness and unpredictability of human affairs.

Even if Iser's thoughts first of all circle around literature and its protean qualities, they are also instructive for a general understanding of narrative as a subjunctive mode of experience. For if we accept that at stake is an universal potential of narrative, which has gained special prominence in literature (to the point that it dominates an entire part of literature appropriately called fiction), it appears as an inherent quality of narrative that its inroads induce us to imaginatively populate the factual and fictive worlds in which we live—whether these are the scenarios of my everyday life or Kafka's castles. The particular potential of narrative imagination then, is, in Iser's words, its "staging of the human condition in a welter of unforeseeable patterns" (p. 297), which is as much the expression as the realization of the extraordinary plasticity of human beings themselves. It is for this reason that the storyworlds of narrative offer a unique "panorama of what is possible," Iser concludes, "because it is not hedged in by either the limitations or the considerations that determine the institutionalized organizations within which human life otherwise takes its course" (pp. 296–297).

If we understand the word "anthropological" in more than a disciplinary sense, that is, in a wider, philosophical sense, we can call this an anthropological argument. It qualifies narrative not just as a linguistic genre or practice but as a fundamental human potential. Rom Harré and I have used this argument in a hermeneutic sense to show that narrative can serve as an experimental laboratory in which possible and sometimes even impossible realities can be envisioned and tested (Brockmeier & Harré, 2001); and this holds true not only for literary critics and students of the human condition but for all members of storytelling communities. Because narrative is such an open and flexible structure and practice, it allows us—Harré and I have suggested—to examine precisely these fundamental aspects of our existence, its openness, fleetingness, and plasticity, traditionally neglected by the human sciences. Narrative can operate as a sensitive guide to the changeable and fluid nature of human life because, to a significant degree, it contributes to it. It can be crucial to our effort of realizing our action possibilities because it is, in part, constitutive of them. "The study of narrative," as we summarized this argument, "invites us to rethink the whole issue of the Heraclitian nature of human experience because it works as an open and malleable frame that enables us to come to terms with an ever-changing, ever reconstructed reality" (Brockmeier & Harré, 2001, p. 53).

Consider, for example, a situation in which diverse versions of experience—present, past, and anticipating the future—are competing with each other for a rationale of action. Something has to be done, but what? Recall the heavy burden that Madame Ranevskaya cannot shake off her shoulders, the stream of conversations, soliloquies, and ruminations in which she incessantly plays through different versions of her present and her past. What would it mean for her life immersed in memories—to remind us only of the options Chekhov indicates—if she turned her country house, both palace and cage of her past, into an economically viable estate? What if she sold it? What if she would do nothing, letting it be auctioned and ultimately destroyed? In this respect Madame Ranevskaya is all but special, as we feel immediately. We all continuously sort out real and fictive, contrasting and competing versions of actions, or inactions; we play them through and reflect on them, imagine possible and impossible scenarios and speculate about their implications. There seems to be something about narrative that makes it particularly capable of "critical and reflexive engagement with ... competing accounts of the world-as-experienced," Herman notes (2009a, pp. 150–151). For him, what comes to the fore here is one of narrative's special qualities: Stories afford "an environment in which versions of what it was like to experience situations and events can be juxtaposed, comparatively evaluated, and then factored into further accounts of the world, or a world" (p. 151).

If we take this point, then the construction of meaning—viewed as options for acting within particular social and cultural contexts—is a much more complicated enterprise than commonly assumed. Therefore, I have referred to this "environment" in terms of an experimental laboratory of human meaning-making, an aspect that also had center stage in the discussion of the interpretive nature of narrative experience earlier in this chapter. One part of the accumulative complication involved in this kind of meaning-making is bound up with its discursive dynamic. The critical and reflexive engagement with competing accounts of the world-as-experienced is typically not the business of a single person alone but part of more extended social interactions. In one way or another this dynamic is even manifest if one single person reads or writes or otherwise is involved in a storytelling event. Discursive-psychological theorists like Harré (1998; Harré & Gillett, 1994) and Derek Edwards (2005; 2006) have put much emphasis on the function that interaction with others plays in elaborating the significance of putatively individual experiences as well as many other psychological processes and states.

Discursive psychology resonates with several other recent approaches to language, narrative, and mental or psychological phenomena in Linguistic Anthropology, Linguistic Ethnography, and Gender Studies. These approaches add weight to the idea that people work up the meanings of events, actions, and their own accountability (including what they then refer to as their intentions and emotions) through "talk-in-interaction," rather than carrying them around in their heads in the form of scripted experiences, memories, thoughts, feelings, and so on, ready to be represented or externalized on cue. As a consequence, language forcefully appears as a constructive and action oriented form of life. Talking and narrating are constructive, as Edwards explains, "in the sense that they offer a particular version of things when there are indefinitely many potential versions, some of which may be available and alive in the setting"; and they are "action oriented in the sense that they are constructed in ways that perform actions in and for the occasion of their telling" (2005, p. 260). On this account, referring to a particular experience as, say, an autobiographical memory, appears to be an act of meaning formation that is always interwoven with a particular discursive dynamic, a dynamic in the present. That is, it is defined less by independent cognitive or neurocognitive operations than by the interactional, institutional, and ethical constraints of a given cultural situation. Viewed in this light, the identification and labeling of a cognitive phenomenon—in our case, a memory—appears as the result of the discursive event, and not as its starting point, as held in traditional psychological theorizing. Rather than emerging out of an inner-individual and inner-psychological process, a memory always intervenes in a field of discourse already established.

To sum up the strong narrative thesis we can say that it draws attention to the constructive, imaginative, and discursive qualities of narrative—as emphasized by Herman, Harré, and Edwards from different angles. Closely related to this, it exposes the world-creating qualities of narrative as a form of agency, a form we use in a wide spectrum of actions. Again the autobiographical process is a case in point; it simultaneously unfolds several temporal scenarios that are not conceivable, in fact, not even imaginable, without the forms and practices of narrative.

Several authors have brought into prominence the constructive and creative meaning potential of narrative as a "way of worldmaking," employing an expression by Nelson Goodman (1978).[13] Herman, for example, has suggested reorienting narrative theory around questions of worldmaking, and, in turn, situating the inquiry of storyworlds at the nexus of narrative and mind. This implies bringing the study of narrative into a closer dialogue with psychology and other sciences of mind. By the same token, Bruner has approached the goal from a psychological vantage point, shifting his discipline closer to humanistic scholarship in general and narrative theory in particular. At the same time, he has widened the idea of worldmaking by integrating a more psychological focus on what he has called narrative "self-making" into the larger trajectory of cultural "world-making" (Bruner, 2001). In my reading of Bruner's argument, this is to maintain that there are no special, autonomous psychological processes or narrative practices of *self*-making, which is another way of underlining narrative's crucial role in the cultural fabric of meaning that makes up humans' self or identity projects.

There are many phenomena in which narrative experiences mingle with what some see as "pure" psychological processes, with the autobiographical process being only one of these phenomena. Keep in mind that narrative has been proposed as an alternative "root metaphor" for all psychology (Sarbin, 1986), and particularly for the psychological study of human life (Schiff, 2013). A similar status has been claimed for narrative as a central category for the study of humans' social existence (Andrews, Squire, & Tamboukou, 2013; Gubrium & Holstein, 2009), history (Roberts, 2001), human action in general (MacIntyre, 2007), and political action in particular (Andrews, 2007). It also has been recommended as our most appropriate way of understanding the experience of illness, somatic and mental, and disability (Charon, 2006; Hydén & Brockmeier, 2008; Lewis, 2011), the experience of aging and dying (Gunaratnam & Oliviere, 2009; Randall & McKim, 2008), and our existence as civic and legal subjects (Amsterdam & Bruner, 2000). More than this, narrative has been expounded as paradigmatic notion for the whole of the human sciences (Hinchman & Hinchman, 1997; Polkinghorne, 1988; Kohler Riesman, 2008) and, on a philosophical plane, for the understanding of the human condition (Arendt, 1998/1958; Ricoeur, 1992; Schapp, 1954).

Whereas these approaches have advocated the significance of narrative for our psychological, social, and cultural reality, narratologists, in turn, have argued that narrative depends on and interacts with fundamental mental functions and psychological practices. Herman, besides putting forward narrative as crucial for our understanding of human consciousness, and as our unique mode of articulating the what's-it-like property of human experience, maintains that narrative world-making and self-making are "imbricated with"—that is, both support and are supported by—a broad spectrum of basic psychological processes (2012). Furthermore, informed by Oatley's studies on the relationship between narrative and emotion (2012) and Keen's (2007) inquiry into the modern history of empathy and the novel, we may say that there is, and has always been, a seamless connective tissue between narrative and the emotional dimension of meaning-making.

This view is increasingly shared by a new generation of narrative scholars, both in the social sciences and the humanities. Combining a critical view of the classical, structuralist narratology of Genette, Greimas, Barthes, and others with more recent developments in psychology, cognitive science, sociolinguistics, discourse and media studies, these "postclassical" theorists strive to develop a new conception of the interplay between mind and narrative (e.g., Alber & Fludernik, 2010; Fludernik,1996; Herman, 1999a; 2013). Some of these ideas are reminiscent of Iser's (1993) approach to narrative discussed earlier; some others have already been touched on in the discussion of narrative experience at the beginning of this chapter. On the whole, without the work emerging from this new domain of narrative studies the alternative, narrative approach to autobiographical memory outlined in this book would hardly be possible. Therefore, let me mark what I see as the three important assumptions of postclassical narrative studies that, it is safe to state, have radically challenged the traditional idea of story and storytelling (and hence also explain the "post" of their postclassical claims and poststructuralist foundations).

The first assumption is that there is no fundamental divide between the psychological-hermeneutic underpinnings of narrative meaning constructions in fictional and nonfictional discourses. That is, there is no qualitative difference between practices of psychological understanding in literary and nonliterary narrative within the same cultural world. The second assumption is that the traditional concept of narrative, based on the Aristotelian idea of a well-structured, closed, and sequentially organized plot (given again paradigmatic status by 20th-century structuralist narratologists), captures only one particular type of story, an isolated and self-contained story. This concept not only fails the enormous cultural multitude of narrative forms and practices across a variety of media, but also their openness, flexibility, and embeddedness in diverse local traditions, their belonging to specific cultural storyworlds, fictional and nonfictional. This, however, is an essential element of the modernist and postmodernist experience: the challenge to find narrative forms and techniques that are able to manage contingency, incoherence, and the many loose ends of life (Klepper, 2013).

The third assumption is that there is no basic divide between narrative as representation and narrative as action and social interaction. Stories, *all* stories, are ways to do things with words, to use Austin's (1962) influential formula of language as action. Stories are strategic interventions into ongoing activities. They are forms of action, employed by social actors. Yet keep in mind an important insight by Austin's teacher, Wittgenstein (2009): In humans' everyday life there rarely are isolated linguistic actions. Human beings carry out and are involved in many activities, one is language. A similar qualification applies with respect to communication. Humans communicate by many different means, including verbal means. All of this is to say that verbal activities of communication take place contemporaneously with and not independently of other symbolic and material activities, including bodily, performative, and media supported activities. It is this differentiated—that is, not juxtaposing or opposing—view of language and activity that shapes the notion of narrative as action. I should add, though, that this third assumption is a conclusion most theorists and scholars of narrative do not draw explicitly. The view dominating both the "classical" and the "postclassical" field is first and foremost that of narrative as form of *representation*, of stories as a mirror of the world (e.g., Ryan, 2007).

My project builds on these three elements of a new understanding of narrative. In repudiating the supposed divides between fictional and nonfictional, literary and nonliterary, representational and action-oriented narrative it seeks to open a space for formulating novel perspectives on the connective tissue between narrative and the mind; and it is here where I also localize memory. One of these perspectives is the strong narrative thesis.

I hinted at the growing recognition of narrative's importance beyond the traditional purview of literary texts and, in particular, fiction, which is an essential proposition of the postclassical view of narrative. This tendency reaches across various disciplines and has led many to reconsider basic categories relevant in all human sciences, such as consciousness, mind, and memory. As a consequence, capacities and dispositions of the mind traditionally defined in mentalist and individualist terms have been re-described with respect to the narrative fabric of meaning that underlies them and binds them into a wider social and cultural world. Hand in hand with this, individualist ideas of the narrative mind, widespread both in classical and postclassical narrative theories, have been reframed in social and cultural terms.[14] This new attention to a more situated vision of the narrative mind also underscores its historical dimension. By this I mean the fact that the narrative web of meaning in which our minds, as well as our concepts of mind and memory, are entangled has evolved over longsome historical and culture-specific processes. Obviously they are not simply part of our biological equipment.[15]

Against the backdrop of these recent shifts in the conceptual architecture of our knowledge my focus now moves to a clearly more specific subject, the autobiographical process. This subject, although cutting through traditional fields of memory, mind, consciousness, and identity, is marked in more concrete and special terms, both conceptually and empirically. To bring to a close these remarks on the significance of the narrative, including literary narrative, for my exploration of the autobiographical process, let me underline a last point. As has become clear, I share Bruner's (1986; 1990a) and Herman's (2012; 2013) conviction that the study of narrative worldmaking can inform, and not just be informed by, our understandings of mind and memory, just as the study of mind and memory can inform our understanding of narrative meaning-making.

But this is not to say that I plead against the experimental and quantitative forms of investigation so common in the social, neuro-, and medical sciences. The subject at stake defies any kind of reductionism. As Schacter put it, "a science of memory has room for both laboratory and everyday studies" (1996, p. 310). It also has room, I would add, for narrative studies of mind and memory, in fact, for all studies that help us understand humans' often messy acts of meaning-making. My intention, therefore, is not to restrict but to complement the repertoire of scientific approaches and methods both in the lab and in real life investigations by advancing what I propose as narrative hermeneutics. This is all the more imperative when the aim is, as formulated at the end of the last chapter, to explore narrative as an alternative metaphor and model of memory. For this purpose, I once again zoom in—in the next chapter—on the autobiographical process.

CHAPTER 5

Dissecting Memory

Unraveling the Autobiographical Process

What manner of theater is it, in which we are at once playwright, actor, stage manager, scene painter and audience?

W. G. Sebald (1998, p. 80)

So far I have used the term autobiographical process broadly, referring to the process in which remembering and interpreting are intertwined in a way that can only be separated artificially. In this chapter,
I specify this concept as my basic unit of analysis, unfolding and explaining it in an exemplary case study. In what may be called, with a term
from Geertz's interpretive cultural anthropology, a "thick description"
of an autobiographical process, I show how we navigate the mishmash of
experiences—past, present, possible, and anticipated—and its mixture
with our sense of self and efforts toward identity formation, all of which
are inextricably fused with emotions. In reformulating the traditional
subject matter of autobiographical memory in this new conceptual framework of narrative meaning-making I want to move away from the archival
idea of memory. The focus on the autobiographical process is meant to
further concretize my narrative alternative to this model of memory.[1]

The starting point of my case study is a sequence from an autobiographical process in Ian McEwan's novel *Saturday*. Literature, as I said earlier,
provides us with a powerful magnifying lens to examine the fabric of
the native mind. McEwan's *Saturday*, published in 2005, might be seen
as the lens of a microscope. Many novelists investigate the human mind,
but the British writer pursues the matter with perhaps more scientific

rigor than the job strictly requires, remarks Daniel Zalewski (2009) in his review of McEwan's novels. At the heart of McEwan's writing is less a concern with plot or with postmodernist narrative constructions or their deconstruction than with the psychology of the protagonists. Psychology, as Zalewski demonstrates, has always been McEwan's presiding interest, even if he, like many scholars and scientists of his generation, has shifted his intellectual allegiances: In his early works he studied perversity, in his last novels (including *Saturday*) he studied normality, even if with a keen eye for the extreme scenarios of ordinary memory.

Clearly McEwan has a special affinity for dissecting the human mind—and this we can say not only because *Saturday*'s protagonist is a neurosurgeon.[2] It seems that his extraordinarily developed narrative "fellow feeling" has aligned itself with an almost scientific curiosity about what makes people tick. His surgical approach to the landscape of consciousness, as well as to our unconscious mental life, makes itself felt in all of his novels. And it is true, privileging the landscape of consciousness over the landscape of action, a distinction introduced by Algirdas Greimas (1987), has been a hallmark of much of modern literature (Bruner, 1986). In numerous instances of European and North American narrative discourse we see the emergence of the modern mind as intimately linked to the emergence of modern consciousness-representing and consciousness-creating forms of writing (Herman, 2011a). It, therefore, should not come as a surprise that a writer born into the midst of the 20th century is deeply familiar with these forms. More than this, McEwan has cultivated a pronounced sensitivity for narrative strategies representing and creating subjectivity. In an essay examining the role of the individual artist and the individual scientist he compares literature to science because both advance "however minimally [. . .]—in subject matter, in means of expression—our understanding of ourselves, of ourselves in the world" (McEwan, 2012).

Of course, for a writer widely held to be at the height of his powers this advance of understanding is not a straightforward enterprise. Even though *Saturday* has been read as celebrating scientific progress, especially in the medical and neuroscientific domain, this celebration is paradoxically being conveyed in the form of a novel, as Dominic Head (2007, p. 187) remarks. Does this mean McEwan endorses the equation of a scientific-paradigmatic and a narrative mode of thought? This might be too strong a claim. What is obvious, however, Head writes, is that McEwan makes the interplay of narrative and scientific logic a central feature of his book—for example, by linking the heroic status of his protagonist, the neurosurgeon, to the failure of his literary imagination, a capacity of which he actually is downright contemptuous. At the same time, though, the widespread appreciation of the novel both by critics and a broad international readership may speak to the assessment that it "succeeds in ridiculing on every page the view of its hero that fiction is useless to the modern world," as a review in *The Guardian* put it (quoted from Head, 2007, p. 187). In fact, there seems to be little disagreement about the sophisticated narrative makeup of *Saturday*. In the wake of literary modernism and postmodernism, McEwan appears to have developed an accomplished mastery in using a repertoire of literary techniques and strategies that allow for a profound psychological analysis of the mind—that is the narrative mind of a Western middle-class professional whom we encounter in the years after 9/11.

THE AUTOBIOGRAPHICAL CRISIS OF A NEUROSURGEON

We can't retreat to the nineteenth century. We now have a narrative self-awareness that we can never escape.

McEwan (quoted after Zalewski, 2009, p. 51)

The narrative sequence I want to look at in close-up covers only a few minutes, whereas the novel tracks on 280 pages a whole day in the life of its protagonist. So some words about the place and the context of this extract are needed. It offers us a short insight into the world of Henry Perowne, the neurosurgeon, the novel's main character. And although we face an eventful and at times even dramatic landscape of action, the focus again is on the landscape of consciousness: on Perowne's psychology and how it is entangled with the world at large. This puts the book in the tradition of the 24-hour consciousness portraits of Joyce's *Ulysses* and Woolf's *Mrs Dalloway*, a tradition of which McEwan no doubt is fully aware. Literature, as he practices it, is a conversation not only with the reader but also with other writers, a conversation conducted through the generations.

Perowne lives and works in London, and the novel follows his actions and thoughts on a Saturday in 2003. Perowne is a man at the top of his game. He is in a leading position in one of the country's most prestigious hospitals, and he is married to a beautiful wife, a successful lawyer. Two promising teenage children, an elegant townhouse in London's posh Fitzrovia neighborhood, and a high-end Mercedes in which he drives soundproofed through the city complete the picture of the next-to-perfect life of the upper-middle class. A certain distance from the rest of the world seems indeed important to Perowne, especially on this day. Saturday, the 15th February 2003, is a historic day when London is crowded with more than a million demonstrators for an antiwar rally, the largest demonstration in British history. It is the time when the government is planning the invasion of Iraq.[3] But Perowne, himself more of an apolitical man of science used to thinking and operating in controlled and controllable environments, tries not to get involved. He seeks to go about his everyday chores with his usual care and preoccupations. After all, engaging in the routines of the day seems to be an efficient way to ignore the noise of the outside world. This, however, appears to be more and more difficult. We are shortly after the 11th September 2001 and there is the lingering fear that as the country is getting ready for war something similar might happen in London. As the day goes on, Perowne's well-established social capsule cracks. And so does the capsule of his mind.

Emblematically, the day starts at a nightly hour. Perowne gets up and steps to the window, discovering what he believes is a descending airplane on fire. For long it remains unclear whether this alarming appearance in the sky of London is an accident, an act of terrorism, or a hallucination fuelled by some kind of subliminal fear. Watching the television news does not solve the puzzle. But the thought of it stays with Perowne for most of the day, foreshadowing the tension, fear, and insecurity that gradually will take over. It is this threatening atmosphere that increasingly dominates the course of events. In a review, Richard Rorty (2005) describes McEwan's book as a quintessential example of a novel that makes vivid the sense of threat that many in the Western world have felt after 9/11. At the same time, it articulates the uneasiness about the future, a dark awareness of the unequal and unjust distribution of wealth and options on which much of the splendid life in cities like New York and London depends. To Rorty the true tragedy of the modern West is that it has exhausted its ideals, especially the hope that these, perhaps, originally great ideals could make the world a better place. As this hope diminishes, it is increasingly replaced by fear—and by concerns about the "little things" of everyday life and consumerism. "The problem for good-hearted Westerners like Henry Perowne," writes Rorty (2005), "is that they seem fated to live out their lives as idiots (in the old sense of "idiot," in which the term refers to a merely private person, one who has no part in public affairs)."

Although the nature of the strange phenomena in the sky of London—and the ensuing sense of threat—remains disconcertingly unclear, Perowne goes back to bed and tries to get some more sleep; but in vain. After shifting for some time back and forth between night and day he eventually finds himself busy facing the day's chores, an unmistakable sign that the struggle for sleep is lost.

> Perowne's plan is to cook a fish stew. A visit to the fishmonger's is one of the simpler tasks ahead: monkfish, clams, mussels, unpeeled prawns. It's this practical daylight list, these salty items, that make him leave the bed at last and walk into the bathroom. There's a view that it's shameful for a man to sit to urinate because that's what women do. Relax! He sits, feeling the last scraps of sleep dissolve as his stream plays against the bowl. He's trying to locate a quite different source of shame, or guilt, or of something far milder, like the memory of some embarrassment or foolishness. It passed through his thoughts only minutes ago, and now what remains is the feeling without its rationale. A sense of having behaved or spoken laughably. Or having been a fool. Without the memory of it, he can't talk himself out of it. But who cares? These diaphanous films of sleep are still slowing him down—he imagines them resembling the arachnoid, that gossamer covering of the brain through which he routinely cuts. The grandeur. He must have hallucinated the phrase out of the hairdryer's drone, and confused it with the radio news. The luxury of being half asleep, exploring the fringes of psychosis in safety. But when he trod the air to the window last night he was fully awake. He's even more certain of that now.
>
> He rises and flushes his waste. At least one molecule of it will fall on him one day as rain, according to a ridiculous article in a magazine lying around in the operating suite coffee room. The numbers say so, but statistical probabilities aren't the same as truths. *We'll meet again, don't know where, don't know when.* Humming this wartime tune, he crosses the wide green-and-white marble floor to his basin to shave.

(McEwan, 2005, p. 57)

Approaching narrative texts, scholars have long used the distinction between story or *fabula* and discourse or *sjuzhet*. The story is the chronologically ordered sequence of events told in a narrative, the discourse is the actual way in which these events are presented, which often is far from being chronological (Chatman, 1978). This well-established distinction, as neat and plausible as it may appear, does not come without problems. One is the unquestioned assumption that underlying all narratives we find a chronological order of events, or a chronology that gives order to the events. This comes in tandem with the equally unquestioned assumption that there is an objective Newtonian clock and calendar time providing an independent background to all events in the universe, including one's mind. This idea may travel well in the domain of everyday common sense; it is, however, hard to sustain when it comes to the autobiographical process, not to mention other creative and imaginative potentials of the narrative mind (I mentioned a few of them in the last chapter discussing the strong narrative thesis).

Nevertheless, let us postpone the problematic premises and implications of the distinction between story and discourse for a while (I return to them in Chapters 8 and 9) and, vis-à-vis McEwan's text, take advantage of what has made this distinction so widely accepted; that is its promise to turn every narrative, as messy and incomplete as it may seem, into a chronologically ordered sequence, a story with a clearly laid out structure of action.

So what is the story? And if the adage is true that every story continues with another story, what is the story that is continued here? I already said that *Saturday* is located in the wake of the events of 9/11 and their consequences for what Rorty (2005) called, pondering on Perowne's turmoil, the "spiritual life of secularist Westerners." As readers of the novel, we also are already told that Perowne's preceding week was as busy and stressful as could be, which might explain why he woke up in the early morning hours, in diffuse anxiety.[4] We also have learned that after watching that burning plane—and noticing that, with it, something extraordinary, something from the "outside" had begun to intrude in his so far well-protected "inner" world—he went to the kitchen and watched the news with his son, who had just come home. And we also know that he then returned to bed where he made love to his wife. All this has prepared us to follow effortlessly what happens next, and this brings us to the sequence just quoted. After his wife got up (to what for her is a normal working day), Perowne slips into an unquiet state between sleeping, waking, and daydreaming. When he starts mulling over the errands the day will bring for him—things like shopping for the fish dinner he wants to cook that evening—he at last gives up and accepts that the night is over. At this point the story sets in. Perowne gets up and the narrative moves back to the landscape of action, as unspectacular as it is. Indeed, there is not a whole lot in the way of external action: He enters the bathroom, sits on the toilet, flushes and turns to the basin to shave. To be sure, these actions can be easily aligned in a chronological way. More convoluted, however, are the events that take place in the landscape of consciousness. It is here where the real drama unfolds, and it does so in the form of an autobiographical process.

At first sight it appears somehow strange to call this sequence an autobiographical process. Linked to mundane bathroom routines, it hardly seems of interest. Yet, although these actions are rather unspectacular, including the apparently not quite culture-conforming use of a toilet, they trigger a sensation. This sensation is only peripherally connected to what set it off. Psychological memory researchers would call this kind of mediated recall "priming," whereas narrative scholars may speak of a "metonymical chain" that connects to sensations of shame or guilt. When Perowne tries to calm himself down—"Relax!"—and get a handle on it, he realizes instantly that it would be too simple to reduce this sensation to "wrong" toilet practices. Its source appears to be something different, perhaps an embarrassing memory, something that, in any case, he would rather like to avoid or to repress, as we would say in a different vocabulary. Yet this does not make the sensation less burdensome. Clearly what is about to unfurl now is some kind of self-examination. But does he want this? Now and here? What further impedes this self-questioning is that the feeling it seeks to localize has detached itself from what originally has elicited it. This is a well-known phenomenon, carefully described by Sigmund Freud, William James, Marcel Proust, and many others. In fact, all of us are familiar with it: Something passed through one's mind and a minute later all that remains is the feeling without the sensation or experience that aroused it.

Still, for a moment Perowne remains uncertain as to whether to continue this inquiry that, he senses, could turn into an unpleasant self-inquisition, or just leave it alone. Who wants to trace a sense of oneself having behaved embarrassingly or laughably? What adds to the conflicting feeling is that if he does not nail down the concrete source that might have provoked it, he cannot rationally convince himself to dismiss it. That is what he did with the first idea suggesting that his way of using the toilet would be the source of his unease. Obviously there is more to it—a memory perhaps besieging and threatening enough that it would be better left unexamined, as Perowne, Rorty's "good-hearted Westerner," eventually decides to do, precisely because there seems to be more to it, too much to it.

Interestingly, at the moment when Perowne's stream of consciousness abruptly stops, before it could turn into a more extensive autobiographical self-interpretation, the narrative style changes. It shifts from free indirect speech (the third-person narrative that reveals a subjective mental state as though it were a first person narrative) to a direct voice, Perowne's voice: "But who cares?" This shift marks a straight intervention into the process of mnemonic sense-making; indeed it transforms it. Metaphorically speaking, it brings the labor of remembering to a halt. What so far appeared as an act of remembering now can be taken as an act of forgetting or, perhaps, of concealment and silencing. "Mnemonic silence" is a term used in experimental memory psychology to indicate that a memory is not "expressed" (Stone, Coman, Brown, Koppel, & Hirst, 2012). Mnemonic silence is viewed as leading to forgetting because it allows the memory to "decay" (Hirst & Echterhoff, 2012; Wixted, 2004). On closer examination, we realize, however, that this forgetting is quite proactive. It is itself an interpretive act and, to stay with the metaphor, it is not really silent. It consists of suppressing, or even repressing, one act of remembering with another; it means supplanting an emerging memory (that, although still unclear, already feels potentially threatening to Perowne) with other memories. These memories seem to be more reassuring, even if they appear to be a bit searched for (as that of the operating surgeon's sense of "grandeur") or downright banal (as the drone of the hairdryer Perowne's wife used just a short while ago). But they do the job, clearing the mind from an emerging worry, a potential memory of which so far only the emotionally irksome flavor looms ahead.

Some memory researchers speak of "retrieval-induced forgetting" to qualify the kind of selective forgetting prompted by "mnemonic silence" as a form of selective remembering, of remembering something in order to forget something else (Barnier, Hung, & Conway, 2004; Brown, Kramer, Romano, & Hirst, 2012; Hirst, Cuc, & Wohl, 2012). So do we have here an instance of "retrieval-induced forgetting"? It depends on how we understand these terms. If remembering and forgetting are taken as ontological categories with a clear scope substantiated by assumed (neuro-)cognitive mechanisms underlying the encoding, storing, and retrieval of information, then they miss the inherent subtlety of the interpretive dynamic at stake. In fact, they miss the interpretive dimension of this process altogether. In this case, the critique would be correct that the focus on the putative *mechanics* of memory tends to ignore the *meaning* a memory has for the rememberer (Randall, 2011, p. 22). That something is perceived as a memory is, as discussed before, already the result of an interpretive process of meaning conferment. A memory is not just there, a given entity waiting in some hidden archive to be expressed or, in the case of "mnemonic silence," not to be expressed. As the Perowne episode illustrates, there may be just an indiscernible shift in the interpretive stance and its affective coloring (which is, as we saw, also a shift in the intentional stance) and this is all that is needed to alter the character of the entire process: allowing one of its aspects—in hindsight called forgetting—to dominate over another of its aspects—in hindsight called remembering—or the other way around. More than this, it allows for the entire episode to be wiped out in a second: as a figment of imagination or a scrap of sleep; "what remains is the feeling without its rationale."

An ongoing interplay of interpretive, reflective, and creative acts

In light of such shifts, which in the kind of autobiographical processes under examination are more the rule than the exception, I have suggested understanding this process as an ongoing interplay of interpretive, reflexive, and creative acts. These acts, as we have also seen, are far more than purely cognitive ones. In contrast to its conceptualization in much of the cognition-focused psychological and neuroscientific memory literature, the autobiographical process appears as an enterprise in which both cognition and emotion are intimately entwined. How else are we to understand Perowne's autobiographical process if not as deeply affective labor, as a project of emotions that drives, orients, and permeates all cognitive operations to which autobiographical remembering and identity construction so often have been reduced? Once the investigation of the autobiographical process exits the memory lab, recollecting past experiences can no longer be understood in terms of purely cognitive operations, as is the case when it is conceptualized in terms of mechanisms of encoding, storing, and retrieval.

A second key problem I strive to overcome with this conceptualization is that the interplay of interpretive, reflexive, and creative acts traditionally has been conceived of in exclusionary terms of either remembering or forgetting, whereas both are, in fact, integral parts of one process, even though they can be labeled differently according to the perspective from which they are approached. But not only has this complex dynamic been reduced to just these two components, remembering and forgetting; what entails an additional complication is that most of the literature focuses on just one of them, the isolated act of recall or retrieval, while dismissing forgetting as the villain, and the results of his deeds as failures, suppressions, or sins (Brockmeier, 2002a).

Perowne, for one, tries hard not to get into a reflection of this dynamic. He quickly fends off even the semblance of an autobiographical crisis in his bathroom. This instantly becomes clear in the already identified shift of narrative perspective to a direct voice: "But who cares!" (even if it is true that this clause could also be read as free indirect discourse). This shift also changes Perowne's self-positioning from a half-sleeping and brooding "perceiver" of events (such as potentially troubling memories) to an active and sovereign protagonist who, of course, also has the memories of an active and sovereign protagonist. Perowne is a man used to such acts of self-positioning. Yet this is nothing special; self-positioning is part of a cultural grammar that all of us learn from early on. We are permanently positioning ourselves and others in a moral space of good and bad, right and wrong, agentive and passive, as Harré (2012) has argued. Positioning, in this sense, is an act of claiming certain rights and duties, of being entitled to something. If we look at the bathroom scene from this positioning theory perspective, we notice that it is about Perowne's self-assurance of his right to reject even a hint of the unsettling thoughts that haunt him at this early hour. What in this act of positioning, in the course of one or two sentences, enters forward from behind the films of sleep and doubt is a self-confident protagonist, a surgeon in the operating theater cutting through brain membranes, deciding about life and death, about remembering and forgetting. We could call this act of positioning "The grandeur." The remainder of the sequence likewise appears as under the control of a subject again restrained and sovereign ("fully awake" and "certain"), without hesitation giving rational interpretations to even the strangest memories, weighing up their "truths" and "statistical probabilities," identifying their "ridiculous" sources.

Memories like these, presenting Perowne as a self-controlled and self-possessed surgeon, obviously have a strong self-defining quality. "Self-defining memories"—similar concepts are "vital memories" (Brown & Reavey, 2014) or memories of "momentous events" (Pillemer, 1998)—have received special attention in the literature. Like all personal memories, "self-defining memories" concern specific and memorable past events and experiences but can be distinguished from others in being particularly vivid, emotional, and familiar; fusing affective scenarios and themes, they configure an individual's most important concerns (Singer & Salovey, 1993). Drawing on Freud's concept of the *Ich-Ideal*, Jacques Lacan (1994) spoke of an ideal ego resulting from a mnemonic process of narcissistic identification. From still another position, self-defining memories are viewed as a central feature of the autobiographical self because they are essential for what some call the internalized life story (Thorne & McLean, 2003). If we consider such memories as part of an overarching autobiographical process, then they appear inseparable from identity-confirming self-interpretations that allow an individual to neutralize, as it were, other memories, even potential memories, especially if they are troublesome and menacing, as in our case. Confronted with the powerful memory of the ideal-ego surgeon, a memory tested and confirmed in thousands of successful operations, they cannot compete. That is, they do not acquire the interpretive power of self-defining memories—at least not yet.

Keep in mind that the dialectic of remembering and forgetting we have traced appears in McEwan's sequence almost underhandedly. It is something pervading, but not identical with the blend of interpretive, reflexive, and imaginative acts that make up the overall dynamic of the autobiographical process. So let me sum up this dynamic that starts with an emotional trigger, a strange feeling, which becomes the subject of attention, entailing an interpretive inquiry that is to define whether at stake is a memory at all or just a strange sensation "without a rationale" and, if it is conceived of as a memory, whether it is worthwhile to be traced or rejected and ignored, perhaps in light of a stronger self-defining memory.

FORTUNATELY WE FORGET

A further peculiarity of the autobiographical process should be pointed out, namely, its quicksilver nature. A circular phenomenon—because its very fluidity and swiftness make it escape our attention—it affects our perception of events in both the landscape of action and the landscape of the mind. Consider that the sequence I have described in terms of the dialectic of remembering and forgetting might be closer to seconds than minutes in chronological time. This means that, in order to study it, we have to find a way to inhabit the ephemeral moment—which is, as we recall, the challenge for the writer McEwan. In contrast, envision a longer period of time, say, an hour or a day or a week. What an inconceivable number of events pass through the mind in such a period of time!—feeding an incalculable stream of consciousness. But then we know that much of what flows in this stream is without any relevance for the experiencing individual, which is to say, the stream of consciousness is of differing autobiographical density or intensity.

Since its introduction by William James in 1890, the concept "stream of consciousness" has sometimes been used as if there were a more or less compact entity called consciousness. However, there are quite diverse forms and degrees of consciousness, and some of them are relevant here, especially those linked to or overlapping with forms of "narrative consciousness" (Brockmeier, 2007; Herman, 2011b; Oatley, 2007). I want to foreground only one aspect of narrative consciousness, and for this the Jamesian concept of stream of consciousness might suffice. James's (1981) concept is very broad. In covering the whole of our mental activities, emphasizing their transformative flow as a continuous stream, it also comprises acts and states that are anything but conscious.[5] This can also be said about the stream of consciousness as it is understood in literary and narrative theory, where the concept was soon adapted from psychology but then developed a life of its own (Humphrey, 1968). Commonly, literary and narrative scholars use the term to refer to the continuous flux of perceptions, thoughts, memories, and feelings in the minds of fictional or real characters—and to the narrative modes of presenting or enacting such a stream. (I already discussed some aspects of this in terms of narrative experience.) Both literary and psychological authors agree that only a fraction of our innumerable sensations, perceptions, and mental activities becomes the subject of attention. And only an even smaller portion remains present in our consciousness, that is, in common parlance, it stays in our memory, at least for a while. This is what we are concerned with most of the time.

Yet what happens when we want to consider more of our consciousness than what sticks out of the sea like the tip of an iceberg? How can we get hold of what is invisibly below the surface? What happens to those countless events that swarm our minds without ever, or only to a limited extent and for a short time, reaching the center of conscious attention, from where they could possibly turn into the stuff of autobiographical reflection? After more than a century of research in several disciplines we are well aware that much more is going on in our minds and brains than what reaches the attention threshold and becomes the subject of conscious reflection and autobiographical interpretation. In James's classic words, "Millions of items ... are present to my senses which never properly enter into my experience. Why? Because they have no interest for me. My experience is what I agree to attend to" (1981, p. 380). To James, only meaningful phenomena shape one's mind. In turn, my mind is only interested in what appears to be meaningful to me. So what then is meaningful to me? James is unambiguous about this: "Interest alone," he writes, because it "gives accent and emphasis, light and shade, background and foreground—intelligible perspective, in a word" (p. 381).

One answer to the question of what happens with all the rest of it, the millions of items that remain outside of any intelligible perspective, is: we forget. Fortunately enough, as advocates of forgetfulness like Nietzsche have argued.[6] Others see the advantages of forgetting in more pragmatic terms. Oliver Sacks remarks about the creative side effects of some kind of forgetting:

> while I often give lectures on similar topics, I can never remember, for better or worse, exactly what I said on previous occasions; nor can I bear to look through my earlier notes. Losing conscious memory of what I have said before, and having no text, I discover my themes afresh each time. This type of forgetting may be necessary for a creative or healthy cryptomnesia, one that allows old thoughts to be reassembled, retranscribed, recategorized, given new and fresh implications ... [so that] one's memories and ideas can be born again and seen in new contexts and perspectives. (2013, p. 20)

Yet sometimes we also believe ourselves to be fortunate if we do not forget, if we manage even to expand the domain of things we remember beyond the sphere of "interest for me." An excellent memory capacity is commonly regarded to be a sign of great mental powers, a virtue, a blessing. Yet is it really? There are many stories of individuals with extraordinary mnemonic capacities, people who cannot forget—from Luria's (1987) report of *The mind of a Mnemonist* to Borges's (2000) study of *Funes the Memorious* (also translated as *Funes, the Memory*). They all are sad stories. They demonstrate that human brains and minds have not evolved to function like enormous archives of information. And when they do so, due to some curious anomalies, people get into serious trouble. It seems that it is easier for humans—at least for their sense of self and identity—to cope with certain neuropathological restrictions to their mnemonic capacity than with its hypertrophic extension (Medved & Brockmeier, 2008; 2015). In his case study of the neuropsychology of hypermnesia, Luria described his patient Sherashevsky, a professional memory artist, as a person with a prodigious, indeed incredible memory. At the same time, he was unable to go beyond the isolated elements, the endless bits and dots of knowledge that he flawlessly recalled. He seemed to keep everything in mind—in his desire to forget, he would write down his memories and then burn the paper, hoping they could be destroyed—without, however, ever envisioning an overarching whole, a structure of embracing meaning that lasted beyond the here and now. "Everything he did in life was merely 'temporary,'" Luria (1987, p. 157) noted.

I should mention that Luria's book became famous not only because it compellingly captured the mind and memory of an exceptional mnemonist. There was also the book's style, the sensitive narrative portrait of a person it offered, instead of a report of what commonly would have been labeled as "a case." The book extended the traditional focus on peoples' disorders and anomalies to the interpretation of the entire mind of a person and, even more, to his personality and way to cope with his fate. In a word, there was the attempt to bring all of this "back to some fullness of life" that made the book unique, as Bruner (1987b, p. xix) remarked in his foreword. "This is not a cold, clinical account," Bruner went on to write, "but a humane interpretation of what it means for somebody to live with a mind that records meticulously the details of experience without being able, so to speak, to extract from the record what it means, 'what it's all about'" (p. x).

In ordinary life, our ability to direct our attention and interpretive activities to the question of what it's all about is in general highly reliable. We are very good at selective attention, James remarked, and this is particularly true for overarching issues of meaning and interest. We have learned to skim through and then ignore the multitude of sensory memories that emerge in every passing moment, and then carry on. The overwhelming portion of what keeps our minds busy is without interest and thus immediately forgotten—if we still want to use the term in this context. It seems that it is one of the central functions of our mind, both in its conscious and nonconscious activities, to protect us from the overflow. Even Freud, although better known for insisting on the need to remember, to look behind the scenes of "screen memories," and to dig up and analyze the hidden events of the past, emphasized the psychological advantages of certain kinds of forgetting, for example, when occurring after successful psychoanalytical treatment. Before such treatment, however, Freud saw forgetting of important personal experiences not as a benign phenomenon or as the result of "mnemonic silence" but as potentially pathological in as far as it is linked to unconscious operations such as the repression, distortion, dissociation, and condensation of memories that reveal central psychological concerns of troubled individuals (Habermas, 2012; Terdiman, 2010). And this forgetting Freud took, in contrast with Nietzsche, not as a healthy and liberating process but as a complicated creation of the autobiographical process.

Writing and narrative

This brings us back to the question of how we can know about these items and their strange life of which, for the most part, we never become aware, or only to the point at which Perowne turns away. How then do we get access to them and, what is more, how do we examine them? In attempting to answer these questions several possibilities have been explored. They range from methodical self-examination of thought processes (Wundt, Fechner, and Tichener) and the stream of consciousness (James) to Freud's psychoanalytical tradition. The psychoanalytical tradition has yielded further dialogical or discursive approaches to the kind of self-observation and self-interpretation that emerge in the interaction between analyst and the analysand. More recently, the study of "inner discourse" has joined these approaches. What is called "inner discourses" or, more traditionally, "inner speech," is a heterogeneous class of discursive practices that have become the subject of interactional and pragmatic inquiries building on Vygotsky, Bakhtin, and Vološinov (e.g., Larrain & Haye, 2012; Stam, 2010).

All of these approaches may help in understanding the autobiographical process, particularly the invisible parts of the iceberg. In view of my analysis of McEwan's passage, however, I would like to add a further approach to this list: the study of life writing. This study is indispensable for our purposes because it comprises all perspectives just mentioned applied to a wide spectrum of everyday, documentary, and fictional practices of life and identity narrative. Paul John Eakin (2008), in explaining why his interest in self and identity formation has kept him working with published autobiographical narratives, writes that most of these materials (or "data," as some would say) are, to be sure, literary. But, he goes on, they are much more than that because they offer "a precious tangible record of an otherwise evanescent process of identity construction" (pp. 85 86). What Eakin means is that we do not have any other way to take a close look at the quicksilver reality of the autobiographical process than through written or otherwise materialized records. It is the production of a durable record on which all of McEwan's virtuosity as a writer is targeted because only this allows him, as Head (2007, pp. 192–194) points out, to inhabit the immediate and ephemeral moment.

I already touched on another reason for my focus on this kind of autobiographical record: There is a long tradition of sophisticated narrative self-examination by life writers. Writers are not only literary authors but also ordinary human beings who, like all of us living in a "culture of autobiography"—a concept by Folkenflik (1993) that I discuss in more detail in Chapter 7—have become increasingly engaged in narrating themselves. Life writing is the umbrella term for a broad spectrum of genres and media, as well as for reflective and critical discourses revolving around them; it embraces many forms and experimental spaces for all kinds of narrative self-presentation and self-exploration (Saunders, 2008; 2010). The field is multicolored, reflecting the diversity of contemporary ideas and practices of self and identity. And so there are a number of different ways to order it. Theorists of storytelling, for example, have distinguished between narratives of self and identity that are informal, inchoate, and mostly conversational ("small stories"), and narratives told within larger formats such as literary or interview-based life accounts ("big stories") (Bamberg, 2007; Freeman, 2007). "Big stories" point to the other end of the spectrum where literary and cultural theorists and critics of biography and autobiography identify a number of highly differentiated genres and media of life writing (Smith & Watson, 2010, have listed 60 of them; cf. pp. 253–286). In this part of the spectrum, we also find a tradition of self-narration that seems to answer an existential need to localize ourselves in the larger scheme of things; Eakin (2014) speaks of "autobiographical cosmograms."

I also mentioned that many modern life writers occupied with the project of autobiographical self-resolution, whether literary or not, not only have investigated themselves and their place in the world but also turned their attention to the very narrative makeup of their efforts. There is one factor that I want to highlight as particularly conducive to this, and this is writing itself. Writing appears to be especially suited for examining a phenomenon as ephemeral as the autobiographical process because it arrests the stream of oral discourse, even if only to a degree. That we are able to arrest the stream of consciousness is, of course, not only due to our ability to write and read; it is a key function of language in general. A word, an utterance, a symbol, they all mark a fermata of attention. In directing our communicative and mental focus to a moment in the flux of events, a moment that is held on, if only transiently, they also create a fermata of time that makes the present available. It is by the linguistic sign that we insert a constant into the flight of events and noises, a gestalt of meaning that can be double checked, communicated, and thought about. All of this reaches an even more stable and durable status in the domain of written language and, culturally speaking, literacy. Writing provides a framework of communication and thought that presupposes and evokes distance and reflexivity.[7]

The emergence of this framework is also momentous from a historical point of view. It has been argued that writing played a crucial role not only in the emergence of Western conceptions of mind and memory (Danziger, 2008)—an issue treated in Chapter 3—but also in the formation of modern ideas of life and self. Carolyn Steedman (2009) has pointed out that it was a result of the expansion of literacy, and reading in particular, in most of late 18th-century Western Europe that "life—the idea of a life—was infinitely and inextricably bound up with *having a life story*. To tell, to write, to live a life was an act made by the word; or, to put it another way, the life-narrative, verbal or written, was the dominant (by now, possibly the only) way of imagining or figuring one" (Steedman, 2009, p. 226).

Perhaps the most important aspect of writing in this context with respect to my investigation of the autobiographical process is that it can bring the ongoing stream of consciousness to a halt. It can freeze it in a way that enables us to scrutinize the fleeting and meandering details that would pass by in a blink of an eye in a real-time autobiographical process. Writing leaves a trace. It gains an existence that survives the event of its production, and merely by its lasting presence creates new possibilities for its communication and interpretation, as well as new problems. "Writing," in Susan Stewart's words, "serves to caption the world, defining and commenting upon the configurations we choose to textualize" (1993, p. 31).

The configuration of the evanescent in writing is one more reason I have used McEwan's text as an experimental setting that permits us to access the otherwise elusive dynamic of the autobiographical process. Writing brings into existence a version of this process that can be explored in various states, from slow motion to still. It also can, to use another metaphor from film, be rewound and fast-forwarded, affording further possibilities to thoroughly inquire into its narrative fabric.

As a technology of the word, writing, however, does not simply re-present speech or translate it into a more permanent form. In contrast with a long held view, written language is not oral language put down. From the very beginning, writing—or more exactly, the numerous writing systems that have coevolved with the development of human languages—have not been secondary symbols depicting oral discourse but complex sign systems in their own right. Although related and intermingled in a multitude of ways, oral and written discourses differ in various respects. One of them becomes clear by the fact that we owe our understanding of language in general to the existence of alphabetic writing. Consider the view of language as composed of distinct units such as words and sentences. Before people learned to write and read, as Olson (2001) explains, their sense of language was not shaped by the rules of semantics and syntax; the "conceptual perception" of single words only came into being with literacy. Relating this argument to narrative prose and, specifically, literary writing, Oatley and Djikic (2008) notice that talking and conversing occur in a domain of utterances and bodily performances, whereas literary writing takes place in a domain of sentences and grammar. In the domain of spoken language, they write, "there are speech acts—to warn, request, inform, and so on, and the pragmatics of conversational turn-taking. . . . In the domain of literary writing, the laws are of syntax and semantics, and the purposes are to engage attention and offer cues ... that enable the reader to create an imaginative construction" (Oatley & Djikic, 2008, p. 11). Writing, then, can engage our attention, bringing to our awareness things otherwise unnoticed. "Writing," in the words of Rita Charon, "reveals things to us that we know but didn't know we knew" (2006, p. xii). Charon points out that writing a personal story, especially about dramatic and intensely meaningful experiences such as severe illness, often entails a new quality of reflection because it is coupled with the effort to explore and convey the meaning of what has been experienced.

In localizing writing and narrative on a common map we should keep in mind that we deal with different linguistic and cultural formats, but not with fundamentally different domains or orders of linguistic discourse. That linguistic discourse can extend to and incorporate other than linguistic components (for example, visual and enactive ones) is an issue to be treated further on in this chapter. Here the focus is on writing and narrative, and both, in fact, overlap and intermingle in many ways, which is also of relevance for our understanding of the autobiographical process. In general terms, writing and narrative both stake out particular discursive and cultural economies of meaning construction; indeed, unfolding and understanding meaning is at the heart of all practices of literacy as well as storytelling.

A more specific common feature of writing and narrative is that they afford frameworks to arrest and examine the stream of oral discourse and consciousness, as I just pointed out in terms of writing. How can we characterize this quality in narrative? Narrative is a mode of thought that allows us to gain a more detached vantage point on the world and on ourselves. Perhaps the most powerful way to distance ourselves from the passing immediacy of events and experiences is to convert what we have encountered into story form, Bruner (2002) noted. Taking this argument one step further, Freeman (2010a) suggests that we owe to narrative our specific human ability of hindsight, of interpreting and reassessing the past; in other words, narrative "has at its core a dimension of distance" (p. 175).

In their respective manners, both written and narrative language enable us to use this distance, to stand apart from what we are doing—for example, when we are writing or telling—and think about what it is we are doing. They draw attention to language and language practices themselves, and to areas of our mind and memory that otherwise would not enter our consciousness. And they do so all the more if they are interlaced with written narrative prose. To avoid a misunderstanding, a last qualification is needed. I do not want to make the point that understanding writing and narrative as a material configuration of autobiographical discourse means they represent a deeper reality of mind or memory. The notion of language and writing just outlined is far from sharing an illusion widespread among commentators of neuroscience, namely, that the electronic simulation of an fMRI displays the biophysical reality of the mind, "the mind made flesh," as Nicholas Humphrey (2002) put it. Neither writing nor narrative is a prelinguistic mind "made flesh." Yet, if we grant that a written autobiographical process is not simply a representation or depiction of a prelinguistic entity but rather offers a window on the inherent narrative reality of this process, could we then say it is a *model* of such a reality? Surely the narrative enactment of an autobiographical process, as in McEwan's writing, can be described in terms of model and modeling. Some authors consider it a central trait of all written literature that it provides us with models and simulations of the human mind. Oatley (2008; 2011), an established researcher in this field, maintains that fiction—that is, written narrative—is a simulation that "runs on minds." Oatley even views it as a kind of model program that, like a flight-simulator, allows us to exercise and deepen our understanding of minds and emotions, of others and ourselves.

There is, however, an argument that cautions against understanding either writing or narrative as a model and simulation of the autobiographical process in this strong representational and computational sense. In this sense—prevailing not only in Oatley's cognitive psychology of narrative, but also in semiotic, logical, and epistemological model theories—a model represents or models something else; and it does so in a simpler and, perhaps, more ideal way. But this does not apply to our Perowne passage, which neither simplifies nor idealizes the autobiographical process. Considering the traditional meaning of model, autobiographical narratives like Perowne's do not model anything; they are performative, that is, they do not provide us with a representation or with a model of the autobiographical process, but they enact this very process.

This enactment comes as close to our everyday autobiographical process as it gets—and McEwan's sequence is a compelling case in point—because both share the same fabric: the language of narrative, which here has been materialized in writing. In other words, operative at the heart of both the "model" and "what is modeled" is the same narrative dynamic. More than being simply a model of the world (or of a part of the world), narrative *is* a part of the world. As an implication, the traditional idea of narrative as a model becomes questionable, indeed misleading, for in this case "the model does merge with the thing, the map with the territory," to use Herman's (2009a, p. 53) words. This is a further reason why the narrative enactment of an autobiographical process is an altogether different matter than the simulations of computers and the electrophysiological models of the brain (which all too often are also taken as models of the mind).

NEUROSCIENCE MEETS NARRATIVE

Scientific observation is not merely pure description of separate facts. Its main goal is to view an event from as many perspectives as possible.

(Luria, 1979, p. 77)

What in epistemology and semiotics is called a model is a condensed version of a theory, a theory of what is to be modeled. Even if models are often understood in a narrower sense as representations of something else—an object, concept, idea, or interpretation—they involve far-ranging ontological presumptions about what they claim to represent. Memory models are a case in point. They present a defining perspective on what "memory" is supposed to be, and they do so all the more if they presume there is a naturally given entity they simply re-present.

This has consequences for my line of argument. Because I have suggested McEwan's narrative sequence as an enactment of the autobiographical process, I need to further explain the presumptions and implications of this view, which may be called the narrative enactment model or simply the narrative model.[8] So let me expound further the narrative model by comparing it with the dominant memory model in neuroscience, the so-called systems model. Moreover, putting both models side by side provides us with two different perspectives on our subject matter—autobiographical memory from a neuroscientific perspective and autobiographical process from a narrative perspective. Sure enough these two do not offer us "as many perspectives as possible," as demanded by Luria, but they bring into play the two arguably most distinguished fields of inquiry into autobiographical remembering: neuroscientific memory research and autobiographical narrative and its critical reflection.

The systems model or systems approach came into existence in psychology and neurology of memory toward the end of the last century and has since formed memory's conceptual shape. Given that I already pointed out the claims and scope of this research field in Chapter 1, I only want to underscore here some essentials of the systems model and relate them to the narrative model. The systems model replaced a view of memory as an undifferentiated process of information processing, which was assumed to exist in a unitary fashion throughout the animal kingdom. Within cognitivism, the information processing function was considered to be common to all living matter; what was different was the information processing capacity, of which storage capacity was an essential element. All of this was conceived of as analogous to the development of computers. On the same grounds, the systems approach was established in tandem with the development of new digital processors that afforded unprecedented brain imaging technologies. It is an ironic point that these technologies at the same time decisively contributed to replacing the lead model of old-school cognitive psychology, computer-based information processing, transforming "cognitive science" into "neuroscience."

Conceptually, the shift from "processing approaches" to "systems approaches" was prepared by Tulving's (1972; 1983) introduction of two different memory systems meant to process different information, one called episodic memory (in charge of events or experiences localizable in time and space), the other semantic memory (in charge of facts and general knowledge). An updated older distinction between long-term and short-term memory complemented the picture. This was in accordance with a definition of memory brought up early in the history of its experimental study in psychological laboratories where memory was defined in terms of the time during which its very existence was measurable, the retention time. The three basic units of retention time used today are sensory memory, short-term memory, and long-term memory. Sensory memory refers to sensory processes that occur in a physiologically automatized way and are pretty much outside of our conscious control. To get an idea of sensory memory we might think of the impression of a simple figure drawn by a twirling flashlight at night that stays for a moment in our sensorial "iconic memory" even if the light has been turned off. The second unit of retention time is short-term memory, sometimes also called primary memory, which is sensory experience that remains active and available for up to a few minutes before it turns either into the third category, long-term memory, or disappears because it is of "no interest for me."

However, even here the notorious problem of the systems approach is salient because it appears impossible to draw a clear border line between short-term and long-term memory systems. Some memory researchers thus have rejected the entire idea in favor of the view that memory is a unitary continuum operating in the same fashion over all periods of time, short or long. If we were to confine our concerns exclusively to a cognitive domain, then I would agree with Katherine Nelson's (2006) point that experiential memory and general knowledge are always inextricably interrelated and "are kept separate only arbitrarily" (p. 183). As all system models are highly speculative, despite an abundance of detailed empirical studies carried out to demonstrate their respective validity, it is not surprising that there are many diverse views and beliefs among researchers and theorists. In Chapter 2, I referred to Tulving's concerns that neuroscience tends to mistake hypothetical assumptions with empirical evidence. In Tulving's words, "we can talk about memory systems and memory processes, and we can name them, but we have little idea how 'real' these systems and processes are" (2002a, p. 323).

For those who nonetheless accept the distinction between short-term and long-term memory systems, it then is easier to agree on the differentiation between two further memory systems: declarative or explicit memory and nondeclarative or implicit memory. Within this grid, Tulving's episodic and semantic memory are part of the declarative memory system, for both are concerned with explicit memories, that is, events and information about which we can talk and which we can recall even after a long time. This now brings us closer to our main subject, autobiographical memories, to which these criteria apply. So where exactly is the place of autobiographical memories on this map? Because they are understood as memories that can be localized in time and space, they are part of the episodic memory system. But because they also have personal relevance and are often vivid and emotionally charged, some researchers view them as constituting a further episodic memory subsystem, the autobiographical system.

The 1990s were proclaimed by the U.S. Congress and the National Institutes of Health the "decade of the brain." By then, the categorical memory distinctions had established themselves as the core tenets of neurocognitive research and became the gold standard of memory psychology. In Schacter's summary, memory is "composed of a variety of distinct and dissociable processes and systems. Each system depends on a particular constellation of networks in the brain that involve different neural structures, each of which plays a highly specialized role within the system" (Schacter, 1996, p. 5). This view has been canonized in text- and handbooks of memory research ever since, and with it the assumption that memories can be distinguished by their content (or type of information), and that different contents (or types of information) can be stored in partially or wholly different memory systems.

Under the hegemony of this model, recent research has centered on the neurocognitive dimension of memory systems, or more precisely, on how specific neuronal circuits and parts of the brain can be related to specific psychological memory processes. The identification of such relations or correlations is taken to demonstrate the existence of the various postulated memory systems. Considering the institutional research economy of established "normal science," the patent circularity of the theory-model-evidence implied in this causality is not unusual. The model provides an exclusive perspective on empirical evidence that confirms the theory, which, in turn, explains the model. None of this is specific to neuroscience.

What has, however, come about unexpectedly is that, since the inception of the model, the number of memory systems has increased exponentially. And so has the fragmentation of the subject matter as well as the vocabulary used to define it, to the point that the functions, composition, and the very number of neurocognitive memory systems have become increasingly contested even among neuroscientists; I say increasingly because they always have been (e.g., Schacter, 1990; Schacter & Tulving, 1994; Gabrieli, 1995). Nevertheless, despite critical voices even by towering figures like Tulving—I already referred to his paper "Are there 256 different kinds of memory?" (Tulving, 2007)—it is unlikely that the inflation of memory systems will stop any time soon.[9] Irrespective of this tendency, let us try to separate the wheat from the chaff and distinguish from among the dozens and hundreds of systems a core set of memory systems consented to by most neuroscientific researchers. Notwithstanding a certain tension with what I have pointed out, I want to make the assumption of this core set as plausible as possible, understanding it as an array of functionally distinct forms, practices, and aspects of remembering. All of this is meant to take another look at Perowne's stream of consciousness, following Luria's case for more than one perspective. In short, I want to examine the autobiographical process from the neuroscientific vantage point of the systems model just outlined.

Making sense of the autobiographical process: A neurocognitive point of view

Let me briefly recapitulate the two units of analysis at stake, autobiographical memory and the autobiographical process. The first one is more narrowly defined than the second. Within the systems framework, autobiographical memory refers to an individual's recollected past experience that occurred at a specific time in a specific place, as an episode in which the individual was personally involved. Looking at Perowne's stream of consciousness in the light of this definition, we discern only one indubitably autobiographical memory. This is Perowne's recalling of that "ridiculous article" he read some time ago in a magazine about a water molecule of his own waste that is supposed to fall on him one day as rain. In terms of autobiographical remembering this is not much, especially not in light of our prior analysis that revealed this sequence to be so much more telling. Yet even if one accepts that most of what happens in this autobiographical process does not qualify as autobiographical memory in terms of the systems' definition, we still can make use of the systems model in a different way: we can use its diverse categories of memory systems as lenses that, from an autobiographical perspective, give attention to other, non-narrative forms and practices of remembering and forgetting in this process. In this way, we can consider how the various memory systems are interlaced with the autobiographical process, even if they are not autobiographical memories in the strict sense of the systems model. This may not be categorically perfectly clean, it also is against the spirit of the systems approach and the intentions of its proponents, but it still may help us to deepen our understanding of Perowne's autobiographical process. So let us turn again to McEwan's narrative (quoted on p. 133).

There are indeed several memories on Perowne's mind during his time in the bathroom that can be described as episodic. One example is when he recalls that there was an embarrassing or otherwise unpleasant episode in his past that might have been responsible for the awkward feeling of uneasiness he experiences while using the toilet. Because he stops inquiring after its source, it cannot turn into what would be, on the systems view, an autobiographical memory proper, one that can be localized in time and space. The same holds for semantic memories; Perowne clearly remembers a few of them. Think of his idea of how it feels to cut through the arachnoid, the gossamer covering of the brain. Because he does these operations "routinely," this memory is determined by anatomic facts and generalized knowledge, which lack the specificity of a particular autobiographical episode. As such, it would be commonly classified as semantic memory.

In reviewing these forms of explicit and declarative memory there should be, though, no doubt that much more occurs in this autobiographical process than what reaches the threshold of Perowne's conscious reflection. A question we already struggled with is how the realm of nonconscious and nondeclarative memory can be approached. In this respect, the core distinctions of the systems model offer some revealing perspectives that draw attention to important practices of "implicit" remembering. One is the "procedural memory" inherent in nonconscious motor and cognitive skills—the skills, for example, Perowne needs for shaving. An unspectacular everyday activity, shaving nevertheless requires highly developed motor skills, which Perowne remembers "automatically" every morning. Similarly implicit is a form of memory better known as "classical conditioning," which underlies the gender-specific toilet practices that seem to trouble Perowne.

The importance of bodily incorporated remembering, which is for the most part unconscious, has also been emphasized from different angles of memory research. In an influential study on collective memory, Paul Connerton (1989) pointed out that many social memory practices are performative, and that a substantial portion of performative remembering is bodily. Connerton, who applied a notion of performance to societal memory practices similar to the notion Judith Butler (1990) applied to her theory of performing gender, argued that bodily practices of remembering constitute a particularly effective system of social mnemonics. "In habitual memory," as Connerton (1989, p. 72) has it, "the past is, as it were, sedimented in the body." Many societies, for example, have clear cultural rules defining the way in which women are expected to sit (which is the case for men only to a lesser degree). These rules are handed down from one generation to the next, shaping the bodily behavior of women from early on. "Postural behavior, then, may be very highly structured and completely predictable . . . and so automatic that it is not even recognized as isolatable pieces of behavior" (p. 73). On this account, incorporated practices of remembering are cultural practices whose significance results from their particular systemic stability and persistence that reaches far beyond any individual memory. It is easy to destroy a book, a monument, or the institution of a public archive. But what about habitual memory routines that lead, as it were, bodily lives of their own?

Social communities constitute mnemonic systems that, Connerton maintains, "entrust to bodily automatisms the values and categories which they are most anxious to conserve. They will know how well the past can be kept in mind by a habitual memory sedimented in the body" (1989, p. 102). Further examples of implicit, socially incorporated memory are culturally habitualized modes of perception that trigger certain memories, in a process psychologists call priming. Obviously, the multimodal experience of the water flushing the toilet has a priming effect on Perowne remembering the "ridiculous article" he recently read. All these memory categories throw into relief important qualifications of the autobiographical process, a process that, as we have seen, is both conscious and nonconscious. And because it is notoriously difficult to access the nonconscious, the focus on implicit memory practices allows us to get a better sense of the multiform interplay of explicit and implicit practices.

Yet in using the categories of the various types of declarative and nondeclarative memory for a comprehensive understanding of the autobiographical process, we should bear in mind that this process does not really show up on the radar of the systems model. I already broached this before, so let me dwell for a moment on the question as to why this is so. Why does our comparison of the neuroscientific model and the narrative model confirm that they are compatible only to a limited degree?

One important reason is that they are designed for different purposes. Models, as was our starting point, only make sense within the context of a theory, and the theories involved are clearly very different. The conceptual architecture of the systems model has come into existence in academic research environments. Psychological and neuroscientific laboratories are predicated on "operationalizing" memory into a number of aspects and subaspects that can be experimentally controlled, self-contained, and clearly distinguished from one another. In contrast, the concept of the autobiographical process is meant to capture something else. It aims at envisioning the overarching interplay of the different components, aspects, and contexts of autobiographical remembering and interpretation. It, therefore, seeks to bring into prominence the comprehensive process character of the autobiographical process as a whole, its meandering and pervasive nature. In this way the entire conceptual frame of reference transforms. Shifting from neurocognitive (or inner-mnemonic) systems to the remembering subject, the person (in our case, Perowne), his identity construction, and the context of his life, presents the very notion of autobiographical memory in a new light. It appears as a process inextricably embedded in trajectories of meaning and meaning formation, and it is only along these trajectories that the mnemonic forms and practices categorized in the systems model reveal their psychological significance.

Talking about these trajectories of meaning, we must not imagine them as stable systems. Often enough they appear as fluid, blending several forms of individual and social experience, present and past—as in Perowne's autobiographical crisis, which unfolds against the wider political and historical backdrop of a post-9/11 world. Such cultural embedding of memory phenomena in forms of life and personal significance cannot be "operationalized" within the systems model whose ontology (what *is* memory) and epistemology (how is it to be investigated) are anchored in a divergent set of premises. This makes it difficult—but, as I have tried to show, not entirely impossible—to see the two models as comfortable bed fellows.

A cultural Möbius strip

I want to touch on another insight into the autobiographical process suggested by the combination of the two models. Even if we can subdivide implicit and explicit forms, functions, and practices of remembering and forgetting, and arrange them according to a grid of different memory systems (with autobiographical memory being one of these systems or subsystems), we should be clear that these distinctions are predicated on one essential assumption. This is the assumption that there exists an independent memory process of encoding, storing, and retrieval, which is operative in each system on a different (episodic, semantic, procedural, etc.) content. As soon as we question this assumption and, with it, the idea that there are autonomous mnemonic operations or causal mechanisms in isolation from the interpretive contexts of mind, self, and culture—contexts that not only give meaning to memories but also lay down what counts and what does not count as a memory at all—the plausibility of the systems model dwindles drastically.

If we instead include these interpretive contexts into a comprehensive conception of the autobiographical process, then all the different forms, functions, and practices of remembering and forgetting appear as intimately interrelated components of one happening, a happening that, admittedly, is quite complex. Well beyond taxonomy borders, such a conception requests us to pay particular attention to the connections and transitions among the various meaning components, to the effect that we recognize that something seemingly as bizarre and accidental as Perowne's memory of a molecule from his waste water falling down on him as rain can turn out to be a meaningful moment in a larger autobiographical process. It may be viewed as an expression or, more precisely, as *one* expression of the experience that there is no protected refuge, no private mental sphere where one is out of reach of the world at large, not even in one's bathroom.

Many observers have stated that one of the implications of September 2001 is that there is no longer a safe place in the Western world, neither in its political, economic, and symbolic center, nor in its center of private life, the bathroom, as McEwan seems to indicate. In this view, even the nondeclarative memory system of perceptual priming appears as a significant moment of a larger context of meaning comprising the entire mind, the acting person, and the history from which no one and nothing escapes.

The systems model aims at human memory as an exclusively individual capacity that is compartmentalized into separate units. Why have these distinctions played such a prominent role in memory psychology? An answer to this question leads to some of the basic assumptions of a discipline that has put so much emphasis on its own scientific status, on a scientificity that is taken to be modeled on the methodology of the natural sciences. One of these basic assumptions is the conviction that scientific research is measurable research, that the study of human experience and psychological life is only scientific if it is quantifiable. Thus, instead of seeking to understand the complexity of autobiographical remembering or its psychological, phenomenological, ecological, and cultural richness and sophistication, the goal is to transform it into measurable "data." This might explain the propensity in psychological research to continually fractionalize its subject matters—which means, in this case, to increase the amount of distinct memory systems. "A main advantage of having individual [memory] systems," writes Rubin, "is that the degree to which they are active can be *measured* behaviorally and neurally" (2012, p. 18; my italics, J. B.).

In contrast with this approach, the narrative model suggests that in order to understand the autobiographical process it is crucial to understand how its cognitive, affective, and linguistic dimensions operate in concert, and how they do so in the social life of persons and within their cultural worlds. Understanding these dimensions as dimensions of one synthesis of meaning is also to broaden the second key feature of traditional memory research, its individuocentric focus, and instead conceive of the autobiographical process as enveloped in what Pierre Nora (1989) called a Möbius strip of the individual and the social.

NARRATIVE SYNTHESES

To conclude this chapter, I want to take a closer look at how this synthesis of meaning is created. How is it that narrative, as I argue throughout this book, can play such a crucial role in the autobiographical process, tying together a multitude of components, aspects, and contexts in a dynamic synthesis? And how can narrative carry out processes as fleeting and transformative as those described above? Kyoko Murakami (2012), discussing an earlier version of my outline of a desubstantialized notion of autobiographical remembering and forgetting (Brockmeier, 2010), offers a compelling picture of the fluid and transient nature of the act of remembering. She compares it to an elastic band, a band of *durée* or duration in Bergson's (1946) sense that expands the past into the present and, in the process, constantly moves and changes (Murakami, 2012, p. 10). Seizing Murakami's suggestion, I want to raise the question how, then, can we envision narrative to expand Bergson's band of duration into the present of the telling?

To approach this question I turn once more to Perowne's autobiographical sequence and analyze it into a number of different narrative processes and operations; each of them contributes in a specific way to the overarching autobiographical dynamic. At the same time they also have something in common. They realize shifts—quick moves, in equal measure linguistic and psychological, that increase the mercurial dynamic of the whole. Although closely interconnected, the following types of such shifts can be distinguished.

First, *shifts between fabula and sjuzhet*. I pointed out that McEwan's sequence, as any narrative sequence, can be described in terms of story (the chronological order of events) and discourse (the way in which these events are narrated, typically, in a nonchronological manner). Both orders are, however, mingled. A reader infers the fabula from the sjuzhet. In a sense, both are abstractions between which the act of reading moves back and forth. Looking at the fabula or story of our sequence, we find that it is relatively plain in terms of external action—Perowne wakes and goes to the bathroom. The complication comes because the story is interspersed with various additional discourses unfolding layers and fragments of a much more complicated landscape of consciousness. In reading the sequence, we thus continually oscillate between the two landscapes of action and consciousness.

Second, *shifts between various levels and orders of time.* The sequence is interfused with various times and tenses, and with continuous shifts between these different time frames, so-called narrative anachronies. Beginning with a brief "flashforward" (when Perowne thinks of the errands he will do later in the day) and ending with a—suggested— "flashback" (when he is humming a tune from the wartime about 60 years earlier, symbolically connecting to the theme of war that pervades those days in 2002); remember, this is the day of the big antiwar demonstration. These sudden shifts evoke a quite heterogeneous temporal scenario. Rather than offering a stable background for the events, time becomes an inner factor of them, a factor of instability. What is more, there are moments in which Perowne acts in just one time (such as the very here and now when he enters the bathroom) that alternate with moments in which he finds himself simultaneously in multiple times—for example, when he is trying (in the present) to locate the source of that awkward sensation aroused by a memory that passed through his thoughts a few minutes ago (past 1) but is still on his mind, and which refers to an experience longer ago (past 2), which also is still with him, although in a more vague and intangible way.

Third, *shifts between foregrounding and backgrounding.* Foregrounding and backgrounding are narrative operations that define what is figure and what is ground in a given sequence. In film, one well-known technique of foregrounding and backgrounding is zooming. In our passage, the description of such a move figures centrally. Perowne, floating through various mental states between day and night, finally manages to turn his full attention to his memory of the burning plane he believes he saw earlier that morning, a memory that he hopes may explain his strange restlessness. Blurred as things may appear now, "when he trod the air to the window last night he was fully awake. He's even more certain of that now." In tandem with such changes between foreground and background, the narrative includes sudden shifts between abstract and concrete thought. In the twinkle of an eye an abstract idea like the "diaphanous films of sleep" turns into the image of a concrete object like the arachnoid sheath of the human brain. In a sense, even the shift from remembering to forgetting can be understood, as we have witnessed, as a sudden transformation of the effort to foreground a particular, though nebulous, past experience to an attitude of letting it go and glide into the background.

Fourth, *shifts between different mental states*. It is amazing how many distinct mental states Perowne passes through in such a short period of time: from deep sleep and being half asleep to phases of daydreaming, hallucination ("exploring the fringes of psychosis in safety") and, eventually, being fully awake—at least that is what he considers himself to be. And even more astonishing, the shifts through these various states, mood-switching as they may be, take place within one fleeting movement, one flow of consciousness. It has often been pointed out that autobiographical memories tend to be idiosyncratic and quirky. Some details take on a conspicuous shape, others remain foggy; they may even disappear when we try to get a clearer idea of them and couch them in the terms used in these pages, that is, when we try to make interpretive sense of them. And we may think how bizarre it is that the most picturesque memory is the least significant, while a life-changing event appears as relatively trivial; that the memory nearest at hand is pale, while the one dating back for decades seems sharply etched.

What has, however, attracted less attention is that memories cannot only be odd and enigmatic, but also float through various psychological states. Would we be surprised if Perowne's burning airplane reappeared in his dreams and daydreams after he went back to bed? It certainly was on his mind when he watched the news in the early morning to find out about what happened in the sky over London; he also might have described the scene to his son and, later in the day, conjured it up here and there wondering what it meant and means. Eventually, he might have concluded it was a memory. But a memory of what? Even if it was a hallucination so realistic that it could easily be taken for real, for something that would have been quite likely after all, the important thing is that it indeed became a memory. As a memory of a perceived memory, it was recalled again and again, under different circumstances and in different psychological modalities. Each time it might have been envisioned in a slightly different light and emotional state, newly interrogated, evaluated, interpreted—and again remembered, each time enriched by some of those emotions, interpretations, and evaluations. What kind of burning airplane, then, would Perowne have before his eyes when he would go to sleep at the end of that long day?[10]

Fifth, *shifts between various narrative perspectives*. Although, on the surface, the sequence creates the impression of an ongoing stream of consciousness, the narrative actually vacillates among several perspectives. In a social-science context we would qualify them as different sources or data, as contributions or accounts of various participants; narrative theorists use concepts like focalization and multiple narrator.[11] Clearly, though only shortly, there is a first-person perspective marked by a direct voice ("Relax!" "But who cares?")—irrespective of the fact that this voice could narratologically also be understood as part of a free indirect discourse. More eloquent is a third-person narrator who tells us about what the first-person narrator does, thinks, and feels. Still, although the third-person narrator does not know much more than the main character, he at least finds the time to comment on what goes on in the character's mind. He is the one who notes that something "passed through his thoughts only minutes ago, and now what remains is the feeling without its rationale." And obviously he is a better rememberer than the first-person narrator, given that he keeps in mind the many transient sensations, ideas, associations, and feelings that go by in a normal mind—say, Perowne's mind—from one moment to the next.

Following on from the comments made above about the nature of written language, we may be tempted to say that the third-person narrator is a writer, or at least a special variation of an "implied narrator," to modify slightly the narratologically more common term of "implied author" (Phelan, 2005). In viewing McEwan's text as an experimental scenario, we can take the third-person narrator as the one who keeps the records. He is the clerk who takes the minutes that provide us with the ephemeral details of the autobiographical process that typically sink below sea level. Finally, there is a further voice: the wartime tune. It well illustrates the idea of multiple voices or, to use Bakhtin's terms, the inherent polyphony of language. For one, it marks a first-person perspective (because it is hummed by Perowne); but it also suggests a third-person perspective (from which the lyrics, the tune, and its historical background are identified); and lastly, it is an historical quote, a cultural voice that originated neither in the head of the first-person nor the third-person narrator.

So far we have looked at the first- and third-person perspective. Yet narratives can also be seen, on a slightly different level, as being in second-person mode. In one, narrow way this applies to narratives that speak to their recipients or narratees by use of second-person personal pronouns and other forms of address; in everyday conversational storytelling *you*-narration is mostly embedded in acts of narrative co-constructions of shared experiences or is used as a strategic form of interaction and positioning (Mildorf, 2012). In literary fiction, second-person perspectives often round out what has been called "multipersoned narratives" that oscillate between first-, second-, and third-person narrative positions (Richardson, 2006). In another, wider sense, it can be said that every narrative realizes a second-person mode because it is meant to speak to a recipient or narratee whom it tries to draw into a different world, a storyworld—even if this is as personal and intimate a world as the bathroom of an unknown person. From this perspective, the same dialogical nature of all language also applies to narrative. Since the rise, a few decades ago, of reader-response theories, literary pragmatism, and communicative, conversational, and dialogical models of fiction, many narrative scholars have come to see the addressee as actively involved in the making of a narrative or, at least, in the construction of narrative meaning. That is, participants in a "narrative event" act as co-narrators, whether they are involved in the telling and understanding of oral (and that mostly means, conversational) stories or of written stories. In both cases, narrative works as a process of communication and joint meaning construction, an idea I situated in the last chapter within the context of a postclassical understanding of narrative. A written narrative—like the one under discussion—is typically composed with a certain reader in mind, an audience whom the author wants to involve, often in a kind of dialogue. The reader, in turn, engages in a similar dialogue to figure out what the meaning of the story is, interpreting the actions and intentions of its characters, narrator, and author. In this way, the "intentional stance" (Herman, 2008) moves to the center of the literary, sociolinguistic, social-scientific, and psychological study of narrative, a further move linked to the postclassical trend in narrative studies. Drawing on these considerations, we can also incorporate the interpretive activities of a second-person narrator in our already lively picture that shifts among several narrative perspectives.

Sixth, *shifts among various styles of narration.* The repertoire of narrative modes that enact Perowne's stream of consciousness encompasses all three forms of thought presentation that are discussed in today's narratology: thought report ("Perowne's plan is to cook a fish stew."), free direct thought ("But who cares?"), and free indirect thought ("There is a view that it is shameful for a man . . ."). All three modes of narrative merge into one process. Despite this multitude of mind styles and, as indicated in the previous category of shifts, of voices and perspectives, what the sequence lacks is a guiding authorial narrator, that is an omniscient narrator. There is no comprehensive point of reference, no integrating principle of textual organization, no "inner self" that would emerge as "the center of narrative gravity," to borrow Dennett's (1992) formulation. If there is a synthesis, it is only evoked by the narrative flow of the autobiographical process.

Seventh, *shifts between individual and cultural memory.* When Perowne remembers, for whatever reason, a popular song from World War II we clearly encounter not only an individual but also a cultural memory, thoroughly entwined as they are. But this is only one, almost peripheral aspect of the cultural scenario unfolded here. We cannot understand the entire sequence of events in Perowne's bathroom on that Saturday morning if we leave out of account the wider political, social, and historical landscape in which the narrative landscapes of action and consciousness are nestled. This has been the gist of my analysis. Even an unassuming personal memory can be fused with a larger cultural memory, akin to the sight of a jetliner in flames over Central London in the first years of the 21st century, which will inescapably be reminiscent of the dramatic images from Manhattan in September 2001. Following Perowne's stream of consciousness, we cannot help but move back and forth between an individual and a historical trajectory of remembering.

Eighth, what supports all these shifts and moves is a number of *figurative expressions or tropes* that lend themselves to swift and meandering associations (and that I also list here though they indicate, strictly speaking, not narrative but rhetorical devices). What is the tropical or rhetorical fabric of our passage? It comprises metaphors ("diaphanous films"), metonomies (flushing—rain molecule—magazine in coffee room), similes and comparisons (half asleep—"exploring the fringes of psychosis in safety"), and images ("the wide green-and-white marble floor"). The idea that a water molecule from the bathroom will return one day as a rain drop lends itself to a further rhetorical figure, a synecdoche (a part that stands for a whole): there is no entity, no space as personal and intimate it may seem that is not connected to larger cycles of events. These tropes are the glue that keeps the narrative together, the threads that weave it into a whole, the air that lets it breathe. What I have referred to as the quicksilver nature of the autobiographical process is, not least, owed to this psycho-rhetorical texture.

The ninth and last category of the shifts that make up this scenario regards the interplay between *images* and *language* in the autobiographical process. This is a complex category, for it demands a certain understanding of the general nature and role of imagery in autobiographical remembering. And as this is an important issue in the literature—it is often taken to be the defining feature of autobiographical memory—I must say a few more words on this category than on the previous ones.[12] After this excursion, a short summary will conclude this chapter.

IMAGES AND WORDS

Obviously imagery is paramount in Perowne's short narrative sequence: from the scene of the man sitting on the toilet to the pictures of the neurosurgeon cutting through the arachnoid and the green-and-white marble floor on which he walks in his bathroom, Perowne's world and mind are strewn with images—as are the worlds and minds of all of us. But are we talking about images, or linguistic expressions of images? The distinction between imagistic and linguistic structures of the autobiographical process is not an easy one and has often been subject to misunderstanding, especially, if related to the assumption that personal memories are first and foremost pictorial. Augustine, one of the first and most influential authors on the subject of autobiographical memory, stated the matter, in Book 10 of his *Confessions*, in classical terms—terms that have often been repeated and variated ever since: "Memory preserves in distinct particulars and general categories all the perceptions which have penetrated . . . Every one of them enters into memory . . . and is put on deposit there. The objects themselves do not enter, but the images of the perceived objects are available to the thought recalling them." (Augustine [10, viii, 13], 1991, p. 186).

In the same context, Augustine went on to also formulate the question that has remained unanswered until today: "But who can say how images [in our memory] are created, even though it may be clear by which senses they are grasped and stored within" (p. 186). In other words, how are we to understand the pictorial assumption, the claim that autobiographical memories are primarily visual scenes or images with personal relevance, which, once recalled, can (or perhaps cannot) be translated or otherwise transformed into language. Although I look into some concrete examples of present psychological theorizing based on this assumption in the next chapter, I want to situate it here in a more general context, namely, as a consequence of the traditional notion of autobiographical memory.

The locus classicus in our days is Tulving's (1972; 1983; 2002b) distinction of two different memory systems, episodic and semantic memory (Augustine's "distinct particulars" and "general categories"). Whereas other theorists have conceived of autobiographical memory as a subsystem of episodic memory, Tulving himself did not distinguish between the two, identifying autobiographical memories with episodic ones. The paradigmatic case of an episodic memory is a scenic or imagistic episode that happened at a specific time and place and, in the autobiographical instance, has personal significance. Although Tulving changed his definition of semantic and episodic memory over time, it was never uncontested. Especially in view of autobiographical memories, it has been objected that it is difficult if not impossible to distinguish the general knowledge of an event from its recollection as something unique. Some researchers, like Rubin (2012), thus reject the existence of semantic and episodic memory systems in autobiographical memory (pp. 22–23).

Nevertheless, Tulving's distinction became the key to the subclassification of declarative memories and the way they are encoded, stored, and retrieved. (Declarative or explicit memories are viewed as one of the two kinds of long-term human memory.) Yet, this distinction also became the key to some fundamental problems of the entire memory model. One problem with Tulving's model is the same as many other psychological memory models building on his distinction: It is designed from the point of view of classical cognitive research (based on the information processing paradigm) and according to the exigencies of quantitative measurability. This means it misses out on the reality of autobiographical remembering and forgetting outside the laboratory, a reality that is more complex, messy, and colorful than the cognitive models can capture (and that the distinction between general knowledge and unique event recollection permits to imagine). This problem is an ongoing one, often addressed not only by memory researchers in the social sciences and the humanities, but also within psychology (e.g., Bruner, 1994; Danziger, 2008; Neisser, 1967) and the neurosciences (e.g., Rose, 2006; 2010). Even earlier psychologists of the first generation such as James (1981) and Wundt (1900–1920) compellingly argued that if we conceptually and experimentally reduce the complexity of human consciousness in order to be able to isolate and measure some presumably "pure" mental states, we lose the essence of the mind, its complexity, or—to put it in slightly different terms—its capacity to help us create and cope with the complexity of our lives. And there are good arguments suggesting that these two complexities, although not identical, are mutually predicated on each other.

This is not to deny that it might be possible experimentally to create conditions under which pure memory images can be retrieved—if we assume for a moment that such an act of retrieval can be envisioned without interpretation. Even without a laboratory, I remember a number of photographs of my parents and myself, and I think I also recall the situation under which the pictures were shot. I also am able to recollect some paintings from a recent museum visit, and I believe that I can recall a traffic accident I witnessed by chance a few weeks ago. Yet already when I list these imagistic memories, I note that all of them are, in fact, highly contextualized. They are contextualized both at the level of the lived experiences from which they emerged and at the level of the act of remembering. Both levels are involved when I try to make sense of them—right now in the process of laying out this argument. At both levels my sense-making is mingled with reflections, feelings, stories, and history. To cut my memories out of this weave and isolate them as "pure images" that are kept clear of any interpretation surely requires quite an effort. It also requires a convincing reason why I should take this effort and ignore, for example, my knowledge of the peculiar situation in which the photograph of my family was taken. After all, this is the main reason why this otherwise boring black-and-white picture means something to me, why it has become part of my autobiographical "imagistic memory."

One part of the story that has moved Tulving and many other cognitive memory researchers to cut out such context-free memories that match the idea of pure imagistic episodes and are free from "semantic memories"—that is, from what I know about them and what makes them meaningful—is based on the supposition that there is something like a pure cognitive layer of the mind: a presemiotic and precultural domain of mental (or neuronal) raw material. This domain is conceived of as being deeper than language, communication, culture, and history. In the area of autobiographical memory, mnemonic mental images are considered an essential part of this domain.

Now, if we do not want to omit interpretive meaning-making as a constitutive part of the autobiographical process, the idea of a pure imagistic memory episode obviously creates a problem. This problem, posed by the assumption of a clear-cut distinction between images and language in the autobiographical process, can be considered from various points of view. One brings to bear that there is an inherent move from images to words whenever we are concerned with their meanings. Whether visual perception, visual imagination, or visual remembering, all of them present invitations to sense-making. They are "affordances" of meaning construction, to borrow the central term of James Gibson's (1979) ecological approach to visual perception. To be sure, we do not sort out and realize the meanings of all visual perceptions, images, scenes, and many other things, including feelings, moods, and concerns, that cross our mind and keep our mental and affective life busy. Immersing us more often than not in a messy state of being, this meaning overflow is an essential part of our narrative "sense of self," as Peter Goldie (2012) has argued. Perowne, as we saw, turned quite decisively against this onslaught, choosing to leave in the dark some dodgy issues and, presumably, images. But if, at one point, these issues and images took center stage in his consciousness—and McEwan's novel is exactly about this: how they move to the fore in the course of that one day—they eventually would become the subject of narrative reflection and reconstruction.[13] We might think of Wittgenstein's (2009) deadpan questions: How do you *know* that it is an image? And how do you know what it *means*? Which is to ask: Can we give an answer to these questions without language?

Another problem or, perhaps, another aspect of the same problem is that there also is an inherent move from language to image. This move likewise does not respect the presumed divide between the visual-imagistic and linguistic-narrative dimension of autobiographical memory. It can be seen as an irreducible quality of language—mentioned already under the previous point—that it is shot through with the use of figurative expressions, not least, imagistic, and spatial tropes. By its very nature language uses, creates, and evokes imagery. And it does so in a wide spectrum, ranging from figurative images (metaphors, metonymies, and other expressions evoking some kind of "iconic proximity") to strategies of overarching discourse composition and comprehension. Such strategies work holistically. They often underlie narrative scenarios, drawing on "iconic gestalt transfer" from complex natural or human action patterns (Ungerer, 2007). Remember Perowne: What he glimpses or believes to glimpse is a burning airplane, but he perceives this image as an element of an iconic action sequence omnipresent in the post-9/11 cultural imagination, a terrorist attack on London. It is the memory not of the burning airplane but of this complex scenario, composed of perceived and imagined visual elements of a comprehensive gestalt of meaning that is going to haunt him over the entire day.

What is called imagery or iconicity in this context generally refers to the use of language that appeals to human senses of sight, hearing, touch, taste, and smell, among others. Having said that, it is, however, the pictorial power of language that mostly is singled out. *A picture is worth a thousand words.* Perhaps it is because of the assumption of a basic divide between words and images that it has often been overlooked that this picture, even if it might be worth more than thousand words, is itself made of words. Take metaphors and similes; most of them, as Wood (2008) puts it, "do pretend, of course, to sail close to the wind, and give us the sense that something has been newly painted before our eyes" (p. 108), in immediate, tangible presence, that is. Yet even if we can see before our eyes how the oil paint drips from the canvas, make no mistake: it is words that make it drip. Even the author who follows the tenet that *the writer must show, not tell* shows by means of words. Put differently, the pictorial power in question—the capacity to sail close to the wind—is part of the power of language, of its constitutively multimodal nature. Thus, language might be more adequately conceived of as a multimodal symbolic system, which resonates with Bruner's (1991) proposal to understand stories as a symbolic system intertwined with domains of knowledge, perception, and imagination. Building on these reflections, it is fair to conclude that it is not the specific senses or modalities of perception, imagination, or remembering, but rather meanings and practices of meaning-making that are organizing this symbolic system.

A further aspect exacerbates the misperception just mentioned. Words have always been mistaken for what they seem to refer to or conjure. When cognitive psychologists examine the imagistic content of episodic or autobiographical memories, they typically have their participants describe (or identify according to a questionnaire) the scenes they remember—implicitly taking them for prelinguistic or nonlinguistic images. Given the imaginative power of language, it often escapes our attention that what we take to be a suggestive picture is conjured by expressions and narrative accounts saturated with imagery, especially with metaphors, metonymies, similes, and many more visual tropes. In this case, language appears to be transparent and we lose our sense of its mediating role. This effect might even be more compelling in narrative discourse; some authors speak of "narrative transparency" (Joyce, 2011).

Being open-minded and sensitive to the "reality effect" of language is not necessarily a flaw. From early childhood on, perceptive and pictorial imagination develops as part of our comprehensive activities of sense-making, as components of a holistic ability to reach out for meaning. This ability encompasses the coordination of pictures and words as well as many more senses and abilities; it also is linked to the comprehensive meaning-making capacities that have developed socioculturally with humans' narrative imagination (Andrews, 2013). If we thus widen our view to encompass the sociocultural world in which we learn to understand and use words and images, this becomes even more evident. That the reality effect of language itself is a sociocultural creature that has its historically distinct forms and functions is a lesson to be learned from 19th century fiction,that is, from the novel. Many literary theorists and historians have pointed out that one of the most momentous innovations of the realist novel was its discovery of the visual, which anticipated the photographic and filmic perception of the 20th century. Never before had detail and imagery become so crucial as in the great novels of the 19th and 20th centuries. The texture of the visual that emerged in the novels of Gustave Flaubert, Thomas Mann, or Virginia Woolf is comparable to the texture of what Henry James called our very experience: "Experience is never limited, and it is never complete; it is an immense sensibility, a kind of huge spider-web of the finest silken threads suspended in the chamber of consciousness" (1988, p. 17).

True, *words and images* is the label of a commonplace distinction between different types and aspects of representation, media, and modalities, a shorthand way of mapping an extended cognitive, semi-otic, linguistic, art- and picture-theoretical field. But under close exami-nation, the distinction between word and image is anything but such a deceptively simple matter, as W. J. T. Mitchell (1994) maintained from a further angle. Investigating the simple juxtaposition of a supposedly linguistic and a supposedly imagistic medium, such as the book and film or television, Mitchell concludes that "books have incorporated images into their pages since time immemorial, and television, far from being purely a visual or imagistic medium is more aptly described as a medium in which images, sounds, and words 'flow' into one another" (1994, pp. 3–4). This does not mean that there are no differences between these media and semiotic environments, or between words and images, or that vision and visual images are completely reducible to language, or that the imagistic is prior to the linguistic. What it means, according to Mitchell, is only "that the differences are much more complex than they might seem at first glance, that they crop up *within* as well as between media, and that they can change over time as modes of representation and cultures change" (1994, p. 4). It goes without saying that even the semblance of a plain opposition between word and image disappears completely if we turn to the mixed media environments of communicat-ing and remembering that have emerged with the digital age, creating new multimodal compositions that simultaneously involve a number of semiotic modes, such as oral and written language, sound, graphic text, and static or moving images (cf. Grishakova & Ryan, 2010; Hoffmann, 2010; Page & Thomas, 2011).

The autobiographical process is just one example of a meaning-making process that entangles and fuses more than just one modality. Perowne's sequence displays how images, reflections, evaluations, feelings, and moods are part and parcel of the same process; how they intermingle with acts of interpretation and, in particular, self-interpretation; and how these acts of making sense include words and images and episodes (imagined and remembered) and more—for example, the humming of a tune. The interplay and interfusion between images and words makes up the last of nine categories of shifts discussed in this final section of the chapter. All categories contribute in particular ways to the narrative dynamic of the autobiographical process. Many of them, as well as the figurative and imagistic language that carries them out, overlap and mingle, evoking a synthesizing effect that once more enhances their efficacy. As a result, each individual memory is inextri-cably inserted in an ongoing narrative flow of interpretive, reflexive, and imaginative acts.

This notion also brings into sharper focus the claim that narrative is not just a resonant metaphor of a different, perhaps, less reductionist view of autobiographical memory and identity construction. Rather, it offers a differentiated, comprehensive, and sensitive alternative to the traditional memory model, and it does so because the very dynamic of the autobiographical process itself is that of a narrative process. The point of narrative, then, is that it allows us to realize, first, the plethora of interpretive, reflexive, and imaginative acts involved in the autobiographical process; second, their ongoing interplay and intermingling; and third, their rootedness in larger contexts of mental and emotional life, personhood and identity, and culture and history. What I have called the strong narrative thesis is meant to sharpen further this argument in proposing that the autobiographical process only exists because of this narrative dynamic. It is only in the form of narrative that we are able to navigate the mishmash of the complex experiences at stake, experiences that mingle past, present, future, and possible and imagined times of our lives.

The emphasis put on this vision of narrative as a process and dynamic event leads to a further qualification of what I have called narrative synthesis. The idea of such synthesis is based on the argument that narrative is a ubiquitous social practice that combines linguistic, cognitive, and affective modes of human activity. Whereas these modes, as the argument goes, are often (and in psychology typically) investigated separately, my point is that everything depends on understanding how they operate together, forming one complex synthesis. Creating this synthesis is an essential practice of human meaning-making, with the autobiographical process enacting exactly such a process. Now we see that this is not about just one synthesis of meaning but an array of unstable, indeed fluctuating syntheses. Bergson's elastic band of remembering constantly stretches, collapses, and twists. Still another way of making the same point is to say that the narrative syntheses we encounter in the autobiographical process only take on temporary shape. And they do so according to the interpretive frameworks in which they are meant to make sense, with the additional complication that these frameworks are themselves in a continuous state of change. One of the most imperative interpretive frameworks of the autobiographical process, as the Perowne sequence demonstrates, is that of identity formation—which will be at the center of the next chapter.

With this prospect in mind, recall another claim made at the beginning of the book and now further substantiated in the analysis of McEwan's narrative. It is not brains that interpret the world and themselves, but persons. The case study of this chapter has made it clear that meanings and processes of meaning formation cannot be reduced to special cognitive operations or neurocognitive memory mechanisms. In trying to understand individuals and their intentions, affects, and quirks we cannot but take into account the wider contexts of the cultural and historical worlds in which they live. It is in this way that Benjamin's color of people's life worlds can be said to enter the project of a narrative hermeneutics, and stay.

CHAPTER 6

Creating a Memory of Oneself

Narrative Identity

In this chapter my goal is to take a closer look at narrative self-making. The previous two chapters sketched an outline of the autobiographical process; I now turn to the role, scope, and limits of this process in the narrative formation of individual or personal identity. A brief review might be helpful. Chapter 4 started with examining the blending of narrative and experience and then shifted over to the interpretive dynamic of the autobiographical process, a subject that became the main issue in Chapter 5. In a case study drawing on a narrative by the British writer Ian McEwan, I offered a "thick description"—a concept borrowed from interpretive anthropology—of the narrative dynamic of the autobiographical process. The aim of that study was to elucidate how we navigate the mishmash of past and present, of possible and anticipated experiences. Ultimately, this navigation appeared to be driven not by cognitive mechanisms but by affective motives and concerns, by emotional entanglements rooted as much in individual lives as in the social and cultural worlds in which these lives are lived. This emotional dimension will again be an issue in this chapter. Yet the case study of the last chapter has also permitted me to consider further what gives narrative and, not least, literary narrative its particular hermeneutic quality and why it can serve as an investigative lens to examine core features of complex human experience, an issue that continues to concern us in this chapter.

As I concentrate on how the identity–memory nexus looks if we redirect our attention to the autobiographical process and the ways it relates to the narrative form of life that we call our identity, I am aware that this is not the whole story—neither about identity and memory nor about the autobiographical process. For that reason, in various parts of this chapter, there will be an ongoing examination of the limits of the notion of autobiographical identity, ultimately resulting in what I call a postautobiographical perspective on narrative and identity. These limits are particularly evident when we look at some examples of that subgenre of life writing called illness narratives and consider the ways of self-making and the sense of identity of individuals who have only restricted autobiographical memories. There can be a number of reasons for such restraints; a few of them will be treated further on in the chapter. Yet before that, my goal is to bring some clarity to where the thickest gun smoke lingers, the debates on narrative identity. Like the issue of human experience investigated in Chapter 4, the formation of identity has attracted much attention in narrative studies and narrative–psychological investigations. An extensive literature revolves around the notion of narrative identity, and it is indeed this notion that is at the heart of this chapter. I pointed out previously that interpretation is an experiential mode constitutive of the human existence; and now I want to highlight the particular kind of interpretation that is *self*-interpretation. Human beings are self-interpreting animals, as Taylor (1985b) succinctly put it. In this chapter, I now want to zoom in on the narrative fabric of the human animal's autobiographical self-interpretations, a focus that I use to make sense of the notion of narrative identity.

I should emphasize, however, right at the beginning, that my interest in the idea of identity and narrative identity in particular is a specific one: I question the role of autobiographical memory that traditionally is taken to be crucial for personal identity. One reason for this is that the idea of the autobiographical process unfolded in these chapters radically challenges the concept of autobiographical memory in general, and this entails the revision of some widespread assumptions regarding the autobiographical dimension of identity.

LIVES AND STORIES

If adventures happen only to people who know how to tell them, as Henry James famously remarked, this is even truer for memories. The adventures of autobiographical memories and the mysterious ways they relate to what we take to be our identities have always fascinated me. This fascination has grown as I have become more aware of what it means that not only our memories but also our identities are not given to us but made by us and that narrative is pivotal to both enterprises. By this I do mean that we live our lives as stories, or that our lives *are* stories, sometimes is maintained. Even if narrative and life, life as told and ... as lived, are inseparable from each other—as Bruner (1987c), in his essay *Life as Narrative*, has summarized a consensus shared by authors in various fields—there are several reasons that prevent us from identifying one with the other. Alasdair MacIntyre (2007), Paul Ricoeur (1992), Charles Taylor (1989), and a number of other philosophers and theorists of human identity have expounded upon why narrative is so significant for our efforts to give meaning to our lives and identities and to understand our being in the world. And although phenomenological and hermeneutic traditions loom large in this debate, it also has extended to quarters of analytic philosophy; for example, in discussions of what Christine Korsgaard (1996) has called humans' "practical identity," which includes experienced, embodied, and relational aspects and thus goes beyond the traditional analytic focus on identity as metaphysical issue (cf., e.g., Mackenzie & Atkins, 2008). But as far as I see, no one concerned with narrative and identity in more than a merely metaphorical sense has questioned that there is a difference between narrative and language on the one hand, and life and identity on the other.[1] Although language is essential for the formation, elaboration, and negotiation of self-understanding and identity, the issue of identity belongs to a picture that is more extended than that of language. It also comprises pre- and nonconceptual modes of meaning-making and identity that draw on bodily, intersubjective, and other cultural forms of life. Thus, as sociolinguist John Edwards (2009) states, we must recognize even from a linguistic point of view that any study of the relationship between identity and language which considers *only* language will be deficient and limited. And this is also true, as Edwards goes on to argue, when "the single most important fact in the social life of language is its relationship to identity" (p. 13).

Living a life might be said to have a narrative structure (or, as some say, a proto-narrative structure) because it typically is mingled with interpretation and intentionality and thus with meaning-making operations that depend on narrative, irrespective of whether we talk about present, past, future, or possible scenarios. But when it comes to the stories that give shape and gestalt to our identities, they do not simply grow by themselves out of the events and experiences of our lives. It is true, however, that there are many tropes and expressions that suggest exactly this: that our lives *turn* into stories, *lend* themselves to stories, or even *are* stories. Take Ricoeur, for example, who claims that "It is the identity of the story that makes the identity of the character" (1992, p. 148)—a claim that reflects Ricoeur's Aristotelian sense of narrativity, in which character and plot, event and time form the composite ("emplotted") whole of a life (cf. Klepper, 2013). Or take Dennett who maintains that "Our tales are spun, but for the most part we don't spin them; they spin us" (1991, p. 418)—a claim that reflects Dennett's sense of objectivist and, for the most part, naturalist determination. But make no mistake, it is we who account for our actions, experiences, and lives in narrative terms, which sometimes are the terms of a life story. The themes, experiences, and relationships "that are the stuff of our lives can't by themselves take on the form of any particular story. We have to *make it* a story," as Hilde Lindemann Nelson (2001) put it, building on an argument by Mieke Bal (1985).

Likewise, William Randall and Elizabeth McKim (2008) have argued that, in understanding our lives or what people tell us about their lives, it is we who have to *read* these lives as stories. Influenced by literary models of narrative and reading, Randall and McKim place a great deal of emphasis on this particular kind of interpretive "reading," which they see at the heart of narrative identity formation. Accordingly, we should read our lives like readers of literary texts, with the corollary idea of the self as a reader or "inner editor" of narrative, overlooking and editing the many perceptions, reports, thoughts, and "storylines that are swirling around inside of us" (Randall & McKim, 2008, p. 35).

This adds an interesting reader-centered (or perhaps more precisely, reader-response-centered) variation to the spectrum of narrative identity conceptions that is mainly narrator-centered. To conceive of "lives as novels-in-the-making" (Randall & McKim, 2008, p. 49) and to understand the self as a novelist is a prevalent topos in literary quarters, already unfurled by 19th-century writers like Nietzsche (Nehamas, 1985). Bakhtin (1981) saw a kind of selective affinity between the literary form of the novel and the multi-voicedness or polyphony of individual consciousness, especially, if the mind is taken to be a social and societal ensemble of relations and connections; as though it were a continuously rewritten and ever uncompleted text echoing and being echoed by the countless texts of one's cultural world (Brockmeier, 2005). Yet although Randall and McKim take the life-as-narrative (or life-as-text) analogy as far as possible—namely, to put it in my own words, as a life-long interplay that extends to multiple levels of enacted and symbolized narrative activity—they, too, admit its limits. One is that in contrast to readers of literary stories, readers of lived stories likely have less confidence that "the story" makes sense, all the more as they "may feel themselves adrift on a sea of possible plots" (Randall & McKim, 2008, p. 71). In fact, what dweller in a modernist and postmodernist world can ever be sure there is a plausible and coherent interpretation of his or her life? That there will be an overarching unity or, at least, a coherent narrative, which will eventually emerge if we only search, or read, for it thoroughly enough?

Another significant difference Randall and McKim mention is that the text of a lived life story is steadily laid down, without a break, whether the reader is editing and interpreting it or not. In fact, often enough we do not interpret our experiences, and even less often our life as a whole, and rather we live it in the thick of ongoing events and entanglements, emotions and moods. Add to this the possibility that there may yet be more profound reasons why we do not want to engage in committed acts of self-interpretation. Still, Randall and McKim believe that reading literature and the "deliberate cultivation of that activity" (p. 6) not only makes us better readers of our lives; it also allows us to imaginatively develop, cohere, and ultimately deepen our identities, and make our lives "quasi-literary works" (p. x). In this way, the argument goes, one's life story—and, based on this, one's identity—can become "a really great story: coherent and rich and teeming with meaning" (Randall, 2011, p. 36).

I wonder whether this account is not just inspired, but perhaps even overwhelmed, by a vision of literature and its reading that is surely appealing. Nor am I sure whether I share confidence in the generic identity-enhancing potential of reading literature and, as a consequence, of the creative reading of the "text" of one's life. I suspect there are some specific sociocultural circumstances such as education, class, ethnicity, and health that need to be included in the equation. But it is no doubt important to keep in mind that we make and remake not just one but many stories about our lives and ourselves—"we are inveterate revisers of ourselves," note Randall and McKim (2008, p. 27), alluding to the idea of the self as editor—and that these stories, small or extended, spontaneous or carefully drawn out, potentially "cannibalize" all kinds of cultural models and genres of storytelling. These include those articulated in literature, but also in film, theater, art, journalism, and digital settings of life writing and self-presentation. Obviously we are not the only master in our house of stories, and this appears to be particularly true for identity stories or self-narratives. We are never more, and sometimes much less, than co-narrators of our own life stories, wrote MacIntyre; "only in fantasy," he went on to say, "do we live what story we please" (2007, p. 199).

So far in my work, I have not recognized any generalizable, not to mention universal, rules that underlie the interplay between the collective resources of narrative in the cultural world at large and the individual selection of "tellable" events and experiences from one's autobiographical past, present, and future. Rather, I have come to believe that accounts of narrative identity and the autobiographical process are prototypical of what could be called the "principle of narrative singularity" (Brockmeier, 2012a, pp. 455–456). The singularity of stories makes it notoriously difficult to apply quantitative methods of investigation that are widespread in psychology, medicine, and the social sciences. Part of the singularity of stories, and of identity stories in particular, stems from a further complication: their shape also depends on the highly variable social and cultural situations in which we tell them. Finally, what particular language games we are involved in is influenced by the semiotic environments—oral, written, digital, mixed-media, performative—where our stories take on form.

All this explains why it can be such a complicated and indeed messy undertaking when we engage in interpreting and negotiating our lives. In this process there is little if anything predictable or replicable. Quoting Wayne Booth, Randall and McKim (2008, p. 20) refer to a further difficulty of traditional methodologies vis-à-vis the study of narrative identity: "There can be no 'control group'," as Booth remarked, "consisting of untouched souls who have lived life-times without narrative so that they might study unscathed the effects of others" (1988, p. 41).

I mentioned MacIntyre (2007), who emphasized that for the most part the narrative models and constraints according to which we interpret and account for our and others' identities are not freely chosen but culturally and historically given. This argument holds for narrative form and content. As Judith Butler (2005) has it, "My narrative begins in medias res, when many things have already taken place to make me and my story possible in language. I am always recuperating, reconstructing, and I am left to fictionalize and fabulate origins I cannot know" (p. 39). Yet even Butler's fictionalizations and MacIntyre's fantasies are anything but open to fancy-free fabulation; they, too, are subject to the cultural rules of a historical episteme. "History does not belong to us"; as Gadamer put the matter, "we belong to it. Long before we understand ourselves through the process of self-examination, we understand ourselves in a self-evident way in the family, society and state in which we live" (1989, pp. 276–277).

Varieties of narrative agency

There is a dialectic in this interplay between history and individuality that must not be overlooked. Cultural and historical rules do not work like natural laws that we cannot break or change. In fact, we break and change them all the time, adapting our autobiographical identities and adventures to the shifting ideas of what we believe to be a "good life" while, at the same time, adapting these ideas to our changing projects of identity. That this lived and experienced dialectical movement is closely intertwined with the dynamic of our life narratives is an argument that Mark Freeman and I have elaborated elsewhere (Freeman & Brockmeier, 2001). There is, however, an important qualification to this point, namely, the "sociocultural circumstances"—to which I already alluded in terms not very precise and which need to be made more explicit. Lindemann Nelson (2001, p. 62) stated that the "we" that we often find in discussions of this issue can refer to very different people. People might have quite diverse narrative options. There are many individuals and communities in our societies—refugees, migrants, and other ethnically marginalized and economically disadvantaged people, as well as persons with chronic illnesses, injuries, and disabilities—whose storytelling options (including Randall and McKim's "literary competence") are more restricted than those of narrative agents with, say, a well-established educational and professional profile. Clearly, the professional profile tends to lend itself to linear and rounded autobiographical genres such as the *Bildungsroman* and to the storytelling skills necessary for them. I have previously discussed this aspect of narrative identity in terms of narrative agency, a term that refers to narrative as a form of action, which is understood as constitutive of subjectivity. "Narrative agency" puts the accent on a slightly different aspect than the kind of agency I attributed to narrative imagination, which I characterized, in Chapter 4, as a way of exploring possible actions (or action possibilities) carried out in the subjunctive. In foregrounding the constructive and imaginative qualities of narrative, Chapter 4 was meant to expose the world-creating qualities of narrative—which was the point of the "strong narrative thesis." Yet this is just one form of narrative agency that, on the whole, has a wider and more fundamental scope. It can be described both with respect to specific linguistic options of narrative (such as endowing characters in storyworlds with different forms and degrees of agency), and with respect to how a storytelling subject can agentially position itself, which is particularly interesting in acts of narrative self-construction (cf. Bamberg, 2005, p. 10).

What has made the narrative approach to identity so compelling, notes Andreea Ritivoi (2009) in view of this agentive charge, is that it foregrounds potential acts of empowerment. The focus on narrative as a social practice turns people into protagonists—including oppressed, marginalized, and disadvantaged people who often have their rights and voices denied. For Eakin (2008), autobiographical narrative is always an act of self-determination, no matter what the circumstances. It thus is no coincidence that an abundance of contemporary novels in many languages reflect and indeed demonstrate peoples' ability to resist regimes of power, whether through real or imagined political action and subversion or through linguistic transformation of ruling narratives and the power relations in which they are embedded. How does this relate to one's identity? Taking a narrative stance empowers the individual, writes Ritivoi, because "it affords her the ability to control her identity—by choosing strategically which events get recounted and how—through the story she tells" (2008, p. 27). Narrative, as Lewis and Sandra Hinchman (1997) put the matter, "emphasizes the active, self-shaping quality of human thought, the power of stories to create and refashion personal identity" (p. xiv). And it does so, in De Fina and Georgakopoulou's (2012) words, by agentially "conjur[ing] up a double world": the "taleworld" of the told narrative and the "storytelling world" of the telling and the narrative event (p. 79). This power is particularly manifest whenever people turn into social and political protagonists, when they "become participants in their own history," as Molly Andrews (2007) points out, drawing on case studies on the political nature of personal identity narratives. Andrews's studies are based on narrative interviews with political activists in England, the United States, the former East Germany, and South Africa, with people "who have consciously engaged with the key political movements of their day and who have tried to help shape the future of the societies in which they live" (2007, p. 206).

It is interesting to see that the stories told by these activists assume a specific understanding of what narrative is and how it works. For most of them, narrative is first of all a mode of acting and interacting, of doing things. All see their storytelling as a form of life in the strong Wittgensteinian meaning of the term; it is realized as an option of action. One could object that Andrews's participants were special people, and this certainly is true. All of them were experienced and eloquent political activists. They knew a thing or two about political commitment and personal agency, and they knew how to tell moving stories. But does this mean that the view of narrative and narrative agency as a form of life is limited to activists and their life stories?

Of course not. As we investigated the stories of Ann, a girl with Fragile X, a genetic disorder leading to various intellectual disabilities, Maria Medved and I observed that there are various nuances of narrative agency (Medved & Brockmeier, 2004; 2015). Fragmented, syncopated, and unimposing, the stories Ann told were no doubt quite different from the stories of the political activists. Sometimes they were only hinted at, inviting us to fill in small and big gaps imaginatively or, perhaps, just accept their enigmatic quality. Still, they were clearly told as acts of agency and empowerment, enabling this girl to give herself the contour *she* wants, or at least hopes for, not least by choosing which events got recounted and how. This also was the case when Ann's stories merely projected elements from a fantasy or fairytale world into a bleak story from her own life, as in this one about her family, the narrative arrangement of which is reminiscent of the fairy tale format of Cinderella:

> I had to cook, clean, and vacuum while they are all sitting around the house. My step-mom, she's nasty, a rotten mood. When I was there, I did *all* the house-work. . . . [But] a nice person will make things better. Will help out. Everything will be fine. . . . My sister's doing nothing. The bags are heavy, it's not fair. . . . My dad to scream at me. . . . (3 seconds pause) Then a nice person will come and make things good. (Medved & Brockmeier, 2004, p. 751)

Even such a mingling of storylines from various genres that gives shape to a long-wished-for turning point in one's own life—be it only one's imaginative storylife—opens a space for an agentive protagonist-narrator who envisions her life in a different, brighter light. In contrast to the highly audible life stories told by Andrews's activists, the stories of this girl need, however, a special effort to make themselves heard, both by their teller and listener. In fact, they need a different, cooperative practice of storytelling in which both teller and listener actively engage in a joint narrative effort. Moreover, these stories need a different, interactive conception of narrative, an understanding that defies traditional definitions. Without this conception, many of Ann's stories would not even be recognizable. The traditional concept of narrative as a disembodied account given by an individual that provides an interviewer/researcher with information about an interviewee—typical for much research in psychology, the social sciences, and medicine—focuses the investigative framework on the isolated utterances of an individual and thus fails to recognize forms of interactional narrative performances as well as the involved moves of agency and empowerment (Medved & Brockmeier, 2010).[2]

Taking an agentive perspective on narrative as an interactive and cultural practice also throws new light on what Lindemann Nelson calls *counterstories*. Counterstories are narrative redefinitions of people that permit them to "refuse the identities imposed on them by their oppressors and to reidentify themselves in more respectworthy terms" (Lindemann Nelson, 2001, p. 22). Such stories do not necessarily have to be explicitly directed against other stories that they defy.

Sklar (2012) makes the case that graphic life stories of individuals with intellectual disabilities (as he calls them), told from a first-person perspective, already by their sheer existence constitute counterstories, because these individuals have for long been considered to be unable to tell their own stories at all. That the study of narrative identity can help us understand these and, in principle, all human individuals as agents of their identity might also explain why this approach has been particularly attractive to theorists, researchers, and activists "interested in rescuing agency as a category of analysis and in documenting individuals' efforts to control the representations in which their experiences are featured" (Ritivoi, 2008, p. 27).

The autobiographical focus

One feature of the picture of narrative identity that emerges in the work of Lindemann Nelson, Ritivoi, and other researchers (such as Bamberg, 2012; De Fina, Schiffrin, & Bamberg, 2006; Hyvärinen, Hydén, Saarenheimo, & Tamboukou, 2010) is that it shows no contours of a coherent and continuous self but quite the contrary: an unstable scenario of tensions, contradictions, struggle, and negotiations—a "messy self," as it has been experienced and described by many writers and literary scholars since the early 20th century (Rosner, 2007).

An essential part of the messy scenarios of self and identity is provided, to be sure, by autobiographical memories. Although I consider a number of further factors and contexts relevant for this de-unified and unpacified view of identity, it is particularly the autobiographical dimension that I want to bring into sharper focus. Despite my longstanding interest in the various dimensions and aspects involved in the dynamic of narrative identity, it has taken me some time to realize that what I tried to make sense of was, however, not the relationship between "identity" and "memory" but the autobiographical process and its interpretive and creative interplay with people's narrative constructions of themselves. This may seem an insignificant conceptual shift, yet it gives this book an orientation quite different from other approaches (and from my own earlier drafts) centering on memory and identity.

I have thus come to see my project as an attempt to understand this interplay in terms of a narrative hermeneutics.[3] The interpretive-hermeneutic notion of narrative identity implied here is based on a twofold assumption: neither our understanding of who we are nor our very existence in a cultural world can be separated from the stories that we and others tell about ourselves. In making sense of ourselves we do not start with events, experiences, memories, or what we take to be facts of our lives as a "given" and then construe narratives around them; any more than we start with a pure sensory or bodily given, which we then go on to represent conceptually. We start with a story, or more precisely, with a number of stories, or fragments or traces of stories because we are born into, grow up, and live in the midst of a world of narratives that—a point noted before—for the most part are not our own. In this world, an event, experience, memory, or a fact can only be understood as a segment cut out of a narrative web, a web that would exist even without my actively being involved in weaving it.[4]

The stories we tell mingle in countless ways with other stories, which they take up, continue, imitate, vary, criticize, repudiate, in serious and playful ways. As a consequence, we and our lives are more and more *verstrickt*, entangled, in stories and the storyworlds to which they belong. A first version of this vision was set out by phenomenologist Wilhelm Schapp, a student of Edmund Husserl, in his 1954 book *Verstrickt in Geschichten: Zum Sein von Mensch und Ding* (Entangled in stories: On the being of person and thing). What Schapp dubbed *verstrickt*, Ricoeur called mediated. Irrespective of terminology, the point I am interested in is that the idea of a "kind of identity that human beings acquire through the mediation of the narrative function" (Ricoeur, 1991b, p. 188) intersects with that of the autobiographical process, a process that is likewise mediated through the "narrative function." Whereas the point of critical distinction for the notion of narrative identity is the traditional concept of identity and the history of discussions that shaped it, for the notion of the autobiographical process this critical point of reference is the traditional idea of memory. Narrative identity relates critically to "identity" in much the same way as the autobiographical process relates critically to "autobiographical memory."

Obviously my interest in the autobiographical dimension of narrative identity comes with a particular perspective of which I have sketched so far mainly some philosophical implications. More empirically inclined researchers, therefore, might regard the emerging picture as altogether too vague. How does this perspective relate to, for instance, research investigating the interactional and discursive microdynamic of identity discourses and performances? Moreover, social constructivist authors would reject the whole idea of individual identity construction as perpetuating traditional substantialist and individualist ideas. I thus want to take a brief look at an important approach in this area that helps me characterize my perspective in relation to other, empirical researchers in the field.

There surely is a lot of overlap between the work of Alexandra Georgakopoulou (2007) on narrative identity and the argument I have been advancing. Georgakopoulou is one of the leading researchers in the relatively new field of sociolinguistically based narrative identity studies.[5] The focus in this field is on short narrative sequences that occur in everyday conversational contexts. These "narratives-in-interaction" are considered to be the locus where identities are worked up, take shape, and are practiced. Such "small stories," the criticism is, have been neglected by traditional identity research, which privileged "big stories," of which one example is autobiographical narratives. Understanding narrative identity by investigating it as unfolding in "interactional sites" harks back to Erving Goffman's studies on situated communicative interaction. Goffman (1981) was interested in how people present themselves to others and to themselves, something he called "footing." Reformulated by Georgakopoulou (2007) in a discursive framework, this interest draws attention to narrative identity formation not only as something that takes place within the stories people tell about themselves, but also as something that emerges in the way these stories are told and performed. That is to say, it is the act and action of telling short and often fragmented stories that gives space to manifold forms of social presentations and enactments of one's identity.

For Goffman, everyday life is a stage. On this stage, social actors perform their identities in a myriad of social interactions and face-to-face communications. Now Georgakopoulou makes the case—convincingly, to my mind—that Goffman's (1969) view of life and identity as theatrical performance also affords a more comprehensive approach to the study of the intersubjective nature of narrative identity. The question is how the dramas on this stage shape the structure of our personal stories and, in this way, our selves. With this question in mind, Georgakopoulou (2007, p. 16), drawing on Schiffrin (1990), outlines a differentiated approach to narrative and identity that takes Goffman's studies on the self as story-telling performer one step further. On this account, narrative identity is composed by performances on several levels. One is that of an *animator,* which is the aspect of a person that physically produces talk. A second one is that of an *author,* which is the aspect of a person responsible for the content of talk. Then there is the level of the *figure,* which is the main character in the story told, a character who belongs to the world that is spoken about and not the world in which the speaking occurs. Finally, there is the *principal,* the self of the narrator as established by and committed to what is said. Using these multiple narrative registers of self-presentation, Georgakopoulou writes, storytellers create a "kaleidoscope of selves" through which they "can diffuse their agency or responsibility in the social field, create a widened base of support for their views and beliefs, or, generally, cast positive light on them" (2007, p. 16).

Building on this model, Georgakopoulou's analyses of the organization of narrative in interaction (e.g., turn-taking, turn design, sequence organization) offer important insights into the social dynamic of people's narrative management of the "kaleidoscope of their selves." Georgakopoulou appears, however, not to be particularly interested in the role personal remembering and autobiographical memories play in this kaleidoscopo; in her entire book, both concepts go unmentioned. Nor does she pay any attention to the interpretative interplay between autobiographical memories and people's identity projects, a dynamic that is after all inextricably individual and social, psychological and discursive; it thus, we might think, would well be a part of her project.

Apparently, the sociolinguistic concern with the sequential organization of conversational narratives and with "situational identities" based on the role of storytellers in a specific local configuration of turn-taking leaves some things beyond the field of vision. For instance, what are called "larger identities"—identities that, we may assume, comprise autobiographical memories—only come into view insofar as they "are made visible by and inform local telling roles" (Georgakopoulou, 2007, p. 90). It is, of course, not unusual that different disciplinary protocols entail different "local telling roles" for academic inquiries, even if the subject—narrative identity—is the same. So the sociolinguistic focus on the here-and-now configuration of storytelling and the "local management" of the conversational dynamic of talk surely suggests a different approach to narrative identity than the point of view I have brought to bear in these chapters based on assumptions of narrative psychology and hermeneutics. Identifying narrative and discourse identities as "one of the components of the conversational machinery that circumscribe and make salient the participants' larger social identities" (p. 89) foregrounds a take of identity formation that sets other priorities than an approach that tries to deconstruct the Western notion of autobiographical identity by exploring the narrative-interpretive fabric of the autobiographical process. Still it is hard to see why a discourse based approach to narrative identity could not, in principle (and this includes epistemological and hermeneutic principles), be able to account for people's autobiographical memories and thus for their larger identities. Granted, these resources are what sociolinguists call "extra-situational." They reach far beyond the here and now of sequential turn-taking and "conversational machineries"; they are grounded in people's entire lives, in their experiences present and past (that is, their memories), the experiences of others, and cultural models of meaning-making and narrative self-making. Nevertheless, they are the stuff our identities are made of, and I find it difficult to see why a discursive approach to narrative identity should ignore it.

Consider the narrative dynamic of the autobiographical process that constitutively extends to both the storyworld and the storytelling event, or the "taleworld" of the told narrative and the "storytelling world" (De Fina & Georgakopoulou, 2012, p. 79). Understanding both as intrinsically linked is a central concern of the discursive orientation. More than this, the autobiographical process involves Goffman's entire identity repertoire of storytelling "animator," "author," "figure," and "principal." Why then, we might wonder, should the discourse-based study of identity exclude this complex dynamic? Why should it omit the mnemonic dimension of identity discourse, why "large identities" and their autobiographical grounding, which seem to be a crucial dimension of Western identity discourses? Why should it solely be concerned with the conversational dynamic of short interactional sequences, of micro-stories or "small stories," and discount the discursive reality of human remembering and forgetting which, it is true, oftentimes takes place in extended, complicated, autobiographical stories? Why should we not rather investigate the entire, broad range of narrative endeavors in which individuals engage to make sense of themselves?[6] I believe, in fact, that these endeavors can only be adequately understood if explored in the light of the discursive and interactional dynamic that Georgakopoulou and her colleagues have so compellingly given center stage.

A last consideration. Without unraveling the narrative-discursive nature and dynamic of autobiographical memories it might ultimately remain unavoidable to see them as "just being there," emerging from the mysterious depths of our inner archives. As if there were somehow or other airy entities that suddenly surface, providing the raw material for discursive moves, conversational interactions, and reflexive elaborations in the form of autobiographical stories. Yet from where do these memories surface? From what regions of human discourse (or mind or brain) do they arise? And what do we mean if we call them "memories"? If there is no specific explanation, what commonly holds is the basic assumption of Western discourse, the "world knowledge" of autobiographical memory as storage of the past.

Three problems of autobiographical identity

Because I already reviewed the idea of *memory* in the first chapters, my goal now is the concept of *identity*. To this end, I take up Ricoeur's point that every concept of narrative identity has to be measured against how it resolves the problems of traditional concepts of identity. For Ricoeur, a "convincing plea can be made in favor of narrative identity if it can be shown that this notion, and the experience that it designates, contribute to the resolution of the difficulties relative to personal identity" (1991c, p. 73).[7] So what are these difficulties? In my view, there are three basic problems underlying traditional theories of the relationship between identity and autobiographical memory. The first one, already mentioned, is the longstanding metaphysics of a stable and substantial self. Some have traced back this metaphysics to the religious notion of the soul (Hacking, 1995; Taylor, 1989). Assigning temporal and substantial permanence to the self turns it into some immutable substratum, argues Ricoeur (1991b), who recognizes here one of the main dilemmas of established concepts of identity.

Indeed, this legacy continues to have an impact on important aspects of present discussions in several disciplines. In the first place, we might think of modern psychology, on which the metaphysical assumptions of selfhood have had a strong influence from the beginning, as we know among others from Danziger's (1990a; 2008) studies. Yet these assumptions also have shaped modern autobiographical writing and thinking far beyond academic psychology. For the most part—that is, before the 1970s and 1980s—this has resulted in the view of autobiographical subjectivity as the truthful recording of accumulated individual life events, outlining autobiography as a subcategory of traditional biography. This "*bios* bias" (Watson, 1993) of both autobiographical writing and criticism is complemented by the idea of life and identity of certain people "worth" living and recounting. In the first place, these were great male, white, European or European-oriented individuals who, in the act of autobiography, would take stock and engage in retrospective reflection in order to account for how this greatness was achieved (Watson, 1993, p. 59). Thus, *bios*-centered genres of autobiography unavoidably display the structure of a retrospective teleology, that is, a putative goal-directedness of life that only becomes visible in hindsight, suggesting, however, the more or less intentional development of an early given self or proto-identity (Brockmeier, 2001b). Accordingly, an autobiographical or biographical account means to trace back how the inherent goal of a life—the self-resolution in the narrative present—was reached.

Building on the principles of 19th-century *Lebensphilosophie* (philosophy of life) as formulated by philosopher Wilhelm Dilthey, theorists of autobiographical identity like Georg Misch celebrated this privileged way of self-construction as one of the highest achievements of Western thinking about human life and identity precisely for its fidelity to the truthful representation of a life and the orientation toward the metaphysical idea of a self-substratum underlying the vicissitudes and contingencies of lived life. Misch's *Geschichte der Autobiographie* (History of autobiography) was published from 1907 to 1969 in eight volumes, covering the autobiographical literature of Antiquity, Middle Ages, Renaissance, and Modern Times until the 19th century (Misch, 1985).[8] On this account, the canon of great Western autobiographical works represented the universal and timeless benchmark of identity construction, enshrining the autonomous and sovereign Western individual as an all but transcendent ideal. As Georges Gusdorf (1980) put it, "Memoirs look to an essence beyond existence, and in manifesting it they serve to create it" (p. 47).[9]

Although the modern metaphysics of the autobiographical self has always had its critics—beginning with Montaigne—the last few decades have seen it rejected by most theorists of identity and autobiography, as Sidonie Smith and Julia Watson's (2010) comprehensive review demonstrates. The repudiation of this metaphysics is indeed constitutive for several 20th-century research currents on self and identity that have developed along the lines of pragmatism, social constructivism, deconstructionism, dialogical and discursive theories, and cultural studies. Smith and Watson (2010, p. 194) point out that a further aspect of the decline of the metaphysical model of autobiography might have been its historical use as a master narrative epitomizing not only what has been described as the formation of the accomplished subjectivity of "Western Man" (e.g., Mascuch, 1996), but also of the superiority of Western rationality and civilization. For many critics and theorists of the autobiographical self today, this view is not just limited and distorting; it is a construct of outdated propaganda. As Smith and Watson summarize:

> The focus on self-referential narratives of autonomous individuality and representative lives narrowed the range of vision to the West. That focus also privileged "high" cultural forms, a focus that obscured the vast production of life narratives by ex-slaves, apprentices and tradespeople, adventurers, criminals and tricksters, saints and mystics, immigrants. ... The gendering of the representative life as universal and therefore masculine meant that narratives by women were rarely examined. ... But if we recall the diverse modes of life narrating by marginalized, minoritized, diasporic, nomadic, and postcolonial

subjects throughout the history of life writing, the focus on liberal individuality as both the motive and achievement of autobiographical writing is insuf-
ficient as a determining force. (2010; p. 203)

Besides the metaphysics of autobiographical identity, there is a second fundamental problem of traditional theories. This is the circularity
of identity and memory. This circularity stems from the assumption that
identity's claim to continuity is grounded in autobiographical memory
while autobiographical remembering is predicated on the existence of
a self whose identity is based on its temporal permanence. I have outlined one of the early attempts to question this odd circularity by Samuel
Beckett in Chapter 2 (*Beckett's Memory*). If we take Beckett's objection
seriously, we are no longer able to think of identity and the self as timelessly encapsulated in one's autobiographical past. I have tried to elaborate
the consequences of this view of autobiographical identity over the course
of the previous chapters, emphasizing particularly its always emergent
gestalt, its character as an ongoing undertaking, an interminable poetic
work. Rather than being simply the result of past experiences, identity,
viewed in this light, appears as an inherently unstable and protean project, constantly synthesizing past and present, memories and their interpretation, recollection and imagination.

The third key problem of the traditional approach to identity and autobiographical memory is the assumption of memory as storage. Given that
I discussed the archival model in the first three chapters, I do not have
to repeat it here; instead, I want to consider what comes to the fore if we
bring together all three problems on one canvas. The outcome is the presupposition that one's personal identity is *grounded* in one's autobiographical memory.

JOHN LOCKE'S IDENTITY

The idea that autobiographical memory is foundational for human identity
has played a crucial role in the modern Western tradition. This is especially
manifest in the "identity disciplines" philosophy, psychology, psychiatry,
and the social sciences, but also in many quarters in the humanities as well
as in literature and the arts. It is hardly an exaggeration to say that viewing autobiographical memory as the basis of self understanding has been
the royal road to personal identity in modern times. Some elements of this
view can be traced back to early writers like Augustine and Montaigne,
but the proposition was authoritatively formulated in the 17th century, by

John Locke. The influential English philosopher and physician is not only the patron saint of modern empiricism but also of modern autobiographical theorizing. He has promoted the commonsensical world knowledge of autobiographical memory to a noble intellectual construct.

Locke's theory of mind is considered to be the first conception to conceive of the self as resulting from the continuity of one's consciousness. Repudiating both the soul and the body as anchorage for the self, Locke maintained that one has no other way to establish one's identity as a person than by one's personal memories of oneself: that I am identical with what I can remember about my past. In Book 2, Chapter 27, of *An Essay Concerning Human Understanding*, published in 1689, Locke claimed that I am identical with anything I am conscious of, which includes anything I can remember. More precisely, then, the identity of a person is grounded in his or her existence as a "a thinking, intelligent being, that has reason and reflection, and can consider itself as itself, the same thinking thing, in different times and places" (Locke, 2008, II, xxvii, 9.). That means, ultimately, that I am a person only to the extent that I can relate to—that is, recall—my own distinctive past. My identity, thus, is the result of repeated acts of autobiographical self-identification.

To some, this might be the typical view of a philosopher, abstract and aloof, if it did not smack of debates in drafty 17th-century English castles and colleges. But, as already indicated, the Lockean proposition has had an amazingly enduring career, and this not only within philosophy, where it has been ardently defended by established contemporary philosophers like Darek Parfit (1984) and Galen Strawson (2011). It also has been highly influential within neighboring disciplines like psychology and neuroscience, where it became the explicit or implicit axiom of identity research, as well as in everyday discourses on what makes one the same person at different times. It even has shaped the psychiatric understanding and neuropsychological diagnostics of people with memory and identity troubles, for example, as a consequence of dementia (Matthews, 2006; Brockmeier, 2014).

On a more generic plane, the Lockean perspective has cemented the individualist focus both on identity and the mind/brain as a self-evident axiom of psychological memory research. Take, for example, Tulving's notion of the autobiographical grounding of the self through "autonoetic consciousness," a notion, already pointed out before, that has been influential in several areas of contemporary neuroscience (Tulving & Kim, 2009). Connecting consciousness and (episodic) memory, it makes a strong Lockean case. Autonoetic consciousness or self-knowing is the name Tulving has given "to the kind of consciousness that mediates an individual's awareness of his or her existence and identity in subjective time extending from the personal past through the present to the personal future" (1985b, p. 1). At stake, then, is the awareness of one's continuity in time—something that Tulving (2002b) later came to call time travel—and one's consciousness of this awareness. The Lockean flavor is likewise conspicuous in many explicit conceptions of personal identity. That autobiographical memories are essential for the formation of an individual self and "form the core of personal identity" (Schacter, 1996, p. 93), that they are "crucial for a sense of identity, continuity, and direction in life" (Bernsten & Rubin, 2012, p. 1), that "we are what we remember" (Wilson & Ross, 2003, p. 137)—to quote just a few but representative researchers—is a common, if not the common view in standard psychological textbooks as well as in an extended research literature. It also applies to the developmental psychology of autobiographical memory (e.g., Bauer, 2007; Fitzgerald & Broadbridge, 2012; Habermas, 2011).

This is not to deny that in the wide-ranging multidisciplinary literature on identity there have also been differing and alternative concepts. In philosophical terms, notably Hegel and other theorists of subjectivity in his wake have foregrounded dimensions absent in the Lockean tradition, such as the intersubjective, social, and historical. Hegel's philosophy unfolded a vision of the world in which mind, culture, and history are inseparable. Twentieth-century phenomenologists like Maurice Merleau-Ponty emphasized the bodily or embodied nature of human identity and subjectivity. There also has been strong emphasis on the process-oriented and dynamic dimension of identity formation, what Hegel called its dialectic nature. More recently, many scholars and researchers exploring the cultural, political, discursive, and symbolically mediated nature of human identity have come to view it as an open and unpredictable process; some of them have already been mentioned. Overall in these discussions, we can observe a shift of interest: from a predominant interest in the individual mind and consciousness to one in a person's social and cultural being, their actions, interactions, and forms of life. Having said this, it is, however, perplexing that when it comes to the relationship between identity and autobiographical memory, many of these authors nevertheless continue to share the Lockean assumption. I will give a few examples of this astonishing perseverance in a moment; but first let me sketch, from a more general perspective, the identity scenarios in which autobiographical memory typically takes center stage in the modern Western tradition.

Where and why does autobiographical remembering matter for identity? It matters whenever there is an understanding or sense of personal identity that is to meet two criteria. One is that it is established by a subject from a first-person perspective with respect to himself or herself. Hence sometimes called reflexive or, as in my discussion, interpretive, there are many labels for it, such as self-concept, self-awareness, self-consciousness, or self-identity. The other criterion is that this self-understanding relates to a process in time. As already noted, it relates to at least two different temporal moments to bring about a consciousness or a sense of continuity. Classical Western identity theory takes it that normal human beings have a sense of themselves as temporally persisting, a feeling of continuity or sameness—sometimes to a stronger, sometimes to a lesser degree. Anthony Giddens, for example, summarized it this way: "A person with a reasonable stable sense of self-identity has a feeling of biographic continuity which she is able to grasp reflexively and ... communicate to other people" (1991, p. 54). Accordingly, identity is a figure against a ground of instability, a figure that might be conceived of—or, in Giddens's words, "grasped reflexively"—as that part (or ensemble of characteristics, themes, or stories) of ourselves that appears to maintain a certain degree of sameness even if other things change. On this account, the autobiographical perspective fuses two psychologically and socially intricate constructions, time and identity (Brockmeier, 2001c; 2001d).

What distinguishes Giddens's approach from those of other social scientists and social philosophers is that he attributes such fusion of time (that is, continuity) and identity (that is, self-construction) to the work of narrative, with autobiographical narrative playing a central role. "A person's identity," as he writes, "is not to be found in behavior, nor—important though it is—in the reactions of others, but in the capacity *to keep a particular narrative going*" (Giddens, 1991, p. 54; original emphasis). Giddens further qualifies this narrative in saying that "the individual's biography, if she is to maintain regular interaction with others in the day-to-day world, cannot be wholly fictive. It must continually integrate events which occur in the external world, and sort them into the ongoing 'story' about the self" (1991, p. 54). Giddens draws on Taylor's argument that "in order to have a sense of who we are, we have to have a notion of how we have become, and of where we are going" (1989, p. 47).

It does not come as a surprise in this context that both Giddens and Taylor build on the Lockean premise that the notion of how we have become is based on our autobiographical memories or, more precisely, on a chain of such memories, a chain that, as Giddens and Taylor allow, also can be a narrative one. Again, there is a wide gamut of possible positions. What for Giddens and Taylor may be narrative, is for many scholars of autobiography and life writing inevitably narrative. For Eakin, to name just one, the impulse to write autobiography is "a special heightened form" of the self-reflexive consciousness, which he views as "the distinctive feature of human nature" (1985, p. 9).

Ricoeur has called this *ipse*-identity, or selfhood identity, distinguishing it from *idem*-identity which refers to the sameness of an individual viewed from an "objectifying" third-person perspective (Ricoeur, 1992). *Ipse*-identity, then, is the construct or the sense of one's self in time, and this construct or sense—according to the Lockean proposition—cannot but rely on one's autobiographical memory.[10] This vision has not significantly changed with the arrival of some new players in town. These are the neurosciences, on the one hand, and narrative, discursive, cultural, and sociocultural approaches on the other. Locke's ongoing impact is all the more odd given that these new players have entered the game with the declared intent to overcome traditional shortcomings. As I have reviewed the neuroscientific approach in the first two chapters, I concentrate in this chapter on one of the new developments in the other field, the narrative approach. To highlight what I take to be its essential features I want to distinguish three different, though interconnected claims associated with the concept of narrative identity before I, a bit later, return to the question why the Lockean view has been so influential, in fact dominating modern understanding of the identity-memory nexus.

Narrative identity: Interpretive, subjunctive, and performative claims

All three claims aim to replace substantialist and essentialist conceptions of self and identity, thus trying to resolve one of the traditional problems of identity just described. The first claim, as we remember, is that it is through stories that we make sense of ourselves and others, of our being in the world; this is the *hermeneutic* or *interpretive claim*. The second claim is that it is through these stories that we not only give shape to who we are and believe to be, but also envision what we will and want to be, how we want to be seen, and what we could have been. This is the *subjunctive* or *explorative claim*. It draws on another assumption already discussed: that narrative, as a form and practice of agency, enables us to explore the horizon of our options of action. The third claim is that it is through discursive practices of narrative, through narrative interaction, that we perform our identities in a social arena; this is the *performative* or *intersubjective claim*. In contrast with the hermeneutic or interpretive claim and the subjunctive or explorative claim, this third claim has not been outlined yet; hence a few words are in order.

As has been shown in an extensive sociolinguistic and discursive literature (some of which is referred to above), narratives in the social arena are only rarely fully blown stories. Typically, they occur in random, short, and fractured conversational form. In contrast with what many textbooks on methods and methodology in the social sciences, psychology, education, and the health sciences have posited, few stories unfold in a sequential way following a clear beginning, middle, and end. Most everyday stories are told in casual situations and fluid narrative environments. And these narrative environments do not lack diversity; they range from spontaneous encounters in the family, workplace, and school, to more institutionalized cultural settings such as the talk show or similar formats of public self-presentations, the therapeutic session, or religious confession. I mentioned above Smith and Watson (2010) who have distinguished 60 different genres of life writing.

Yet, that is not all. Not only are there told, written, and recorded autobiographies, diaries, and other self-documents across a variety of performative storytelling media, including drama, dance, film, TV, and video. There also are specific digitally mediated multimedia and multimodal environments in which narrative identities take shape: social networks, web platforms, personal websites, blogs, lifelogs, and the like constitute important venues of self-presentation and self-reflection. Whether we are aware of it or not, we present ourselves not only in multiple narrative gestalts and themes but also in the full panoply of narrative media and modes. We do so because we take pleasure in performing and talking about ourselves, some to a larger, some to a lesser extent.

We also engage in culturally offered options of autobiographical self-explorations because we live in a world suffused with the assumption that we have to establish our autobiographical identity because we do not already know who we are, to recall this thought by Taylor (1989). In fact, we all have been raised in what has been described, in the wake of Folkenflik's (1993) apt formula, as a "culture of autobiography." Unavoidably, we have grown deeply familiar with the prevailing gamut of self-resolution. As we have learned from early on to navigate through a multitude of identity stories, we swim in these stories like fish in water. They are our element. Telling them is our most important autobiographical practice.

The idea of narrative identity associated with interpretive, subjunctive, and performative claims has established itself in a field of like-minded approaches that draw attention to the sociocultural variability of both narrative and identity. Using slightly different vocabularies, they all highlight the dialogical, discursive, and cultural nature of human identity. There are ideas from philosophical pragmatism, Vygotskian, and ethnographic traditions that loom large in this literature. And yet, amazingly enough, under close scrutiny many of these approaches prove to continue the Lockean notion of autobiographical identity, even if they seek to advance theoretical trajectories that are quite different from the individual-centered assumptions underlying this notion.

It is fair to say that the concept of autobiographical memories has not remained unchanged in the hermeneutic and constructivist light of many of these approaches. Memories, in this literature, are often viewed as selected, reconstructed, and reconfigured in the process of their narrativization; they can be related to wrong sources or invented contexts of origin and then adapted when integrated into the plot of one's identity or transformed into the many more or less spontaneous stories permeating our lives and minds. Indeed, as we saw in the last chapters, the perception that memories in the process of their recall are interpreted, reconstructed, and substantially modified, to the degree of distortion and falsification, is compatible with much of contemporary cognitive and neurocognitive psychology and brain research.

However, my point here is that one presupposition has survived unaltered both in traditional and alternative approaches, indicating that, in this area, the cultural paradigm shift in our understanding of memory is a multilayered, in fact, contradictory and heterochronous transformation. This presupposition is the archival premise, the assumption that autobiographical memories ultimately are encoded, stored, and retrieved. The only way to conceive of their reappearing is as arising from the depths of one's mind (or brain or unconscious) from where they provide us with what Freud called the raw material of our identity projects, irrespective of whether these projects are understood in psychoanalytic, cognitive, and neurocognitive terms, or in narrative, discursive, or sociocultural terms. To get a better sense of how, on this account, autobiographical memories are meant to surface from the storage of our minds and brains to be reconstructed, transformed, and inserted into our narrative identity constructions, I want to shift again to psychology and neuroscience and the way this emergence is pictured here.

NEUROCOGNITION OR NARRATIVE: WHAT IS THE EPIPHENOMENON?

When we examine how the relationship between autobiographical memories and narrative is understood in cognitive psychology and neuroscience, we find two principal ways in which memories surface. In the first, they arise at one point, either voluntarily or involuntarily, and it becomes the job of narrative to articulate and perhaps make sense of them. In the second, they are elicited and used strategically, either under experimental conditions or in conversations as part of discursive actions (such as the positioning of oneself or others, or to make a point or challenge one made by someone else). Accordingly, a large portion of studies about self and identity assume narrative discourse as something that either *represents* autobiographical memories or is *imposed* upon them in order to structure, elaborate, and articulate them.

Consider a few representative examples from this literature. One of the first contemporary experimental memory psychologists to address the role of narrative is David Rubin, whose significance in establishing an independent field of psychological research on autobiographical memory I pointed out in Chapter 1. For Rubin it appears obvious that autobiographical memories are usually recalled as narrative and that "language and especially narrative structure are necessary components of autobiographical memory" (1998, p. 53; see also Rubin & Greenberg, 2003). Not so clear, however, is what is meant by "narrative structure" and "autobiographical memory." As already noted, Rubin conceives of complex everyday autobiographical memories as multimodal; that is, they involve visual, auditory, olfactory, tactile, and other sense-specific memory systems, as well as a narrative and language. Within this framework, each modality is related to separate memory systems "that process and store each of these forms of information"; although every memory system encodes, stores, and retrieves information according to its own dynamic, it is the narrative system that "integrates the memory into the life story" (Rubin, 2005, p. 79). In order to become autobiographical, an event needs "a narrative context in which this event is embedded and which helps you understand and share with others ... [its] significance" (Rubin, 2012, p. 11). An example of narrative context is a "cultural life script," which can give location and structure to an emerging autobiographical memory (Berntsen & Rubin, 2004, 2012b). Like many psychological memory researchers, Rubin tends to qualify all aspects of memory—irrespective of their biological, mental, social, cultural, or categorical status—in terms of "systems." Narrative, thus, appears as one of many subsystems of an overarching system Rubin calls the "basic systems model" of autobiographical memory (Rubin, 2000; 2006; 2012). Within this systems model, the narrative subsystem helps organize our recollection, but the recollections as such, associated with sense-specific modalities, are non-narrative or pre-narrative.

In Rubin's and Berntsen's cognitive (and, in part, neuroscientific) vocabulary, narrative is an epiphenomenon. An epiphenomenon is a secondary phenomenon that derives from a primary phenomenon. The primary phenomenon, in this view, is the universal "cognitive mechanisms" that lie behind or beneath the epiphenomenon. This has been the paradigmatic view in cognitive psychology, formulated early on by Brewer: "The cognitive structure underlying narrative is the mental representation of a series of temporally occurring events that are perceived as having a causal or thematic coherence" (1980, p. 223). In superseding earlier cognitive psychology and its focus on information processing as underlying "memory performance," today's neurocognitive psychology (or cognitive neuroscience) of memory has changed the view of the "underlying structure." Now it is neural networks/systems and other neurobiological substrates.[11] What has not changed is the epiphenomenal status of language and narrative. In this respect, the neuroscientific turn has poured new wine into old bottles.[12]

Rubin, for many years a cognitive psychologist who then also has come to use methods from cognitive neuroscience, summarizes the common supposition of both research fields in defining narrative as an "explicit memory system"—Rubin and Greenberg (2003) speak of a "narrative reasoning system" (p. 57)—that encodes and articulates information from other cognitive and neural systems, which are considered to be "more basic." In giving words to recollections, narrative makes "explicit" what is understood as primarily existing in a (neuro)cognitive mode prior to and independent from narrative. Even if it may be universally agreed in psychological memory studies, as Bauer (2007, p. 28) claims, that "autobiographical memories are *expressed* verbally," this does not exclude that it also is universally (that is in cognitive and neurocognitive memory psychology) agreed that their true nature is nonverbal or preverbal.[13]

Unlike cognitive psychologists and neuroscientists, Dan McAdams tackles the relationship between narrative and memories in the tradition of personality psychology (McAdams, 2008). For him, our self-narratives are personal myths that we tell others and ourselves because we "seek to provide our scattered and often confusing experiences with a sense of coherence by arranging the episodes of our lives into stories" (McAdams, 1993, p. 11). Life story, in this view, represents a comprehensive level of personality that encompasses traits and character features. Bringing together different parts of ourselves, including the remembered past, perceived present, and anticipated future, and integrating all of them into a meaningful and convincing whole, life stories give coherence and stability to our identities.

A typical autobiographical memory in this field of research would include an episode from the past that was stored in memory and gets "disclosed" in, say, the course of a conversation between romantic partners, a memory that is understood as something "he or she has never told the other partner before," which then is narratively "elaborated" according to certain personality traits (McLean, 2008, p. 1694; see also McLean & Pasupathi, 2010; 2011). I think Brian Schiff (2013) has a point in his critical review of this kind of personality psychology when he points out that, despite the use of the same vocabulary of "narrative" and "autobiographical memories," it significantly differs from the interpretative approach to human mind and life as suggested by Bruner's (1990a) narrative psychology.

In developmental psychology, an influential research current has studied the interrelations among narrative, memory, and self, following Vygotsky. Viewing themselves in a Vygotskian tradition, Pillemer and White (1989) have maintained that narrative, as part of the child's acquisition of language, is a means for social development. Interacting with adults, the child learns through narrative to "reinstate" and "represent" memories. Yet if memories are to be reinstated and represented, they must already have been present. In fact, this is Pillemer and White's (1989) assumption, which is shared, as already indicated, by the entire research field: memories exist in a prelinguistic mental state—which is for some purely imagistic—before they are narrativized or, more generally, "activated." According to the standard view,[14] this "activation" is caused by a "memory cue" that leads to the retrieval of some "item of knowledge or information" stored in long-term memory in a kind of passive or dormant state. The "activation then spreads to the representation associated with the cue-activated item and as it spreads it dissipates" (Conway & Loveday, 2010, p. 57). That is, autobiographical knowledge is transformed or translated into different forms or states of representation—from sensory to conceptual and affective representation—with narrative, on this account, being just one further rather downstream form (or system) of memory representation.

It is in this sense that Pillemer (1998) outlines the narrativization of a "pure" memory as just one possible form of representation. Memories can be recalled on various "levels of representation." In what Pillemer calls "personal event memories," he sees first of all a sensory level of representation, which then can be "translated" into words. Thus, "A person who wishes to recount a past trauma must translate nonverbal, affect-laden, sensory images into an understandable, coherent narrative" (1998, p. 22). Again, we are faced with the experiential priority of imagistic memories. And again, somewhat surprisingly in the light of these theoretical assumptions, all examples of "personal event memories" reported by Pillemer are verbal examples; as they are in Fiske and Pillemer's (2006) study on "narrative descriptions" of earliest dream memories. At stake are stories or accounts by people who *talk* about their memories using, among others, linguistic images—from figurative expressions to narrative elaborations of mnemonic imagery.

As pointed out in the previous chapter, mnemonic images in real life are typically entwined with words and stories as well as with all kinds of other mental phenomena such as imagination, dreams, moods, or the feeling of pleasure or pain or anxiety: the full panoply of the mind. Many of Pillemer's participants, in fact, give not only very visual descriptions and narrative accounts of their memories, but also extended interpretations of them; again it seems hard, if not impossible, to separate what is memory and what interpretation. One way, the way I have suggested, is to understand these autobiographical stories as narrative blending of several genres of interpretation. Another way, Pillemer's way, is to conceive of them as cognitive "translation" from an imagistic (or sensory) level of representation to a narrative level. The obvious presupposition of the latter view is that there is an original event or experience, be it imagistic/sensory or purely cognitive—Pillemer (1998) calls it a "momentous event"—that is stored in the mnemonic archive of one's mind or brain.[15]

If we recall that, for Vygotsky, higher psychological processes, including autobiographical remembering, are always sign-mediated and that, on this account, language development is closely intertwined with the development of mind and memory, then this surely is an unexpected conclusion for what is presented as a Vygotskian approach.

No memories in the social world?

Moving back to the social sciences, a similarly surprising finding emerges from research on narrative and the mind within social, sociolinguistic, and ethnographic studies of memory. Here socio-interactional orientations similar to Vygotsky's—which are generally missing in traditional psychological research on autobiographical memory due to its focus on the individual mind and brain[16]—are widespread. Accordingly, the attention shifts from mind and memory to conversation and collaboration, that is, to the discursive and contextual contingencies of communication.

Consider approaches like the ethnographically based research on narrative, communication, and culture initiated by Hyme (1964) and Bauman (1986), Ochs and Capp's (2001) linguistic anthropology of narratives, and Gubrium and Holstein's (2008; 2009; Holstein & Grubrium, 2000; 2011) narrative ethnography. It does not strike me as a coincidence that all these studies deal in one way or another with the formation of narrative identity; nevertheless, the issue of individual autobiographical remembering surfaces only peripherally—if it surfaces at all. I tried to understand this "disinterest" in sociolinguistic and discourse-analytical research on narrative and identity discussion in the work of Georgakopoulou and her colleagues earlier in this chapter. By the same token, Gubrium and Holstein describe their narrative method as "attuned to discursive contours and old-fashioned naturalistic observation," a method that is meant to serve as a "procedure and analysis involving the close scrutiny of circumstances, their actors, and actions in the process of formulating and communicating accounts" (2009, p. 22). The authors go on to explain their interest as social scientists in what they see as external, materialized, and thus observable and recordable talk: "We have found that the internal organization of narratives, while important to understand in its own right, does not tell us much about how stories operate in society" (p. 25).

This indifference, if that is the right word, toward the nexus of narrative and mind seems particularly obvious with respect to people's memories and autobiographical narratives, which are widely excluded from the spectrum of phenomena investigated in this field. And this spectrum is no doubt a broad one, ranging from conversational practices (e.g., sequencing, turn-taking, positioning) and linguistic details (e.g., semantics, grammar, repair, lexis, and phonetic features like pauses, volume, and prosody) to narrative features, whether viewed in the tradition of Labov's structural analysis (as abstract, orientation, turning point, complicating action, and coda) or in a narratological tradition (as plot and storylines, focalization, genres). It might also include the study of stylistic features like metaphors and other figurative expression. Considering the wealth of these aspects of narrative discourse, the lack of any attention to its interplay with the autobiographical process is all the more difficult to understand.

Discursive psychologist Derek Edwards (2005) gives this exclusion a positive twist when he states that we "are not endorsing a treatment of these matters as rooted in psychological processes and explanations, and in fact the main thrust of DP [Discursive Psychology] is to avoid psychological theorizing in favor of analysis based in the pragmatics of social actions" (p. 260). It thus stands to reason that the ethnographic, conversation-, and discourse-analytical protocols of these social science research traditions are tantamount to renouncing the study of psychological processes and states altogether.[17] If psychological processes and the sphere of human subjectivity are considered at all, they appear once more as an epiphenomenon—in this case, however, as epiphenomenon of observable practices of discursive action and interaction.

This leaves our exploration of the narrative dynamic of the interplay between narrative identity and the autobiographical process with a peculiar result: whereas traditional memory psychology conceives of narrative as an epiphenomenon of what is taken to be the proper, that is, neuronal or neurocognitive reality of autobiographical memory systems, social science research reverses this relationship and conceives of personal memories as epiphenomena of what is taken to be the proper, observable reality of narrative discourse and the pragmatics of social action.

The view of remembering, identity, and narrative that I put forward differs from both approaches in that it avoids either form of exclusion. Rather, it embraces both the psychological and narrative dimensions of the autobiographical process, and it does so in such a way that they can be grasped as different aspects of one and the same dynamic. In other words, although I see this dynamic as a psychological one in which emotions play a crucial role, I also consider it to be, at the same time, a discursive and cultural one. I believe it is the particular strength of the combined Vygotskian and Wittgensteinian perspectives underlying my vision of narrative identity and the autobiographical process that they defy the precarious distinction between the individual and the social and allow for a culturally thick notion of both psychological and narrative-discursive processes.

In allotting more significance to the psychological dimension and to the entire sphere of human subjectivity than other narrative and discursive approaches, my project is well aware of the dangers of rectifying psychological ascriptions and projections that Middleton and Edwards warned against (1990b, 1990c; cf. also Middleton & Brown, 2005). These authors stress the problems of what they see as the objectifying vocabulary of traditional memory psychology, especially in its ontological assumptions of underlying cognitive and neural systems and mechanisms. It is in language and discursive interaction, as Edwards (2005, p. 261) writes, that people do "the kinds of things for which psychology has developed a technical vocabulary and explanation." Engaging in everyday talk, individuals often claim that they offer causal explanations of their own or others' behavior and thoughts by using those established psychological concepts—such as "repression," "stored in memory," "attention deficit," and so forth. However, when they say they use psychological concepts, Edwards (2005) goes on to argue, "we mean that this is what they may project themselves as doing, rather than that this is what we theorize them to be doing" (p. 261). What they are doing, as the discursive psychologist maintains, is using a certain vocabulary and applying "psychological" models in conversational moves that might be less about probing one's memories than about the unfolding of an argument.

Yet whereas Edwards refers to technical concepts of traditional memory psychology, I look at a different cultural vocabulary, the vocabulary of narrative, both in its everyday and literary usage. My argument is that this vocabulary is more appropriate to understand the autobiographical process—which, I believe, we *can* explore more thoroughly than conceded by behaviorist and empiricist principles—for narrative is anything but external to the autobiographical process; it is, in fact, constitutive of it.

There is little doubt that the assumption of a gulf between the individual and the social (which is echoed in the assumption of a gulf between different epistemological and methodological principles) continues to dominate the areas of research being reviewed here. Domination, though, is not absolute hegemony. There are a number of profound changes in our cultural understanding of memory and remembering, as pointed out in the first chapters. What this means in this context, I tried to capture in describing the gist of a collection of papers on memory as repudiating, in concrete empirical analyses, the separation of individual or personal remembering from social, collective, or cultural remembering (Brockmeier, 2002b). Against the backdrop of the thick cultural fabric that binds individuals to other individuals and to larger social and historical communities, the idea—not to mention the category—of an isolated and autonomous individual rememberer appears as a surreal fantasy. Many researchers and scholars, therefore, have shifted their attention to the forms of interplay and interaction, of interdependence and fusion between the allegedly separate spheres of the individual and the collective, the private and the public, and the timeless and the historical, offering new comprehensive perspectives (cf., e.g., Bietti, 2011, 2014; Murakami, 2014).[18]

I mentioned several major theoretical traditions that have provided conceptual models for understanding these entanglements. One is pragmatism, with its vision of the intersubjective but nevertheless self-reflective constitution of self and identity, as suggested by George Herbert Mead (1934). In his wake, contemporary theorists of the self have emphasized that the intersubjective formation of narrative identity is not at all incompatible with, but in fact predicated on processes of self-reflection (e.g., Giddens, 1991; Kirschner & Martin, 2010; Straub, 2005). These processes have been described in terms of inner dialogues (or soliloquies) or multiple dialogues with a plurality of I-positions that are active even if someone is silent and alone (e.g., Athens, 1994; Nelson, 1989; Randall & McKim, 2008). As Hermans (2000) states: "Even when we are outwardly silent, we find ourselves communicating with our critics, with our parents, our consciences, our gods, our reflection in the mirror, with the photograph of someone we miss, with a figure from a movie or a dream" (p. 27).

Of course, Bakhtin's (1981; 1986) conception of language as a continuous flow of dialogues and correspondences and the mind as a polyphonic novel looms large in this literature. But the field is not restricted to the mental sphere. Sometimes the inner dialogues overlap with another plurality of openly articulated dialogues. "Self and society," writes Hermans, "both function as a polyphony of consonant and dissonant voices" (2002, p. 148). Opening this perspective toward societal life brings into play even more discursive I-positions, indexing, for example, official roles and social positions. Alessandro Fasulo and Christina Zuccermaglio have shown that in environments like the workplace the pronoun "I" used in self-referential talk serves as "a device to highlight the most official of one's selves" (2002, p. 1119), while other selves or more generic references to the same speaker remain less articulated than the official *social persona* of the speaker.

There should be, however, no misunderstanding: mainstream views in psychology, neuroscience, and biomedicine on the one hand, and in the social sciences on the other, are still a far cry from overcoming the idea of a fundamental separation of these two spheres—the individual, inner, and monological, and the outer, social, and interactional—as questionable as this separation has proven to be. I see the disinterest for autobiographical memories in socio-interactional and discourse-oriented social identity research as a side effect of this division of labor.

All of which leaves us with the question of how researchers and theorists in this field account for the emergence of autobiographical memories, especially of memories that are more extended and elaborated than the transient short memories surfacing in ongoing sequences of talk. The question is all the more justified because evidence abounds to suggest that conversationally maneuvered autobiographical memories play an essential role in many genres of identity discourse. This is a claim not only maintained by theorists of autobiography and life writing in general, but also by some discursive researchers of narrative identity practices (e.g., Fasulo, 2004; Murakamy & Middleton, 2006). As an aside, there are even a few narrative researchers, examining the meaning of auto/biographically crucial events such as life-changing accidents and injuries, who conceive of the discursive-narrative, psycho-emotional, and autobiographical dimensions of peoples' identity as inseparable (e.g., Charon, 2006; Smith & Sparkes, 2008; Sparkes & Smith, 2008)—in the same way in which the "wounded storyteller" (Frank, 1995) is inseparable from the wounded body and the wounded mind, and as storytelling is inseparable from the social and cultural world in which it takes place.

What makes it difficult, however, to engage in a more detailed discussion about the exclusion of the autobiographical in most of the discursive, sociolinguistic, and ethnographic literature is that neither the particular nature of autobiographical memories nor their status in the process of individual identity formation are issues admitted to critical reflection; a point on which Edwards explicitly insists. And it is dodgy to speculate about statements that are not being made. Notwithstanding, drawing both on the literature and on "conversational evidence" gained in many years of discussions with friends and colleagues in sociolinguistics and the social sciences, I hazard a guess: the implicit view of memory and identity inherent to these discourses is pretty much the same as we find in the psychology of memory as well as in common sense—that is, the Lockean view. As Geertz (1983b) observed on common sense as a cultural system, if you do not break explicitly and patently with it (in this case the Lockean sense), you remain a part of it.

RETHINKING NARRATIVE IDENTITY

The Lockean paradigm of personal identity, of identity as grounded in the autobiographical memory of oneself, is a variant of the archival model of memory adapted to the Western framework of individual self-construction. Although Locke's proposition can be seen as building on some essential structural features of early modern memory cultures (as pointed out in more detail in the next chapter) and even on premodern notions of memory and conscience such as Augustine's, it has had a strong influence on today's conceptions of autobiographical memory, which has become evident in our excursions into diverse fields of memory research from the natural and social sciences to narrative studies. The narrative focus on memory and the focus on the narrative fabric of memory are of particular interest here; in fact, they are at the heart of most chapters of this book. And from this vantage point, it is all the more amazing how persistent the Lockean tradition has been in the narrative field.

This, however, explains only one set of the problems haunting many discussions on narrative identity. Another complication comes with the representational or referential view of narrative and language in general, which philosophers of language call the realist view. It is linked to a wider representational notion of perception, knowledge, and truth that Rorty

(1979) characterized with the image of a mirror—a mirror that is supposed to depict the world. On this view, the main function of language appears as representational in that it refers to objects, processes, or experiences, which, in principle, are independent from and prior to it. Along these lines, autobiographical narrative is taken to be a re-presentation of events and experiences of a life, with the implication that narrative identity appears as the re-presentation of a person's identity, as his or her self-description—as though there were a prelinguistic, if not pre-semiotic self to be depicted in a story called narrative identity.

After having already problematized both assumptions in several contexts, I conclude this chapter with a look at a particular narrative practice that allows me to demonstrate an alternative way of considering human identity and its entanglement with narrative discourse. This way opens to an understanding of language beyond the representational view. A second purpose associated with the example of narrative I present in a moment is to sensitize the reader to a category of narrative identity practice that is often overlooked; it certainly is in most of the literature discussed in this chapter. And it is so, I suspect, not least because of the representational notion of language. What makes these narrative practices different from those investigated so far is that they serve less of an autobiographical function and more of an immediate function of social interaction and communication, of connecting. In this vein, we shift attention from the mnemonic dimension of identity to the manifold ways our sense of self and our identity emerge from intersubjective and bodily activities.

Although this category of identity practices is not at the center of this book, it is helpful for the understanding of the autobiographical process to be aware of the existence of an important dimension of human self and identity where the autobiographical focus loses its sharpness and determination. Illness, injury, and disability are a part of human life, and in many of these instances, a person can, indeed, lose the capacity to remember and/or speak, capacities that are fundamental for certain forms of autobiographical self-resolution. Astonishingly enough, such loss of autobiographical capacities, which comes with a loss of autobiographical knowledge, does not automatically result in a loss of one's sense of self. This is what Maria Medved and I found when we were working with patients with neurotrauma, studying the stories they told us about their experiences with their trauma and their changed sense of self (Medved & Brockmeier, 2008, 2010). Victims of neurotrauma caused by stroke, accident, anoxia, or infection of the brain, they were diagnosed to have anterograde memory impairments. This meant that many of them experienced the world in which they lived after their injury as fuzzy and confusing. No doubt, living a life under such conditions is difficult: one has to deal with a brain that has been abruptly transmogrified. Both the brain and the mind have suddenly become "strange." And what is more, it is hard to make sense of all those new brain "habits," not to mention dealing with them in everyday life. Now, if we assume that it is in the first place through narrative that people actively try to give meaning to their being in the world, including making sense of their brains, then individuals with neurotrauma are uniquely challenged.

> Neurotrauma almost always affects the very cognitive and communicative abilities one needs to narrate. More specifically, it disorders or reduces one's capacity to remember, to focus, and to organize complex plot structures. If, for example, memory capability is severely limited, obviously it is difficult to remember one's personal past, never mind tell autobiographical stories. (Medved & Brockmeier, 2008, p. 470)

As a consequence, individuals suffering from neurological lesions can be left without one of the most powerful tools in the toolbox of identity practices, namely, narrative discourse and narrative thought. Consequently, we concluded, a person suffering from a neurotrauma is not only confronted with illness and disability, which in and of itself often leads to an existential crisis; they also confront the additional crisis that comes with narrative dysfunction and a sudden lack of any ability for autobiographical meaning-making, just when it is needed most. And if we further presume that the idea of identity and one's sense of self is intimately intertwined with autobiographical narrative, it is likely

> ... that such a radical alteration of narrative competence would have profound consequences for a person's experience of his or her self, in fact, for the entire process of identity construction. If identity construction is understood as the ongoing narrative, that is, the discursive localization of one's self in time ... then serious restriction to one's narrative abilities cannot but result in a serious challenge to one's identity and sense of self. (Medved & Brockmeier, 2008, p. 470)

The surprising outcome of our research was, however, that—in contrast with a widespread view in the literature—none of the patients reported or complained about a diminished or otherwise troubled sense of self. Irrespective of their severe memory impairments and of the obvious chaos in their lives, these people seemed to have maintained a strong sense of sameness, if not of self-continuity. Even as they acknowledged their "really, really bad memory," the essence of the stories we analyzed unveiled a sense of self that appeared to have been largely undisturbed by their brain injury. Regardless of the profound changes in their brains, minds, and lives, their narratives tell us about their persisting intentions and readiness to participate in their everyday life worlds, from managing household responsibilities to attending family weddings.

A remarkable aspect of many stories was that they were not concerned with loss, limits, and adversity. It often has been written that many illness narratives highlight a break or crack between life before and life after sickness. The stories of our participants, however, were different, for they suggested ongoing connections between pre- and postmorbid lives. We, therefore, read them as narratives of an unbroken sense of self. Obviously, all individuals in our study appeared to draw on experiences of themselves that sustained the assault on their brain. One lesson to be drawn from these findings is that autobiographical identity practices clearly are not our only self-practices. Language and narrative, as I have argued, are indispensable conditions for our most complex forms of autobiographical self-reflection, especially, if they unfold multilayered temporal scenarios. But there are many other identity practices. Embodied in a variety of activities and social interactions, they are not dependent on time and temporal constructions and do not necessarily presuppose language. Nevertheless, they are part and parcel of our being in the world.

To substantiate this point further, I turn to an autobiographical story that again is different from the stories previously considered. It is jointly told as a freestanding narrative by a Swedish couple, Oswald and Linda, in the context of a longer conversation. Both are in their seventies; Oswald has an academic background and Linda worked as a secretary. Oswald suffers from mid- to late-stage dementia, a condition characterized not only by severe memory problems but also by language problems in areas such as word-finding, syntax, and pronunciation. In addition, Oswald has a hearing disability and difficulties with his eyes. He also suffers from body stiffness and limited facial expression, comorbid issues in the wake of Alzheimer's disease. All of this is relevant as background of this autobiographical story, lending it, we might say, an existential tension. The storytelling is triggered by an interviewer who asks the couple how they first met some 50 years ago.

1. Linda: where did we meet?
2. Oswald: where we met
3. L: yes

4. O: met on what
5. L: first time
6. O: first time
7. L: yes
8. O: yes (hesitant)
9. (pause 3 seconds)
10. yes
11. first time
12. yes yes it must have been whewhewhen iiiit we was when we were newnewnew
13. Both: (both laugh)
14. O: new new newl
15. what's it called
16. L: but the first time that we met
17. we were at a party
18. O: mebe so (maybe so) yes that was the way it was
19. L: yes
20. O: but then it was
21. then it was like that yes
22. that SOMEONE
23. YOU
24. L: yes
25. O: who met someone
26. L: yes I met YOU then yes
27. O: yes

This story and the conversation to which it belongs is a part of a larger corpus of interviews collected by the Swedish Center for Dementia Research. All audio- and video-recorded interviews and conversations of the corpus were conducted with couples in which one spouse was diagnosed with Alzheimer's disease. When I recently spent a semester at the Center studying the nexus of remembering and narrative in individuals with dementia I came across the conversations with Oswald and Linda and was touched by the warmth and complexity of their relationship even under conditions of extreme adversity.[19] By and large their emotional bond seemed to have been unaffected by the dramatic changes Oswald went through, and despite the often reduced way they had come to talk to each other. Even conversing about simple issues required a great amount of effort and commitment from both partners. It takes, for example, the entire sequence for Oswald to grasp fully that the initial question "Where did we meet?" aims at an event in which they were both involved.

Nonetheless, both co-narrators are still actively engaged in joint storytelling and seem to enjoy it.

Like the conversation with Oswald and Linda, most conversations from this corpus comprised a number of freestanding stories jointly told by both spouses in a familiar environment. Typically their storytelling was slower, more laborious, and heavy-going than that of unimpaired narrators; yet in terms of themes and content many narratives were not different from the plain everyday stories all of us tell one another. With the autobiographical account from Oscar and Linda, we are no doubt in the realm of "How it all began" stories: narratives of the first date or encounter, of the beginning of a relationship, which in this case has lasted a lifetime. This is a classical genre for autobiographical narratives. We might even say that for many spouses and lovers, telling and negotiating "their" stories, often considered to be unique and a kind of personal property, is a constitutive element of the relationship, both as a foundational memory and as story told about the past. Time and again repeated, confirmed, and enhanced in the changing present, they accompany the relationship like a symbolic enactment of the bond. Here, it is told in a format that discursive and sociolinguistic narrative researchers call a "small story," a story that in the first place is *performing* or *doing* identity.

Obviously there is a stark contrast between this everyday conversational narrative and the sophisticated storytelling of a Chekhov or McEwan. However, we must not forget that oral and conversational discourse draws on many more resources linked to the face-to-face presence of the narrative interlocutors. This already became evident when we discussed the stories of Ann, the girl with Fragile X, which displayed a different, cooperative practice of storytelling in which both teller and listener engage in a joint narrative effort. The rich communicative possibilities activated in such interactive narrative formats are visible only to a limited degree in a transcript, however detailed it may be. Not only can oral storytellers use their voice, face, and their entire bodily presence and interaction, they also are connected directly to the situation, the narrative event or, as some say, environment—all of which enriches their expressive and communicative registers. Writing, in comparison, leaves most of this to the imagination, even it can, of course, shape the imagination, to a degree, by the use of narrative cues. Moreover, for everyday oral storytelling, the distinction between narrator and audience does not really apply. Participants in these typically highly contextualized narrative events are interacting in so many ways that researchers of narrative discourse and conversational storytelling prefer to call them co-narrators (e.g., Georgakopoulou, 2007; Norrick, 2000; Ochs & Capps,

2001). "Genuine conversational storytelling," writes Norrick, "is always interactive, negotiated, and not simply designed for a particular audience by a single teller; indeed, it is often hard to determine who is the primary teller, especially when the events were jointly experienced or the basic story is already familiar" (2007, p. 127).

Everyday storytellers like Oswald and Linda can capitalize on a myriad of shared experiences, conversations, and stories, mostly without mentioning them explicitly. Imagine the shared experiential knowledge, including narrative knowledge, of a couple who have lived together for 50 years—the common stock of routines, habits, and tacit assumptions that have come to govern their everyday life, the sense of the bodily presence of the other, the familiarity with his or her moods and idiosyncrasies. All of them have shaped the conversational and narrative style: a story well-known to both is hinted at by a single word; an ironic tone suffices as a reminder of dramatic days; a quick glance brings into play an elaborate counter-narrative.

It is not difficult to see that this subcutaneous understanding is not only a phenomenon of communication and joint storytelling, it is also bound up with the identities of both spouses. Storytelling has become an "embodied engagement," to borrow Sparkes and Smith's (2012) expression, into the joint identities—perhaps the common identity—of the storytellers. Reflecting on their work on stories of men after catastrophic spinal cord injury, Sparkes and Smith have proposed that the route into understanding narrative as a mode of embodied engagement can only be one that makes narrative researchers aware of their own bodily and emotional involvement in the narrative events they investigate. The emerging sense of corporeality, Sparkes and Smith argue, reflects both the embodied nature of their dialogue with the individuals who participate in the research and the dialogue with their own embodied selves.

How can we apply these considerations to our understanding of Oswald and Linda's story? One aspect that stands out is the embodied nature of their narrative interaction. For couples where one has Alzheimer's disease, collaborative storytelling not only means engaging in a conversation but also offers an important way of retaining their very relationship, says Hydén (2011, p. 339), the lead researcher of the Swedish team. Like Sparkes and Smith (2012), he maintains that much of the close narrative collaboration works so well or, perhaps more precisely, works at all, because it draws on all resources of embodied storytelling. What Oswald and Linda perform and enact in many of their stories is a joint identity, a kind of shared couple existence that Hydén describes as "interdependent identity." As lives and life stories have become so inextricably intermingled, so have autobiographical memories—whether storied or embodied—and the sense of self of both protagonists.

Understanding narrative intersubjectivity

In characterizing Oswald and Linda's story as a performative and embodied act of joint or interdependent identity, I have already outlined the gist of my reading of it. Far beyond simply representing or describing identity or related emotions, this narrative ties together and carries out a number of different functions. To unravel these functions we have to revise and broaden the idea of language as a representational or referential operation—an idea widespread in psychology, the social and health sciences, and narrative studies. What is needed is a notion of language's multiple functions that captures an important feature: that the referential function never exists on its own. I already have referred to the argument of philosophers and psychologists of language such as Wittgenstein and Vygotsky that the referential function of language can only be realized *as* a dialogical, that is, social function; it emerges out of and always remains inherent to the fundamental purpose of all language: to communicate and facilitate interaction and intersubjectivity.

There can be little doubt that the story told by Oswald and Linda first of all serves an intersubjective function. At stake is a very personal process of connecting through joint remembering, a process in which the very event to be remembered ultimately demands only little space; the first meeting—which is meant to be the main theme—is mentioned only briefly in lines 17 and 18. As if the journey, and not the goal, is the important thing. Indeed, before that, both need a number of turns and a pause (L. 1 to 10) to come to an understanding on the meaning of the opening question, "Where did we meet?" Hydén (2011, p. 345) suspects that the two might also have trouble agreeing on what actually took place when they first met (L. 20 to 27). What I find remarkable here, however, is less the obvious trouble that comes with this kind of storytelling, which is in permanent need of what conversation analysts call *repair*. It rather is the fact that both storytellers seem to be undeterred in their efforts to continue their narrative and bring it to a close. Although prompted and accompanied by the interviewer, what drives and keeps the interaction on track, despite all difficulties and obstacles caused by Oswald's disease, is an emotional force. As already emphasized in my previous analysis of the interplay of cognitive and emotional components in the autobiographical process, there is no human action or reflection that is not grounded in affect. There is no way to disentangle cognition and emotion, these core elements of our psychological existence, when we face them in real life. Obviously, both Oswald and Linda have a strong desire to connect and to keep the connection alive; crucial for this is the sharing and confirming of an important common memory. In this manner they continue their joint autobiographical story and their consciously lived life as a couple. As if, in the face of the fairly advanced stage of Oswald's dementia, the common ground of a shared life was once more conjured up and affirmed in the present. Such is the experience that makes this kind of high-maintenance storytelling nevertheless so satisfying for both narrators. When, after various turns and failed attempts, Oswald finally grasps the meaning of the opening question, both react with joy and laughter (L. 13), rather than with frustration and despair that it took so long.

Short and fragmented autobiographical stories are, of course, nothing specific to Oswald and Linda or other elderly couples. Often repeated and interpreted relationship narratives tend to get reduced to a few elements, sometimes central, sometimes peripheral. It is fair to say that the least important function of such stories is a referential one; in other words, it is not about autobiographical knowledge but about something else. To take a closer look at this many-layered intersubjective function of language, which complements and encompasses the referential function, some further differentiations are in order.

To this purpose I draw on Roman Jakobson's (1981) distinction of multiple language functions. Jakobson, one of the 20th century's most all-round linguists and polyglot language thinkers, proposed a model of basic functions of human languages that has proven to be amazingly robust and flexible in many semiotic and linguistic contexts. My take on Jakobson's model is selective; I am less interested in the overall theory of language that comes with it, or in its semiotic intricacies. I want to use some of its distinctions in order to reach a fuller understanding of the various aspects of the intersubjective function. More precisely, my reading is oriented by three viewpoints. The first one is Wittgenstein's and Vygotsky's premise—drawing on a long tradition of thinking of language as dialogue—that the communicative and interactional dimension of language embraces and overarches its cognitive or referential dimension. The second is the intention to apply Jakobson's general distinctions among various linguistic and semiotic functions to a special form and practice of language, that is, to narrative. And the third is my aim of getting a better sense of what happens in Oswald and Linda's story.

Altogether, Jakobson divides six different functions of language (for which several competing terms have been used). Five of them are what

I have called intersubjective; one is referential (or cognitive) and, within my Wittgensteinian and Vygotskian framework, predicated on the intersubjective functions. The five intersubjective functions are the emotional (or expressive), the conative (or appellative), the poetic (or aesthetic), the phatic (or relational), and the metalinguistic (or reflexive).

For Jakobson, language always realizes some kind of emotional or affective function which, as we saw, is indeed fundamental to Oswald's and Linda's storytelling. In a strict linguistic sense, this *emotive* (or *expressive) function* relates to the addressee or the co-narrator, for example, by interjections and other peculiar sound changes that are not necessarily tangent to the referential meaning of a statement or a story but express the speaker's own subjective condition, particularly his or her affect state or intention ("What I find scary about it is . . ."). Jakobson rejects the cognitivist view that the emotive function is a nonlinguistic feature attributable to the delivery of the message and not to the message. Rather, he argues, the emotive function flavors language on all its basic—phonic, grammatical, lexical—levels. And we can even go beyond that: narrative can be interfused with a variety of emotions. If we consider storytelling as a complex process that takes place within an extended semiotic environment (possibly consisting of diverse media and sign systems) and involves various bodily registers, the range of a story's potential emotional fabric extends even further. Even if the content of a story might not be explicitly about emotions, or about some specific emotions, the performance and the entire storytelling event can imbue it with them, or even with different or contradictory affective values; as when a story with a happy end is told in sad or cynical fashion. We must keep this in mind when we rely on transcriptions that unavoidably reduce the multidimensional semiotic environment of the storytelling event. Reading only the emaciated transcript of Oswald and Linda's story it is hard to understand the deeply emotional tension that drives its telling.

In the overall count, the referential is the first and the emotive is second function. A third function singled out by Jakobson is the *conative function*. This refers to the role of language in engaging people directly; for example, when Linda, in another part of the conversation, turns to Oswald, looks him in the eye and says "What are you thinking about?" Imperatives ("Hey, tell me more about it!") and vocatives ("Oswald, of course you remember!") fulfill similar purposes. On the discourse level of narrative there are many ways storytelling can exercise such a connecting force, one being the fine-tuning of the story to the addressee's and co-narrator's individual subjectivity. In our story, Linda is tailoring the emerging narrative to Oswald's specific knowledge, storytelling, and comprehension capacities, which she, of course, knows better than anyone else. By focusing on the personally most meaningful or pleasant aspects of the story, she guides him to a path she knows he can go down. Yet even on this path, she needs to support him in the form of repair (e.g., in L. 26, where Linda turns Oswald's "someone" from L. 25 into the correct "you"), and by giving him the time he needs (as in L. 9). This "scaffolding" (Hydén, 2011; 2013) of Oswald's storytelling can be viewed as a particular case of narrative's inherent *second-person perspective,* discussed in the foregoing chapter. In turn, we also can understand the narrative fine-tuning toward the addressee as a particular case of Jakobson's conative function.

In distinguishing the referential, emotive, and conative functions as three basic aspects of all linguistic communication, Jakobson harked back to Karl Bühler's (1934) classical psychology of language. At the heart of Bühler's "Organon model" was the assumption that language, conceived as communication, unites three dimensions: Someone (a speaker), the Other (an addressee or cospeaker), and the World (objects or events to which both refer). In offering a comprehensive conceptual trajectory for both the representational and intersubjective dimension of language, Bühler was a forerunner not only of Jakobson's model. He also provided the starting point for many semiotic, communication–theoretical, linguistic, and psychological theories regarding the inner linkage between cognitive and social aspects of language. Bühler himself saw his work taking up a central aspect of Plato's notion of language as laid out in the *Cratylus*: that language is "an *organum* through which someone conveys something to someone else about things" (Bühler, 1934, p. 24). Given that Jakobson was well aware of this long tradition of thinking about language, he might have felt encouraged to single out three more functions that Bühler's Organon model only implicated.

One of these, the fourth, is the *poetic* or *aesthetic function.*[20] At first sight it seems to be tied to a very special feature of language that belongs to the realm of poetry and literary prose. In reality, however, what is called the poetic is a quality realized in some way or another in every linguistic communication. "The poetic function," Jakobson writes, "is not the sole function of verbal art but only its dominant, determining function, whereas in all other verbal activities it acts as a subsidiary, accessory constituent" (1981, p. 25). In a sense, this is valid for all functions distinguished here. What differs is the degree to which certain functions are present or dominant, which depends on the type of text or discourse (with the exception of short linguistic units where one or more functions can be absent).

That all language is inherently poetic might have been one of Jakobson's most influential propositions. How then can we understand the poetic function more precisely? In short, it stages language for its own sake. It is true that while this tends to be the dominant function in poetry and poetic forms of prose, it is peripheral in more functional contexts of language use to the point that we are not aware of it at all. Yet as all modes of language are fleeting forms of life, the dominance of one function over others can alter quickly, all the more as we are not talking about mutually exclusive aspects. The poetic function can come to the fore in the blink of an eye, and it does so in the most unexpected situations. Take an everyday example, a shopping list. Looked at it in an unusual light or transposed into an unexpected setting, it turns into a poem. Likewise, the cries at a fish market can reappear at a poetry slam, and the promises of a political orator perhaps please the audience because they are told with the narrative aplomb of a fairy tale. Jakobson particularly underlined the importance of the sound dimension of language, the magic of its melodic qualities, its prosody, and rhythmicity; and we surely recognize this in how Linda structures her contributions to the conversation: she divides them into intonational and rhythmical sequences, short units of utterance in which sound shapes meaning ("yes I met YOU then yes," L. 26). These units are functions of contact, bridges of understanding between the two narrators. Providing the most direct elements of comprehension and attunement for Oswald, they serve as what Rita Charon (2012) calls "membranes of the self."

The importance of tonal and rhythmic aspects of narrative's poetic dimension has been buttressed by investigations into the multiple affinities between narrative and music. Scholars in several disciplines have examined the somatic and affective foundations shared by narrative and music and their importance for communication and intersubjective affect equilibration. Drawing on this tradition of research, Richard Walsh (2011) has argued that narrative—and we can include here conversational narrative—has meaning because it has affect: "Much of the power of narratives, even very simple ones, to move and persuade is not specific to whatever those narratives are about; it is the affective potential intrinsic in the permutations of narrative form itself" (p. 63). With regard to narrative viewed as an embodied experience, the poetic function then has an amazingly broad scope: it ranges from pre- and nonlinguistic modes of meaning-making to acts of meaning under standard conditions of everyday and literary storytelling in various semiotic environments.

Especially important, in our context, is that this range also includes storytelling under nonstandard conditions restricted by illnesses or other physical or mental challenges. We might be at first reluctant to take Oswald and Linda's story as a poetic form, and there are good reasons for this reluctance. But we should keep in mind that there is a poetic dimension to much of human communication that has little or nothing to do with artful creation and aesthetic pleasure. Analyzing this story as an everyday "metric text" that, as Jakobson (1981) puts it, "make use of the poetic function without, however, assigning to this function the coercing, determining role it carries in poetry" (p. 28), can help us understand why and how this kind of storytelling works, and why and how it can work as an identity practice.

The fifth function is the *phatic function*. Realizing particular intersubjective aspects of the communication process, it is more specific than the poetic function. Phatic aspects are central, for example, in acts of establishing contact, such as greetings and initial exchanges with strangers. In some cultural worlds, if you get in touch with someone you do not know, unaware of their intentions or concerns and perhaps even without knowing their language, you still can communicate about the weather. The phatic function of language allows people to connect, establish, and prolong sociality, in whatever basic form ("Oswald, do you understand me?"). It is the *hello* function in Jakobson's model. It links human beings to fellow human beings. In fact, it is one of the first verbal functions acquired by infants. Involving voice, glance, face, gesture, and the entire body as an organ of contact, the predominant role of phatic communication is to reach out and set up a connection, and then to sustain and extend it.

This also includes confirming whether the connection is still there—a crucial element in Oswald and Linda's communication. The phatic function is the trace of the body in language. It makes sure that the storyteller is bodily present even if important dimensions of linguistic interaction (such as sound structures, syntax, and semantics) fail—as, for example, in Oswald's turn: "yes yes it must have been whewhewhen iiiit we was when we were newnewnew" (L. 12). The verbal flow at this point (that extends to line 15) seems clearly interrupted. But this does not preclude that the conversational narrative continues, for Linda answers with a repair move that interprets what she takes as Oswald's point: "but the first time that we met // we were at a party" (L. 16–17). Nor does it question the continuous connection between the two storytellers, because Linda first and foremost relates to Oswald, not to his utterances. She speaks to the person behind the voice, to put it in Bakhtian terms, and thus can keep the communication going even if the voice fades. It is in this sense that we can say the narrative voice is embodied in the presence of the narrator; and it is this that explains its powerful phatic qualities.

The *metalinguistic function* is the sixth component of language in Jakobson's model. If we use Jakobson's (1981) definition of the referential function as relating not to a thing but to the thing spoken of (1981, p. 25), then we can take the metalinguistic function as a subtype of the referential function because it qualifies language as referring to, describing, and discussing language itself. Metalanguage is the language speaking of language. It is a reflexive function, establishing mutual agreement on the "code" of the communication. It comes into play whenever we say something like, "What do you mean?" or "What do you want to say by this?" or "I beg your pardon." I have already pointed out the important role of one metalinguistic activity in Oswald and Linda's conversation: repair. Repair re-establishes the code and thus enables the exchange to be continued as a joint narrative. The increase in repair interventions and, as a side-effect, the often slow and meandering flow of the jointly told story is part of what Hydén (2011) calls a change in the "division of interactional labor" in couple conversations in which one narrator progressively suffers from Alzheimer's disease. "The teller without AD," Hydén writes, "will have to make more contributions to the storytelling and be more engaged in quite advanced repair work in order for the participant with AD to continue being an active conversational participant" (2011, p. 341).

A large part of Oswald and Linda's communicative activities aim at carrying out repair strategies. Often one repair entails another repair, a repair of repairs. Without these constant clarifications (questions and answers, repetitions, paraphrases, fine-tuned explanations, and so on) Oswald would not be able to participate in the storytelling, and the narrative that is constitutively a joint activity would not exist. In the process the status of repair interventions seems to change, however. From an originally, perhaps, mere metalinguistic operation it turns into an essentially intersubjective practice. Making the story work becomes the real story; just bringing it to a close is its catharsis. It is the very point of the narrative enactment as a relationship, a relationship that still works, not least through the permanent input of metalinguistic support and repair.

Viewed in this light, a more profound intersubjective dimension of these metalinguistic interventions comes to the fore, especially when we single out Linda's repair moves. What they bring to bear is not only a constant linguistic or cognitive awareness, and a close monitoring and anticipation of all of Oswald's moves, expected and intended ones as well as those that got stuck. These interventions also reflect and realize a stance, an attitude of responsibility and, ultimately, emotional commitment that provides Oswald and the entire joint narrative enterprise with a sense of care and being cared for. Adding a further layer to the dense texture of intersubjectivity that all these functions of language establish, they contribute to interweaving both narrators into an affective fabric of identity.

Some people live through their illness the way they live through their life, Charon (2006, p. 96) has observed. We can take Oswald and Linda as an example.

The postautobiographical perspective

This also might explain why Jakobson did not distinguish a specific "affective function" of language, for it is inextricably embedded in all other functions. If we assumed for a moment the existence of such an affective function, we would have to qualify it in the same way some cognitive psychologists have described "distributed cognition," namely as "distributed emotion," that is, as a quality that inheres to all other language functions and their interplay. This is what I mean when I refer to the "affective fabric of joint identity" realized in Oswald and Linda's storytelling.

By the same token, this lends further support to the claim that the primary function of this story is not a referential one. Drawing on Jakobson, Wittgenstein, and Vygotsky, I have proposed a view of language and narrative in which the referential function never exists on its own but is realized as a function of intersubjective relations. In this respect we can liken the referential function to the "affective function"; both are ubiquitously lodged in the modus operandi of *all* functions. As we saw, Oswald and Linda's story, although revolving around an important autobiographical event, is not really about digging something up in the archive of autobiographical memory; rather, it is about two persons mutually confirming each other in their efforts to connect and to keep their relationship afloat, against all odds. I am not implying that a special focus on the referential function, in general, is without relevance. There are many institutional and situational contexts of narrative where it is of utmost importance, such as in public truth-finding commissions and in police and legal investigations. But the perspective of narrative identity exposed by my reading of Oswald and Linda's story is not an autobiographical one; in fact, their conversational narrative about how it all began is not an autobiographical process but, as I have suggested, a joint narrative identity enactment.

It is for this reason that I have described this enactment in terms of a postautobiographical perspective (Brockmeier, 2014). This perspective, novel to intellectual contexts but common in everyday and clinical discourses, reflects that there are people who live in particular cultural worlds and under particular conditions of health and illness where the Lockean idea of autobiographically grounded narrative identity makes only limited sense, or no sense at all. In a broader picture, this perspective relates to observations according to which the social texture in which our identities emerge is often likelier to be found in personal interactions, such as empathetic conversations and shared emotional involvement in and narrative response to particular experiences, than it is to derive from a common socioeconomic milieu or from agreement on abstract ethical or political principles (cf., e.g., Appiah, 2005; 2006).

Yet what I want first and foremost to emphasize here is that the postautobiographical perspective opens to conceptions of self and identity that clearly go beyond the Lockean horizon of understanding. It resonates with a tendency in dementia research to overcome the perception of Alzheimer's disease as the black hole of a big loss, caused by a general decline of cognitive and linguistic abilities (Hydén, Lindemann, & Brockmeier, 2014). Underlying this trend is a shift in focus of attention from merely individual cognitive and neurocognitive capacities like memory, which so far have dominated the diagnostic apparatus of neurology, psychiatry, and neuropsychology, to social forms of life. These forms, as we have seen in the instance of Oswald and Linda, are conceived of as embedded, embodied, and enacted practices. To couch the implications of this shift in one word, we would have to talk of a de-centering of memory or, at least, of the traditional perception of autobiographical memory's presumably decisive role for identity and sense of self. With this de-centering, a new array of relational identity practices comes into view that allows us to understand better the fundamentally social and interactional nature of the human being in the world.

In this and the previous chapter, I have considered a broad spectrum of forms of interplay between narrative and identity. At one end of this spectrum there are complex forms of autobiographical meaning-making that are not just represented or expressed by narrative but only come into being through and in narrative, what I have called the strong narrative thesis. This thesis applies to forms of autobiographical identity that only exist due to narrative meaning constructions as, for instance, in our scenarios of autobiographical time. The narrative mode involved here is highly reflexive. It requires and induces a mode of experience that, as I have put it, comprises the experience of its own interpretation.

Yet this is just one part of the spectrum of what I described above as narrative agency. Emphasizing the constructive, imaginative, and discursive qualities of narrative, the strong narrative hypothesis marks one specific area of forms and practices of identity. Another group of phenomena situated at the other end of the spectrum of narrative agency comes to the fore when certain preconditions of the autobiographical process are challenged. We saw that individuals' ability to remember and to engage in autobiographical processes can be troubled because they are ill, injured, affected by atypical developments, or mentally traumatized. Although "the body is the passport, the warrant, the seal of one's identity" (Charon, 2006, p. 87), a person's body—including the brain—and his or her identity are not the same. Especially in the sick there are many ways in which they can be distinct and contradictory. In many clinical settings, Charon identifies a "corporeal gap" between the narrating self and the body, where both tell different stories. This requires skills in "stereophonic listening," that is the ability to hear the body and the person who inhabits it at the same time (2006, p. 97).

The pivotal point is that all the individuals who find it difficult to remember and to engage in autobiographical processes due to sickness, whose plights I have tried to grasp in these chapters, can still actively participate in a multitude of intersubjective practices and, in doing so, have identities and live lives full of meaning and stories. That is to say, we are still considering variations on the theme of narrative empowerment introduced at the beginning of the chapter.

To get a better idea of the meaning of these stories for these individuals' sense of self and identity, I have argued throughout this book that we must be aware of the densely affective fabric of identity. This includes bodily and microcontext-sensitive social interactions that have little to do with the proper storage and retrieval of memories from one's past as maintained by Lockean theories of autobiographical identity, whether narrative or not. Still, we have seen that even under the difficult conditions of Oswald's Alzheimer's disease (as well as of the other individuals with neurological challenges whose plights have been discussed in this chapter) a portion of these interactions is realized in narrative form; that is, it is fused with those narrative forms of life that we call our identity.

But the gist of these pages goes beyond this. For the postautobiographical approach clearly defies the Lockean imperative of autobiographical self-construction and invites us to envision the rich repertoire of practices and forms of life—including practices of narrative self-making—that humans use to enact their identities.

CHAPTER 7

Inhabiting a Culture of Memory

The Autobiographical Process as a Form of Life

This chapter takes a closer look at the autobiographical process as a cultural process. Several previous chapters already have addressed the cultural trajectory along which all autobiographical remembering and forgetting takes place, as well as all research and theorizing about it. However, the main focus so far has been devoted to other aspects of the autobiographical process, which—according to the organizing idea of these chapters—is successively examined from different vantage points. In the last chapter, the focus was on its role in the formation of narrative identity; now the cultural aspect moves to the fore. I first frame it historically, offering a tableau of the modern European and North American concern with self and autobiographical identity, and then move on to contrast this cultural-historically specific vision with a different approach presented in a reading of a Chinese American autobiography, Maxine Hong Kingston's *The Woman Warrior*.

What does it mean to view the autobiographical process as a cultural process? What sense does it make to maintain that we do not simply remember and forget but do so the way we do because we inhabit a specific culture of memory? By this I mean a cultural world characterized by particular mnemonic conditions. These conditions consist of a number of things, which I described in Chapter 3 as a historical memory constellation. Elaborating a suggestion by Danziger (2008), I used this concept to outline what I called a *memory episteme*, a historical framework that gives shape and meaning to our practices and ideas of remembering and forgetting. More precisely, a memory episteme stands for the whole of local and societal practices, technologies, and objects of remembering and forgetting; the ideas, concepts, and theories about what it is and what people do when they remember and forget; and the values and norms that regulate, within a given community or political system, which memory stories are permissible and which are not and hence ought to be excluded and prohibited. In Chapter 3, I was especially interested in how many distinct memory epistemes were able to back up the archival model of memory over many centuries.

Whereas the memory episteme is a concept in the wake of Foucault's (1977; 1980) conceptualization of the unity of "power/knowledge," the idea of a cultural economy of remembering, which plays a major role in this chapter, has a different scope. Although it is a concept of the same order—it aims at the historical whole of a memory constellation—it foregrounds the *cultural dynamic* in which all historical mnemonic conditions are involved. The cultural economy of remembering is both wider and narrower than the memory episteme.

Like the economy of money, commodities, and production, an economy of remembering and forgetting brings together a plethora of resources—material, societal, and mental—that tend to disappear behind the final product. Normally, I do not see it when I have, say, a childhood memory that pops us in a personal and private act, perhaps as a quirk of my inner life. One purpose of this chapter is to get a better sense of the involute cultural economy of remembering, in which the autobiographical process appears as just one factor.

Consider once more the Lockean view. Only by using a cultural lens do we notice one of its most significant implications. Locke's notion of autobiographical memory as a reflexive faculty of individual consciousness has become an essential feature of the modern Western culture of remembering, where it has been, as we saw, equally attributed to the healthy and the sick. At the same time, it is based on the assumption that memory is a naturally given capacity of all human beings, irrespective of psychological, social, and historical differences. In classical Enlightenment fashion, memory is conceived of as a universal quality, a quality that even defines identity—the identity of a Western human being, that is—as a likewise universally distributed feature. Although Locke is commonly seen as one of the towering father figures of modern Empiricism, in his conception of autobiographical identity he emphasizes the moment of rational reflexivity, of conscious self-construction, as Matthews (2006) noted. This moment is part of every individual identity formation, or at least has often been claimed to be so in the history of Western subjectivity. After all, for Locke (2008), as we recall, a person is "a thinking, intelligent being, that has reason and reflection, and can consider itself as itself, the same thinking thing, in different times and places" (II, xxvii, 9).

Viewed in a broader historical picture, it is apparent that the Lockean model of memory has been a significant vanishing point in the conceptual establishment of an individualist culture of memory, a culture that, however, is postulated to be natural. From this postulate ensues its universalist claim. It has been forcefully upheld by modern memory sciences from the beginning of their existence, in spite of various traditions of criticism pointing to the great diversity of the world's cultures of remembering. Arguably, neither the intellectual culture of the Enlightenment nor that of modern memory sciences has paid much heed to this diversity. Still, even if this backdrop may help us understand the Lockean view, does it really sufficiently answer the larger question raised in the previous chapters: Why could this view have been so influential as to shape the dominant understanding of the nexus between autobiographical memory and identity until today?

Couching the question in these terms is, of course, not to suggest that there was one person, John Locke, who singlehandedly came up with an idea so powerful as to shape the entire subsequent Western tradition of thought about memory and identity. As shrewd as the English philosopher might have been, this is not about the thought of a single individual and even less about the impact of philosophical thinking on history. Locke articulated a view and offered a vocabulary for it that obviously has been convincing to many in the modern economy of remembering to the degree that it was taken to reflect the role autobiographical memory plays in the constitution of identity. The question, again, is why could it be so convincing?

THE RISE OF THE AUTOBIOGRAPHICAL STORY

I want to link this question to another one. In his inquiry into the history of the modern ideas of memory and identity, Hacking has pointed out that one of the precursors of what in the 20th century became known as multiple identity or personality and, respectively, multiple personality disorder (or dissociative identity disorder, as it is called today) might have been the ability to go into a trance. Today, trance is little appreciated. It has a dubious reputation and has lost the cultural recognition it once enjoyed. "Our ignorance about trance," writes Hacking, "and our wish to make it pathological, probably means that we colonize our own past, destroying traces of the original inhabitants" (1995, p. 146). Why, Hacking asks, has modern science and public discourse marginalized trance, a state in which we lose a clear and precise sense of who we are and, in this way, of our identity in Locke's sense? It is true that the wheels of modern life and the demands of industry insist on constant attention to and reflection of one's self. Danziger (1990; 2008) has persuasively elaborated on this argument to explain the rise of the modern economy of remembering. Yet with respect to trance and similar mental states and behaviors, this alone cannot be the answer, Hacking notes, because our depreciation of such behaviors seems to have preceded industrialization, even if it was less rigid in earlier times. Clearly something must have discredited trance and similar uncontrolled mental states, privileging instead the rise of concepts of conscious, reflexive, and self-controlled identity. But what?

Hacking refers to the work of anthropologist Mary Douglas (1992) who coined the concept of "enterprise culture." What Douglas described as enterprise cultures corresponds by and large to classical West European and North American societies. Typical of these societies are high levels of individual responsibility and correspondingly great opportunities for individuals. Those who succeed stand out prominently but are quickly abandoned if they fail. Enterprise societies strongly differ from traditional and hierarchical structures of society that Douglas found in the African communities with which she worked. In these communities every person has a place that cannot be lost or forgotten: "You may become the lowest among people of your station," Hacking summarizes, "but there is no intelligible way of dropping out or being discarded, short of death" (1995, p. 146).

What makes Douglas's studies particularly instructive for my inquiry into the Western economy of memory is that they are related to an analysis of Locke's theory of personal identity, which appears, in Douglas's account, as reflection and example of a Western enterprise society. It is a significant historical detail of Locke's concepts of person and identity that they were originally conceived as forensic categories. Their function was to establish a connection of responsibility between someone's actions in the past and his or her accountability in the present, the present of a law court. Locke's philosophy was meant to give an answer to the question of how it can be determined that a person standing trial for a crime is identical with the same person who committed the crime, possibly a long time ago. These considerations also might have reinforced the emphasis on conscious self-construction and, in this way, bolstered Locke's case that the continuity of one's consciousness—the warrant of one's identity—is linked to a coherent chain of autobiographical memories.

The notion of selfhood involved here is patently different from the notions Douglas (1992) studied in African societies. Douglas's findings are undergirded by Geertz (1983a), who explored the conception of the person and the sense of self and selves in Morocco, Bali, and Java around the middle of the last century. Geertz's studies fueled a long-standing debate in cultural anthropology on structure and agency, and on collectivities and individualities, to use Rasmussen's (2012, p. 102) terms. In his account, Geertz famously concluded that "The Western conception of the person as a bounded, unique, more or less integrated motivational and cognitive universe, a dynamic center of awareness, emotion, judgment, and action organized into a distinctive whole . . . is . . . a rather peculiar idea within the context of the world's cultures" (1983, p. 59).

Drawing on Douglas, Hacking (1995, p. 146) sees Locke's forensic person with all his or her enhanced autobiographical self-consciousness—a "dynamic center of awareness"—as a relatively new figure. It came into being with the rise of new practices of commerce, property, and law tied to the Western enterprise culture. Whereas, on the one hand, a stable and controlled personal identity over time based on a chain of consciously reconstructed autobiographical memories was to be a central feature of this figure, on the other hand there were states and behaviors, such as trances, to be discredited and excluded, not to mention madness and personality disorders. It was the consciousness and autobiographical identity of this figure that Locke's philosophy put in a conceptual nutshell, anticipating and reflecting autobiographical remembering as what Foucault (1988) would call a discursive "technology of the self."

Yet Locke's new figure is not altogether new. There is a Christian background that shines through the surface of Enlightenment philosophy. Earlier, I mentioned a precursor, Augustine's idea of memory and conscience. Hacking (1995, pp. 156–157) remarks that Locke's forensic autobiographer also plays a role in the divine plan, which again harks back to Augustine's early conception of Christianity, one that determines our destiny either in terms of eternal bliss or damnation. Whether it is punishment or reward depends on the outcome of a trial, the Last Judgment, an assumption entailing the same problem that, centuries afterward, Locke's forensic theory of autobiographical identity tries to solve in the spirit of rational reasoning.

Revealing though analyses of Locke's conception from contemporary points of view are—and authors like Danziger, Douglas, Foucault, Geertz, Hacking, and Matthews all offer decisively contemporary frameworks of analysis—there is a risk of mixing up the theoretical idea of identity and autobiographical memory from the 17th century with the cultural realities of the late 20th and early 21st century, the home base of these frameworks. A long historical process (in which Locke marks only one step) has made Western cultures what they are today: cultural worlds with a wide range of individualistic and individualizing technologies of the self, among which autobiographical practices play a key role. To describe this role, I again use a Foucaultian perspective. It comes with the concept of "episteme," a sociocultural system of categories and knowledge that is both intellectual and material. In light of a historical dialectic, pointed out by Foucault (1970) as central for the advancement of the modern episteme, it appears that the rise of the discourse of individualism—the "discourse of Man"—which has provided the scaffolding for the idea of the autobiographical process, was itself shaped by the emergence of technologies of the self among which the autobiographical process figures prominently. These technologies were essential in inscribing the discourse of individualism in the minds and psychological habits of human beings who, in the process, became modern individuals.

Inscribing is a word with an intellectual and bookish feel. For some, there even is a postmodern and playful ring to it. When Foucault, however, speaks of "discourse" and "episteme" this always includes institutions of power and violence, as noted before. Knowledge, once it gains societal significance, is never merely mental or conceptual; it is anything but an exclusive academic or intellectual affair, let alone a playful affair. The struggle for the right to impose one interpretation of the world over another interpretation is a political struggle. This idea is crucial for Foucault's thinking (e.g., Foucault, 1977; 1980). It suggests a reading of Locke's forensically grounded model of autobiographical identity as a pointed example of the fusion of three different dimensions: structures of knowledge, psychological functions, and power. This fusion is realized with the coming into being of what we might call the autobiographical episteme.

To better understand the formation of autobiographical identity as a technology of the self that is intimately interrelated with the cultural and political rise of individualism, it is worthwhile to look closer at what I have referred to as the Western "culture of autobiography." Obviously, there is a family resemblance between this concept and the Foucault-inspired concept of autobiographical episteme. Recent publications have stressed the enormous diversity of contemporary autobiographical practices and forms of life writing (e.g., Jolly, 2001; Saunders, 2010; Smith & Watson, 2010). I hence use Folkenflik's term in its pluralized form, cultures of autobiography, to avoid any misunderstanding that the term "culture" could denote a unitary and homogenous entity. With this caveat in mind, I have made the case that modern cultures or epistemes of autobiography are advanced and radicalized versions of individualist cultures because they impose the imperatives of individualism onto the domains of personal memories and lifetime (Brockmeier, 2000; 2008b). Viewed in the light of Foucault's conceptual hybrid "power/knowledge," the political charge of this imposition is evident. It is political in as far as it is part of the historical process of emancipation of a bourgeois order, of a rise to power that endorses the comprehensive advancement of individualism and subjectivity, which, again, includes the advancement of the idea and the practice of the autobiographical process.

Imposition is a strong term, but it appears justified if we bring to mind the cultural scenarios that were involved in, and have evolved into, today's autobiographical cultures. Never before have so many life stories, autobiographies, memoirs, and biographies been produced in such a wide spectrum of genres and media, linguistic and otherwise. Since the end of the last century, this spectrum has been broadened further by new multimedia digital technologies and formats of self-presentation and self-creation. Never before have there been so many public arenas of personal confession and display of private and "inner" life. These places of self-presentation are supplemented by innumerable places of display of memory objects, that is, of carriers of personal and communal memoirs giving material or digital shape to significant personal experiences and public events—from coronations and disasters to sports and entertainment highlights. Never before have so many artistic, academic, and professional discourses been concerned with human lives and life stories. And never before have practices of autobiography and other forms of life writing been so intimately connected with the idea of self-exploration and, in fact, of self-construction and self-creation.

Today, autobiographical identity construction is considered to be a common and elementary practice of the self. It is neither bound to a particular age, level of education, or social habitus, nor to the act or linguistic mode of writing, whether in a traditional or digital sense. Rather, it is widely accepted that in countless narrative forms of everyday behavior, discourse, and reflection we give a gestalt to our memories and self-interpretations, exposing our hopes, desires, fears, and obsessions from an autobiographical perspective. This is the milieu, the biotope of the autobiographical story, the cultural economy of memory and identity in which the autobiographical process has thrived and flourished.

That autobiographical practices have been thriving in this cultural milieu is, however, only one way to put it. There also is an enormous pressure on individuals to shape themselves autobiographically, indeed, to live auto-biographically, to use Eakin's expression (2008), a pressure that has per-vaded contemporary Western societies. How are we to understand this continuously growing pressure, the urge to identify ourselves through autobiographical records and documents? I think for an answer, at least for *one* answer, we need to bring to mind an important distinction: record-ing and documenting is not remembering. Often events and experiences are documented in order to allow others to remember; that is, there can be a difference between those who document and those who remember. But if much of what we do—in notes, photographs, log or blog entries, autobiographical stories and memoirs, museums, libraries, and other archives—is documenting, who then is supposed to do the remembering? Who remembers?

In the Jewish tradition, as the Canadian writer Rick Salutin reminded us, martyrdom is said to be incurred *al kiddush ha-shem*, which means, for the sanctification of God's name. Thus martyrs were remembered throughout eternity, documented, as it were, in the mind of God or, that is, remembered by God, as Salutin (1995) put it. Things are similar for martyrs in the Islamic tradition. Christianity, too, has a similar idea: God is not only almighty but also all-knowing. In the Catholic sacrament of the confession, believers do not confess to God, who does not need to know because his mind is the comprehensive memory of everything that has ever happened, including, of course, all sins. Believers make a con-fession to the priests of the Church who, even if they act, according to doctrine, *in persona Christi*, at the end of the day, are *not* God and thus have only the limited knowledge and memory of mortals. For Protestants and Lutherans, the linkage between the Christian and God is more direct, without any intermediary, except for Christ. So believers are always mir-rored in the mind and memory of God, which also means that they are never really alone.

Perhaps the urge to document and remember so exhaustively in our own time has to do with the decline of such religious belief. Salutin (1995) suspects: "In the past, what you did and suffered, however overlooked on earth, was seen and recorded by the eye of God. Now, for most of us, it can only exist in the eyes of others." To create these eyes is at least one function of much of the public sphere of documenting and recording per-sonal affairs. The exponential presence in our life of photography, video, and television might find here one explanation; as do certain accounts of the digital revolution and the expansion of the World Wide Web, which Internet theorists take to be the new universal memory, the memory of everything for eternity, God's new memory.

Salutin allows that there always may have been the need for personal recognition, for being remembered by someone. But it must have helped to believe in being seen from beyond, or in being appreciated during the afterlife. Sure, there have been other social institutions that played a role here, such as strong community and family links that once also provided a sense of being known, remembered, and hence acknowledged. But these, too, have disintegrated in much of the Western world as a consequence of the social dynamic mentioned earlier. In a nutshell, then, the breakdown of lived, enacted, social, or communal remembrance has led not to a devaluation of individual or cultural memory—but to the increasing appreciation of it. It has made it a supreme virtue, a celebrated quality, a hallmark of human identity in an ever-accelerating world of forgetfulness.

I find it stunning how fast the tectonic shifts toward this economy of remembering have occurred. If we think of language not only as reflecting but also creating reality we may find it telling that the word autobiography, although a Greek term, did not exist in ancient Greece. In fact, it did not exist until European modernity made autobiographical subjectivity a central issue. Historical reviews show that the term autobiography, and its synonym self-biography, had never been used in any previous period until first appearing in the late 18th century in both Germany and England. Within just a couple of years, both terms not only were invented but repeatedly reinvented. This is not to say that people in earlier epochs in Europe did not remember and tell stories about their personal past, or that they did not have individual identities. There is an extended field of historical research that demonstrates the contrary (cf., e.g., Muscuch, 1996). But first and foremost, in previous centuries it did not matter so much, if it mattered at all. After what we know, what made up the articulated fabric of what we would call today a person's identity was more of a typified pattern, a cultural definition of what a life was supposed to be according to the social registers of descent, class, gender, ethnic or communal background, education, and religion. After all, there was the comforting idea of God's all-encompassing memory that made sure that no one lived unknown.

Given that this cultural configuration claimed to be grounded in the divine plan of human life, it seemed only consistent that it also circumscribed the layout of possible forms of self-resolution. Of course, even the *individual* view of oneself can and does have its space and occasion within a religious trajectory. The modern Western sense of individuality and inwardness germinated in the Christian tradition where it found its philosophically and anthropologically first full articulation by Augustine, as Taylor (1989, Chapter 7) has argued. And both individuality and inwardness had their space and occasion even beyond the privileged sphere of kings and queens, noblemen and noblewomen, as Natalie Zemon Davis (1995) pointed out in her study on the lives and life reports of three ordinary women—to mention just one example from the extensive historiographical literature on lives and life writing. One of these women was Jewish, one Catholic, and one Protestant, all living "on the margins" in 17th-century Europe, North America, and South America, and all being fully aware of their individual life history. That said, the self-constitutive function of this autobiographical glance—what I have described as the interplay between autobiographical process and identity construction—appears nonetheless to be constrained by quite rigid historical models of life and life course, which for most common people did not leave much room for conscious self-creation (not even for the extraordinary women Zemon Davis has portrayed).

After all, life stories, whether short or long, sparse or detailed, original or standardized, are important means to claim or defend our belonging to a social community. They have to fit in. They are used "to negotiate group membership and to demonstrate that we are in fact worthy members of those groups, understanding and properly following their moral standards," as Charlotte Linde (1993, p. 3) argued, along with many life story researchers after her. Perhaps we can take this to be a basic feature of Western life narratives across different historical periods.

To be sure, what Davis and many other historians have shown in compelling detail is that the project of taking stock, examining, and accounting for one's individual past had been germinating for centuries behind the thick walls of medieval cloisters and in silent castle libraries. It had been flourishing among Renaissance scholars, and in the worlds of poets, artists, philosophers, rebellious theologians, diarists, lovers, and suicides. But it was not until the onset of bourgeois modernity, with its hitherto unseen social dynamics and the erosion of universally binding religious and moral value systems, that the autobiographical story and the project of individual identity construction was to become a pervasive phenomenon. On a sociocultural level, what we witness in this process is a shift in self-responsibility or *souci de soi*, care of the self, to use another of Foucault's (1990) concepts.

In contemporary social sciences it has become common parlance that modern societies have turned personal identity into a self-reflexive project, an enterprise of continuous identity construction and reconstruction that unfolds through a multitude of different self-practices. Associated with the worldview of ontological individualism, which postulates human beings as intrinsically and essentially individualist, it reconfigures the autonomous self as the a priori of the social. Taylor (1989) has maintained that this advanced individualism has increasingly bound the idea of a self-defining sovereign subject into the modern "moral ontology": into the idea of what it is to live a good and ethically fulfilling life. The ubiquity of autobiographical self-presentation has made this moral ontology of autonomous identity so taken-for-granted that it appears, in line with Locke's view, as a natural given: as if autobiographical identity were a biological phenomenon and thus subject to universal, material laws. Cultural sociologist Norbert Elias (1992) pointed out the paradox that many of our ideas appear to be all the more natural the more they are fused with the practices of societal life. Drawing on Elias's observations, we can take this societal naturalization as helping us to comprehend the seemingly self-evident expectation of members of Western societies that their particular ideas of self and autobiographical identity are globally shared by all humans, as well as their surprise when they encounter people from different societies and cultural traditions whose ideas do not follow the same narrative models.

BEYOND THE ANTAGONISM BETWEEN INDIVIDUAL AND SOCIAL REMEMBERING

There is, however, an important critical qualification to the individualist approach to remembering and forgetting, which I spell out in the remainder of this chapter. It has emerged with an alternative vision of memory as a social (or collective or cultural) phenomenon. This alternative has already been present in the previous chapters, though often only in the background. Now it takes center stage, and it does so with a particular focus that should be singled out beforehand.

The emergence of a new field of research on social memory has also provided new perspectives on individual and, especially, autobiographical remembering. In fact, it has challenged the very opposition of "the individual" and "the social" that has been widespread for so long in memory research. I repeatedly have argued that the deeply rooted antagonism between individual memory and social or cultural memory running through the literature and defining the field—that is two fields, as Olick (2011) remarks—is misleading (Brockmeier, 2002a). Building on an integrative vision of memory, one that spans individual and collective processes, I have advanced the argument that there is no such thing as an autobiographical process that exists outside of the economy of remembering and its cultural traditions. These traditions also include the use of certain narrative repertoires, which alone makes the distinction between individual remembering and social context obsolete. If we keep in mind our discussion of the mind-narrative nexus in Chapter 4, there can be no doubt that language (and narrative, for that matter) is not just a "context" of the mind, let alone the brain. We are born not into "contexts" but into cultural traditions within which we learn, in one and the same developmental process, how to autobiographically remember, forget, and tell stories about ourselves and others (Fivush & Haden, 2003; Nelson, 2007a; Wang, 2013).

What then, exactly, is meant by this reference to a cultural tradition? "Tradition," as Wittgenstein remarked in an interesting qualification, "is not something someone can learn; it is not a thread you can pick up when you want to, anymore than you can pick your own ancestors" (1984, p. 558). Wittgenstein was repudiating a behaviorist understanding of learning. Against this understanding, he emphasized that the emergence and perpetuation of tradition is a function of intergenerational meaning constructions. We are not conditioned to follow a tradition; nor is a tradition a given genealogy. It is an ongoing social succession of meaning practices and negotiations, and in this respect it is different from, for example, one's genetic and ethnic descent. Considering memory traditions, it is fair to say that they deal with cultural fabrications in a strong sense—not because they are made by *a* culture but because their semiotic makeup is not natural but cultural. It is "arbitrary," in de Saussure's sense, and that is, it depends on cultural symbol and sign systems.[1] This then moves our attention to a sphere where the demarcation line between the individual and the social dissolves.

A point to be made here is that, of course, it was not this demarcation line that was questioned in the history of ideas on memory in the first place, but something else. Most concepts and theories of social memory have emerged in opposition to the notion of memory as an individual capacity. The Western conceptual history of social memory since Maurice Halbwachs can be viewed as developing *against* an individualist and self-centered understanding of memory, an understanding that has underlain modern philosophy of mind and personal identity since Locke—if we leave out of account the philosophy of Hegel, little known in the Anglo-Saxon tradition, which contended that mind, culture, and history are inseparable. This understanding has also shaped the psychology and neuroscience of memory since its inception by Ebbinghaus, the psychopathology of memory since Freud, and the literary discourse of autobiographical remembering since the end of the 18th century and, even more, since modernism. As a consequence, two distinct traditions of memory research have developed, one centering on the individual and his or her mental and neurobiological capacities, the other on social and cultural contexts, practices, technologies, and traditions of remembering.[2] Both the individualist and the collective/sociocultural camp are well established, conceptually and academically. Organized independently from each other, they investigate their specific versions of memory fairly self-referentially. In other words, memory researchers are typically at home in one camp or the other and hence only rarely need to confront each other.

Despite this orderly division of labor, some troubling questions remain. Are there really two distinct forms, kinds, or entities of human memory, one individual and one social? And if so, how are they linked, overlapping, or mingled? Finally, assume they *are* linked, overlapping, and even intermingled, at which point does their conceptual distinction and opposition—which seems to justify their division, if not fragmentation, into different disciplines—lose its meaning?

Indeed there are researchers and scholars in either camp, who doubt the separation of social and individual practices of mind and memory. That said, it is another issue of how to define them and understand their relationship, an issue that has haunted many human sciences, ranging from the more inside-focused approaches of psychology and neuroscience, philosophy, and psychiatry to the more outside-focused anthropology, sociology, and history. Moreover, the inside-outside gamut is reiterated within each disciplinary context. This is reflected in two fundamentally different approaches to social or collective memory, one individualist and one collectivist; one refers to collective memories as the aggregation of socially framed individual memories (where remembering, though viewed as taking place in some kind of social context, is in itself an individual cognitive process), one that one conceives of collective memories as phenomena sui generis (cf. Olick, 2011).

Take anthropology. Considering the question of how are we to understand the individual and/or social habitation of thought, mind, and memory, Geertz (2000) has described the entire history of the discipline as a continuous struggle to bring, as it was variously put, individual and social, inner and outer, private and public, psychological and historical, experiential and behavioral into an "intelligible relationship." For psychology, Bruner (1990a) has sketched a similar history of the tension between the inner and the outer, the individual and the cultural. Oddly enough, within psychology, memory research has been exclusively concerned from its scientific beginnings with the individual as the site of mnemonic processes, while the social, cultural, and historical dimensions of memory have been explored in quite a different field, that of cultural psychology—a field that, what is more, was for long not considered a part of scientific psychology anyway and rather relegated to the humanities or the social sciences (cf. Cole, 1996; Valsiner, 2012). The conviction of experimental psychologists and neuroscientists that human memory has to be investigated independently from humans' cultural forms of life has, by the same token, strongly contributed to the isolation, if not irrelevance, of traditional psychology of memory within the broader field of social and cultural memory studies.[3]

Another question arises from cultural studies of mind such as those by Geertz and Bruner, and here the answer is more complicated. Is it not precisely this presumption—that what is problematic and needs to be determined is, in Geertz's terms, "some sort of bridging connection" between the world within the individual mind (or brain) and the social and material world outside of it—which brings up the problem in the first place? Differently put, perhaps it is the very juxtaposition of the individual and the social that not only entails the need of "some sort of bridging connection" but also resurrects the Cartesian opposition between the world within the individual mind and the world outside of it.

This question has become even more substantial through research in a number of fields suggesting that humans' mental and neurological capacities, including their mnemonic faculties and practices, coevolved with culture. Michael Tomasello's books *The Cultural Origins of Human Cognition* (1999) and *A Natural History of Human Thinking* (2014) offer a comprehensive synthesis of research supporting this suggestion. "Our minds are not in our bodies," as Geertz put it, "but in the world. And as for the world, it is not in our brains, our bodies, or our minds: they are, along with gods, verbs, rocks, and politics, in it" (2000, p. 205). In line with this view, there has been a growing tendency to treat the biological and the cultural, as well as the individual and the social, no longer as "discontinuous, sovereign realities, enclosed, stand-alone domains externally connected ('interfaced,' as the jargon has it) to one another by vague and adventitious forces, factors, quantities, and causes," to again borrow Geertz's pointed terms (p. 206). Instead, they are constitutive of one another and thus must be treated as such.

In the wake of such arguments, some authors have wondered whether the diverse categories of mnemonic phenomena used in the field—individual memories, social and cultural memories, and social memory representations—really reflect separate things. The term social memory, with its sometimes more, sometimes less clear contrast to individual memory, seems to imply just that, states Olick (2008a; 2008b). Olick, therefore, argues for a different understanding of social memory: as merely a broad, sensitizing umbrella concept, rather than a precise operational definition. What is defied in this latter way is the idea of a clear borderline between social and individual memories, which Geertz so radically problematized. According to Olick, social memory comprises a wide variety of "mnemonic products and practices," many of which fly in the face of the social/individual distinction. Take mnemonic products such as stories, rituals, presentations, speeches, images, records, books, historical documents, buildings, and landscapes. Or consider mnemonic practices such as reminiscence, recall, commemoration, celebration, regret, and autobiographical remembering. Memory practices occur in an infinity of interactional contexts and semiotic environments and through a multiplicity of media, but they only work because they are at the same time individual *and* social, because they have personal *and* societal meanings. "To focus on collective memory as a variety of products and practices," Olick argues, "is thus to reframe the antagonism between individualist and collectivist approaches to memory more productively as a matter of moments in a dynamic process" (2008b, p. 158).

In this chapter, I pursue this line of thought—as suggested by Geertz, Bruner, Olick, and others—by reframing the putative antagonism between individualist and social approaches to remembering with respect to one particular category of mnemonic practices and products. This is the category of autobiographical remembering or, as I have come to reformulate it, the autobiographical process. My case is that the autobiographical process cannot be situated either within the individual or the social camp; nor does it represent some sort of "bridging connection" between the world within the individual mind or brain and the sociocultural and material world outside of it. Rather, one of the main functions of the autobiographical process is to allow the individual to inhabit a cultural landscape and, to localize him- or herself within a historical world. On this account, not only the process of autobiographical self-localization but also the very idea of autobiographical identity—the idea of personal identity as rooted in the conscious remembrance of one's life history—are themselves deeply embedded in a particular cultural world.

To further expound this argument I now shift to a different vantage point, one of strangers and immigrants who face the Western cultural economy of remembering from the outside. In the case of immigrants, this "outside" loses its outlandish strangeness when people begin to blend in with their new life world, when they move to the "inside." Taking a closer look at this experience permits us to gain insight into what happens when different mnemonic traditions meet and possibly mingle, in the process creating new traditions, traditions of mixed memories.

MIXED MEMORIES: THE IMMIGRANT CONDITION

The stories people tell about their lives and the lives of those around them leave footprints across history. Others follow these traces, often without being aware of it. Oral or written, public or private, the telling of and the listening to life narratives is conventionalized by traditions that give more or less importance to autobiographical practices.

That autobiographical memory traditions are multicultural meaning constructions is an experience that has become increasingly bound up with what is called global mobility. To speak of global mobility in view of the many violent manifestations of migration may ring euphemistically. Forced migration, displacement, flight, exile, and social and cultural uprooting have come to determine the existential condition of a steadily growing number of people, "the wretched of the earth," in Frantz Fanon's (1967) famous expression. Experiences of translocation in a global age, where for countless migrants the transitional becomes the permanent, are interwoven with often dramatic experiences of what anthropologists and cultural theorists refer to as permanent cultural transformations (Prentice, Devadas, & Johnson, 2010). Hybrid life forms emerging in the wake of such translocation and displacement have undermined long-established traditions, a phenomenon described as part and parcel of globalization and its creation of "liquid modernity" (Bauman, 2000). They also have generated novel cultural traditions, which comprise new narrative traditions of remembering and forgetting that help in shaping and handing down these new experiences.

There are many stories that recount what it means to leave your home, or be forced to do so, migrate, and try to settle in an unknown world, a world in which you, most likely, will continue a life as a victim of exclusion and social stigmatization. These stories speak to what it means to live in more than one cultural and symbolic universe and not to feel at home in any of them. They report the experience of members of so-called minorities, which is, in fact, the prototype of the postmodern experience. To be sure, we are talking about an array of very different things: oral autobiographical accounts and forms of life writing from many diverse narrative traditions; stories told by a great variety of immigrants, refugees, asylum seekers, boat people, guest workers, adventurers, and many others who have become members of the new tribes of global nomads.

Considering this diversity, we may ask whether there is anything in common, something that suggests the formation of a specific migrant or immigrant culture of remembering. In her study of immigrant self-understanding, Ritivoi (2002) maintains that there is a specific mental and narrative attitude that is brought about by the immigrant condition. We might call it a particular autobiographical sensitivity. This kind of self-reflexivity, if we follow Ritivoi, is essential for making sense of one's past under conditions of radical change and an uncertain present and future. Immigrants are commonly more aware than most people of their ongoing autobiographical efforts. In leaving the original settings of their lives they are led to understand, perhaps more urgently than others, that one's identity is never finished but instead remains an open story. It is a work in progress that produces ever-changing versions of oneself, with autobiographical remembering playing a central role in this work.

Examining personal letters of British immigrants to America from the 19th century, David Gerber (2006) notes about this kind of autobiographical self-reflection that it reveals the self "as a process, fluid and relational, that continuously works at integrating change and continuity" (p. 69)—something that needs to be understood in narrative terms, that is, in stories. In contrast with earlier emigration and immigration, the 19th-century situation was part of an emergent global modernity that demanded people not only meet the material and existential challenges of such a radical break, but also confront a "second project": resolving "the challenge posed to personal identity" (p. 69). For Gerber, the self-awareness that is part of this effort is the awareness of one's self as a process, regardless of whether one's self was once (or was believed to be) stable, rooted, and substantial. Often this is the source of the nostalgic memory of "yesterday's self," as Ritivoi (2002) described it. The immigrant condition is unavoidably bound up with the experience of "self-as-process," the "continuing work of self-making amidst the creative work of living" (Gerber, 2006, p. 70).

A portion of this kaleidoscope of modern experience that has been particularly well examined is the immigrant condition in North America. Investigated for many years by social and cultural scientists, it also is an important issue in literature, the arts, and the study of life writing. One reason for this is obvious: the immigrant condition is, in one way or another, part of the cultural memory of most, if not all people in North America, including the expropriated and displaced indigenous. Again, few possibilities afford us better insights into the subjective side of the immigrant condition than autobiographical accounts told, written, drawn, filmed, performed, and otherwise created and recreated.

But just to say they offer an inside view—a first-person perspective of the experiencing subject—would leave out an essential complication of this view: the "autobiographical self" often did not exist in the indigenous cultural traditions of many immigrants to North America. As described at the beginning of this chapter, this inside perspective is closely linked with the fascination, if not obsession, with the individual self, which is so much a part of Western traditions. However, whereas there are deeply rooted literary and philosophical models of European and North American individualism, subjectivity, and autobiographical self-reflection—take, for instance, the plots of Faust, Don Quixote, Don Juan, and Robinson Crusoe, investigated by Ian Watt (1996) as the only genuine myths of modernity (because they do not stem from ancient and biblical myths)— "Asian-Americans" did not find any narrative genres, plots, and styles allowing them to articulate their specific "hyphenated experience." And those genres, plot structures, and storylines comparable to the Western myths of individuality that were familiar to them from their earlier life were, not surprisingly, unknown to typical Western audiences.

I learned this in an unexpectedly personal way when Nhi Vu and I were studying autobiographical accounts of Vietnamese immigrants to Ontario who had left their home country after the end of the Vietnam war. We noticed that many of these stories were meant to give form and order to often dramatic and traumatic autobiographical experiences by using traditional narrative models such as Vietnamese tales and fables. There was, for example, the story of Mr. Nguyen. Mr. Nguyen told us about his changeful life, framing it along the storyline of "Mr. Tai losing his horse." Mr. Tai and his horse are the protagonists of an old Vietnamese tale that shows how misfortunes can later turn into good fortunes, and the reverse (Vu & Brockmeier, 2003, pp. 458–459). However, when recounted in English and applied to life in downtown Toronto, these models forfeited much of their plausibility and charge. They lost what we called "narrative intelligibility" (Vu & Brockmeier, 2003). While I was puzzled by the ups and downs of Mr. Tai's horse, my bilingual Vietnamese Canadian colleague Nhi smiled and nodded, because she recognized the underlying Vietnamese version of the plot that, for me, was lost in its dry English translation. Without Nhi's explanations, I would have been unable to get a sense of its original narrative vigor.

Obviously, there is a link between place, memory, and language of one's upbringing and the resources for autobiographical talk that Stephanie Taylor calls the born and bred narrative resource. "The born and bred narrative resource is the history implied in references to origins and 'roots,' and to 'home town' and 'nativeness'," Taylor (2010, pp. 13–14) writes. In many ways, this narrative resource establishes and keeps alive a connection to place associated with local or native identities, be it within a specific local, regional (often dialectal), or national context. It binds in, yet it also distinguishes. "It sets up a distinction," Taylor states, "between the people who authentically belong somewhere and others who are newcomers or outsiders" (2010, p. 13). In many of their memory accounts, non-Western newcomers try to get a grip on the dilemma of how to remember one's past when an important part of one's born and bred narrative resource is missing; when one's autobiographical stories lead back to places and times without the self-centered narrative focus that fulfills the expectations of North American individualism. In North America, the land of immigrants, this dilemma appears in countless variations. As a consequence of the global nature of migration, very different forms of autobiographical narrative practices have developed. They vary according to the ethnic and cultural origins of immigrants, as well as in respect to their social and political status and education. For instance, for a long time, part of the experience of Asian immigrants was the far-ranging discrimination they faced—socially, economically, and legally.

It is a remarkable process in which, irrespective of these obstacles, a robust Asian American tradition of autobiographical literature emerged over the course of the second half of the 20th century, as Brian Niiya (1999) has shown.[4] Already in 1988, *Asian American Literature: An Annotated Bibliography* listed at least 50 published unambiguous autobiographies. In addition, there were numerous nonfiction works containing oral histories, reports, and biographies, non-book length autobiographical accounts, and a significant number of autobiographical novels and works of fictions that articulated autobiographical experiences of Asians in North America. Although we know that behind these experiences are the lived realities of millions of people, the question remains how we explain this sudden outpouring of personal memories within a few decades. All the more, in fact, given that this outpouring could not draw on specific narrative forms and conventions, nor was it backed up by institutions in the world of literature, academia, publishing, and media conducive to its emergence.

This question becomes even more interesting if we keep in mind the complication, already noted, that in many of the countries from which the authors emigrated we do not find traditions of autobiographical writing and self-reflection comparable to those in Western countries. In traditional Chinese literature the thematic and psychological focus on human individuality is typically interwoven with a strong concern for social relations, as various literary and cultural-historical investigations have emphasized (e.g., Hegel & Hessney, 1985; Marsella, DeVos, & Hsu; 1985). In resonance with Confucian and Taoist traditions, the focus tends to be on what characters do in their familial and institutional roles and their relationships to others vis-à-vis a set of moral obligations, rather than what they do, feel, and remember as autonomous and "outstanding" individuals, as in much of Western life writing (Wu, 1990). Only recently, the orientation toward these forms of life seems to have lost its moral and aesthetic hegemony and, not least under the influence of Western ideas and models of the self and self-reflections, the autobiographical "I" has emerged in Chinese literature (Dongfang 2001a, 2001b; Wang, J., 2008).

In searching for clues on the Asian American autobiographical tradition, Niiya remarks, we thus must look not at Asia but at America. So let me seize this suggestion and take a look at the literary and cultural history of this tradition. That this history also reflects, and impacts on, political, economic, and institutional constraints—the aforementioned economy of remembering, which also defines how the autobiographical process is supposed to be realized—might be surprising only for those who take the autobiographical process to be an exclusively individual, mental, or neuronal enterprise. There is, however, little surprise when we take the point made in these chapters that there is no individual microcosmos of remembering that is not part and parcel of the macrocosmos of cultural memory, to use an expression by Qi Wang (Wang & Brockmeier, 2002). More specifically, the autobiographical process is not a mental proclivity or a cognitive operation but a form of life, a form of history. I thus first review some of the political, economic, and institutional constraints of the Asian American autobiographical tradition before I turn to its narrative and psychological features.

The Asian American autobiographical tradition

There are a number of specific historical aspects that stand out in the first decades of (published) Asian American autobiographies and memoirs. One is that almost all writings have in common that their authors are known for little else except their autobiographies. Only one author was known to a broader public outside his immediate community.[5] All others represent for the American public what Niiya (1999) calls the idea of a collective self. People read their writings because they spoke for the memories of a group, not of particular individuals. Although this might also be the case with autobiographical writers from other ethnic minorities who speak for their communities, there is something different going on with autobiographers of Asian descent. Most of these Asian Americans were not writing autobiographical books that were intended to speak for their group, as Niiya maintains; rather, "The story of the Asian American autobiography is the story of the collective self *imposed* on writers who never intended it" (1999, p. 430). For many years publishers turned out autobiographies and memoirs that confirmed a widespread picture of the Asian American experience, supposing that the public would read these books as true and authentic representations of lived reality. This meant that only autobiographical memories that lived up to the stereotypical expectations of Americans— or at least, American publishers—had a chance to go into print. According to Niiya's account, the rationale behind this was twofold: a preconceived notion of what Asian Americans should be like and an interest in conveying a particular political message. What was this message?

Nearly all the published autobiographical literature by Asian Americans shares some features. First of all, there is optimism. It is the optimism of America during World War II, the post-war and pre-Vietnam era of the Cold War, a time of unshakable faith in the American way of life with its virtues of hard work and smooth assimilation. During the Second World War, while Japanese Americans on the West Coast were being held in concentration camps, two "explicitly happy" autobiographies by Chinese Americans were published.[6] Likewise during the 1960s, while ghettos burned, racial minorities took to the streets, civil rights and Black Power movements marched, more "happy autobiographies" appeared.[7] "Until the mid-1970s, "nearly all published Asian American autobiographies were books that supported the status quo" (Niiya, 1999, p. 430). It seems that the periods when the most, and the most popular, autobiographical books appeared coincided with periods when the status quo, including that of minorities and immigrants, was questioned the most—by civil rights and women movements, by democratic and liberal critics, by anticolonialism and anti-Vietnam war protesters.

A second remarkable trend, especially among the first wave of Asian American autobiographies (a great number of which appeared in the 1960s) is the profusion of woman autobiographers. This is all the more striking because the number of female immigrants was minuscule compared to the number of male immigrants at the time. Bear in mind that these are the years of large-scale labor emigration from Asia. Most of the immigrants were working class migrants who settled in largely poor ethnic ghettos (for example, the infamous Chinatowns) or in farm or transport worker camps. Thus it is all the more peculiar that almost all published autobiographies of Asian Americans reflected the perspective of female visitors, who were mostly upper or at least middle class.

This preference by the American public and the publishing industry for autobiographies by Asian women becomes more comprehensible if we recall the widespread representation of the beautiful Asian female. Women from the Far East were not just beautiful, they were exotic. And, most importantly, they were shy and deferential, at least in film, photography, and the many sites of popular culture. This marks a stark contrast with the image of Asian men who—after decades of war in and against countries like Japan, Korea, China, Vietnam, Laos, Cambodia, to mention only East Asia—and decades of films, books, and media coverage showing Asian men in contexts reenacting those wars, might have been less inviting (cf. Sato, 2005).

And there is another female linkage. Practically all of the women autobiographers addressed issues of female identity speaking to both the liberal and conservative women of the middle classes. All these women, writes Niiya (1999), "attack their traditional cultures for repressing women and praise the West for allowing women more freedom" (p. 432). Amy Ling (2009), a critic and scholar of Asian American culture, argues that the works receiving the most accolades in their time reflected their audience and its taste rather than the quality of the books themselves. Ling refers not only to autobiographies like that of Jade Snow Wong, but also to the works of Winnifred Eaton, who played a crucial role in setting up the tradition, including the canon of conventions according to which Asian Americans were expected to remember their lives. Born to an English merchant and a woman from Shanghai who had been adopted by English missionaries, Eaton wrote enormously successful books in the first two decades of the 20th century, delineating the template of what she saw as the Asian American experience (Birchall, 2001). Some of her books were written with an explicit autobiographical claim, such as *Me, A Book of Remembrance* (1915). Her *A Japanese Nightingale* (1902) was turned into a Broadway play and, in 1919, made into a motion picture. Its success later led her to write screenplays for the burgeoning film industry.

By selecting these books, films, and plays, publishers, studios, and the entertainment industry apparently wanted to appeal to the taste and cultural prejudices of an audience that, to be sure, was not particularly interested in learning about the Japanese or Chinese and their culture of memory. "The frail Japanese or Eurasian heroines," as Ling states, "romantically involved with dominant Caucasian men in high positions, the Chinese American success story at a time when the United States was at war with Japan, satisfied a public that sought to confirm its own myth, in stories about its superiority, generosity, and openness" (2009, pp. 83–84).

Finally, there is another commonality, namely, Christianity. To different degrees, the majority of the authors remember their Americanization as a journey to the Christian faith. I find Niiya's interpretation convincing that such life stories served to reinforce to the predominantly Christian American readers the idea of Christianity as a cultural bridge. At the same time, they subtly confirmed the superiority of the Western idea of autobiographical remembering as an individual and inward-looking mental operation, an operation that, since Augustine's *Confessions,* had been viewed in the Christian tradition as an act of soul examination.

All these factors contributed to the complex interplay of selection and reinforcement operative in the emergence of the Asian American memory tradition. In synchrony with television and film industry, schooling, and educational programs, a white middle class projection defined what it meant for Asian Americans to live a morally proper life. It also outlined their memory values, the ideas of what they were to remember about their past and consider as their new autobiographical identity. Finally, and perhaps most importantly, it suggested what they were to convey to their children as a central part of their immigrant cultural memory. What this outline came down to, then, was a moral blueprint for growing up as "real Americans," assimilated to what Milton Gordon (1964) described as "Anglo-conformity."

Only in recent years have novel forms of Asian American life writing emerged that break with this tradition. In challenging the inherited scripts of assimilation and hyphenated self-understanding, they have explored more individual approaches to self-representation, cultural memory, and ideas of national belonging (Davis, 2007; 2011). Individuality is a key concept here. The new autobiographers leave behind the traditional idea of a collective Asian (or, at best, Chinese, Japanese, Vietnamese) self that is defined by the expectations of American readers. Experimenting with genre and narrative techniques, they use new ways of life writing such as graphic novel, meta-fiction, and autoethnography to "hybridize," that is, normalize their hyphenated existence (Geok-lin Lim & Hong, 2007).

At the beginning of the 21st century, Asian American autobiographers are committed to what Rocío Davis (2007) describes as two intersecting projects. One is reclaiming history, that is, a particular history that goes beyond the canonical Euro American models appropriated by earlier Asian American writers; the other is building community, a community that differs from what was seen as a merely transitory community of foreigners/immigrants on their way to becoming "real Americans." Despite its heterogeneous composition, the Asian American community—or perhaps more precisely, communities—remembered and evoked by a new generation of autobiographical writers, can be conceived of as part of a larger enterprise. This is the creation and preservation of a new cultural memory, a new shared vision of past and present, both in collective *and* individual terms. Clearly this new social and personal remembrance, as Davis suggests, is linked to a new vision of history at large:

> From a generic perspective, life writing narrativizes memory, reflection, and imagination, as the autobiographer configures his or her past into a shape that takes its formal design from established modes. But because the content of the narration in the context of Asian North American writing necessarily involves racial negotiation, social experience, and political engagement, the narrative becomes "history"—the public story of a past shared with others and assumed to have actually occurred. (Davis, 2007, p. 4)

REMEMBERING CONFUCIUS

Many literary and cultural critics agree that it was one autobiography that first broke with this imposed Asian American culture of memory, one book that triggered discussions that would change this situation decisively. This book was Maxine Hong Kingston's *The Woman Warrior: Memoirs of a Girlhood Among Ghosts*. Whereas in the last section I sketched the structural and political constraints of the cultural discourse of autobiographical remembering, my analysis of Hong Kingston's memoir in the final part of this chapter foregrounds the workings of a counter-narrative. It demonstrates that the rules and conventions of a memory tradition can be challenged, at least sometimes. It thus points out a different aspect of the claim that the individual microcosmos of autobiographical remembering is always part and parcel of the macrocosmos of cultural memory.

What was special about Hong Kingston's *The Woman Warrior*? Published in 1976, it seemed to ignore what until then had been the canon for life writing, defining what and how the Chinese American was expected to remember in order to become a real American. Constituting a novel genre unto itself, this memoir presented a new way of autobiographically understanding oneself within a world of diverse cultural traditions. In carrying out an individual merger of American and Chinese traditions of cultural memory, Kingston created a hitherto unknown form to reinterpret the "hyphenated condition." For Davis, Hong Kingston's *The Woman Warrior* not only revealed an important intervention in the political and cultural understanding of what it meant to be Chinese American, but also challenged established concepts of narrative identity, feminism, and the autobiographical mode; after Hong Kingston, "American autobiography was never the same" (2007, p. 4).

I already have given some cultural and political background. Hong Kingston happened to write her memoir at a particular historical moment in the United States, in the socioculturally turbulent 1970s. A period of political openness, these also were times of new interests, new audiences, and new editors. A novel sensitivity emerged to issues until then excluded from the world of learning, literature, and published autobiographical self-reflection, such as race, class, and gender. A new picture of the immigrant condition came to the fore that was rarely smooth and pleasant but often miserable and brutal. It certainly did not have much in common with the fantasy vision of the exotic Asian beauty and her successful Americanization and Christianization.

In *The Woman Warrior*, Hong Kingston remembers her childhood and youth as the daughter of Chinese immigrants Tom and Ying Land Hong who grew up in the 1940s and 1950s in Stockton, California. Her world is that of a community of Chinese Americans, and her main theme is to strike a balance between her Chinese past that permeates all aspects of her life and her American present and future. Maxine's parents, highly educated people in prerevolutionary China, owned and operated a laundry in California. Having settled among immigrants who also had been their neighbors in the ancestral land, they only spoke Chinese. Their world was a world apart. Living in the midst of their memories, they seemed to never really arrive in the American present. Aside from helping with the laundry business and attending an official American school and, in the evenings, a privately run Chinese school, Maxine immersed herself in reading the Chinese literary classics her parents brought with them. The second big thing was watching movies. The movies were mostly Chinese operas. Presented at the local Confucian Church, the operas turned the place from a merely spiritual to a cultural and intellectual center of the community. "Remembering Confucius" is what Hong Kingston would later call the recollection of these experiences.

And, of course, there was the world of "talk-story," the ubiquitous oral narratives from China that were told in the family, especially by her mother, Brave Orchid. A strong woman deeply rooted in Cantonese traditions, her voice commanded, as Maxine feels, "great powers." With the thermometer in the laundry reaching more than a hundred and ten degrees, Brave Orchid would say that it was time to tell another ghost story so everyone would get some good chills up their backs. The lively family tradition of storytelling and reminiscing about the Chinese past, which involved personal experiences and family histories as well as traditional myths, legends, and Confucian maxims and parables, created a unique space of everyday cultural memory. For the young girl, individual and collective remembering blended, and real characters, imagined figures, ghosts, and other heroes of fantasy became even more indistinct as is usually the case with children. This densely populated space, the space of a "girlhood among ghosts," would increasingly reveal itself as the emotional home of the autobiographical self of the future author, who would incorporate many of the meandering memories of her parents and other dwellers and visitors of this narrative universe into her own memories.

It is easy to imagine the stories from this space as nostalgic reminiscence about enchanted childhood days à la Marcel Proust. But Hong Kingston's tone is different. Her writing is not that of a hundred and ten degrees. She makes it clear that the coming-of-age of a girl in America in the midst of a continually reiterated Chinese family memory, which operates as a pressure cooker of a much larger cultural macrocosmos, comes with irksome uncertainties and threatening contradictions. In contrast to her parents she has, and wants, to enter the outside reality. She wants to inhabit the American America and not only the Chinese America, figuring out "how the invisible world the emigrants built around our childhood fits in solid America" (Hong Kingston, 1989, p. 5); and she wonders:

> Chinese-Americans, when you try to understand what things in you are Chinese, how do you separate what is peculiar to childhood, to poverty, insanities, one's family, your mother who marked your growing with stories, from what is Chinese? What is Chinese tradition and what is the movies? (pp. 5–6).

Not surprisingly, whenever the little girl gets in touch with "solid America" she encounters difficulties. School is the place where these difficulties manifest themselves most obviously. But are these difficulties of the school, of America, or of herself? Kingston's memories recount touching episodes from the classroom. "I could not understand 'I.'," she reports. "The Chinese 'I' has seven strokes, intricacies. How could the American 'I', assuredly wearing a hat like the Chinese, have only three strokes, the middle so straight?" (Hong Kingston, 1989, p. 166)

Like all children learning to write, Maxine wonders about the oddities of the characters, their personalities, and their imagined inner life; an entire comparative folk psychology becomes visible. "Was it out of politeness that this writer left off strokes the way a Chinese has to write her own name small and crooked? No, it was not politeness; 'I' is a capital and 'you' is a lower case" (pp. 166–167). But "I" and "you" is, of course, not only about letters; it is also about who is the Chinese self and who the American self. More than that, who is the self and who is the other? And when and with which voice do they speak?

> I remember telling the Hawaiian teacher, "We Chinese can't sing *land where our fathers died*." She argued with me about politics, while I meant because of curses. But how can I have that memory when I couldn't speak? My mother says that we, like the ghosts, have no memories. (p. 167)

The girl asks herself, is there a difference between "me" and the silent ghosts? An unsettling question, all the more as Maxine has trouble not only writing but also speaking "the other language" at all. During her first three years at school she fell into total silence and the world turned black.

> I painted layers of black over houses and flowers and suns, and when I drew on the blackboard, I put a layer of chalk on top. I was making a stage curtain, and it was the moment before the curtain parted or rose. The teachers called my parents to school, and I saw they had been saving my pictures, curling and cracking, all alike and black. [. . .] My parents took the pictures home. I spread them out (so black and full of possibilities) and pretended the curtains were swinging open, flying up, one after another, sunlight underneath, mighty operas. (p. 165)

Whose memories?

Hong Kingston's memoir is split into five parts. Each section tracks different aspects of the development of the young girl into a woman, and that is: an avenging warrior. Sifting through the surrounding story-worlds, Maxine forms a vision of herself: "I could make myself a warrior like the swordswoman who drives me" (Hong Kingston, 1989, p. 48). Was there any better way to survive the many challenges, both Chinese and American? Playing through different autobiographical possibilities, possible worlds and possible selves, the different sections interweave personal memories with the stories of inspirational female figures. All these figures are autobiographically appropriated and turn, in one way or another, into one: the woman warrior. Three of these role-model women belong to Maxine's family: her mother Brave Orchid, her aunt Moon Orchid, and a mysterious "no-name aunt." Two of them belong to the realm of collective imagination, the original woman warrior Fa Mu Lan and the poetess Ts'ai Yen, both legendary Chinese figures and protagonists of many tales.

In extending the individual frame of her memories, Hong Kingston sets out to simultaneously localize herself within her everyday Chinese American world in Stockton and the imagined world of her family's memories and popular Cantonese stories of ghosts and demons. She remembers when her girl self opens an old metal tube that holds her mother's documents, "the smell of China flies out, a thousand-year-old bat flying heavy-headed out of the Chinese caverns, where bats are as white as dust, a smell that comes from long ago, far back in the brain" (p. 57). In tracing her autobiographical I, as this metaphor suggests, Hong Kingston gets entangled in an uncontrollable network of cultural remembering, oral, written, painted, and otherwise performed—an endless cultural intertext that inextricably mingles with history itself.

Emphasizing the interplay between an individual's sense of self and the community's stories of selfhood, Sidonie Smith (1991) remarked that it is through this oscillation that the narrator in Hong Kingston's narratives brings herself into existence. Smith goes on to write that *The Woman Warrior* offers us the occasion to observe the complex cultural imbroglios "that surround the autobiographer who is engaging two sets of stories: those of the dominant culture and those of an ethnic subculture with its own traditions, its unique stories" (1991, p. 1058). Moreover, we may add, we are offered an occasion to view the merger of these two sets of stories into one stream, the stream of Hong Kingston's own autobiographical process. Again and again, she shows that this process has its own dynamic, which will not stop even if she leaves the times and places of her upbringing: "before we can leave our parents, they stuff our heads like suitcases which they jam-pack with homemade underwear" (Hong Kingston, 1989, p. 87).

No wonder, then, that even the banal aspects of American everyday life appear to be elements of a new plot, as in these early memories:

> But America has been full of machines and ghosts—Taxi Ghosts, Bus Ghosts, Police Ghosts, Fire Ghosts, Meter Reader Ghosts, Tree Trimming Ghosts, Five-and-Dime Ghosts. Once upon a time the world was so thick with ghosts, I could hardly breathe; I could hardly walk, limping my way around the White Ghosts and their cars. There were Black Ghosts too, but they were open eyed and full of laughter, more distinct than White Ghosts. (pp. 96–97)

More than one generation after Maxine Hong Kingston, another Chinese American autobiographical writer, Yiyun Li, wrote that "a foreign country gives one foreign thoughts." In her book *A Thousand Years of Good Prayers*, this is a thought of Mr. Shi, who is visiting his daughter in America. Yiyun Li came to the United States in 1996, at 24 years of age. She describes the same strangeness and fascination of talking, thinking, and remembering in a language and culture so different from the one in which she had felt at home before. Though they share several themes, Hong Kingston's experiences differ from Li's in that they were made within a world of immigrants, a world she perceived from within. The perspective behind the memories of *The Woman Warrior* is not that of an adult Chinese who faces America from the outside, as an individual immigrant or visitor, but of a girl who has developed, from the inside, her own genre that reflects her hybrid point of view as a native Asian American. In contrast, Li's likewise highly acclaimed book, although clearly echoing her Chinese linguistic background, has fascinated critics in the way it ably bows to the forms of the Western tradition of autobiographical self-examination. Colm Tóibín (2006) noticed that Li's collection of stories may be her first book written in English but it shows her utterly at home in a narrative style and a kind of psychological empathy shaped by Chekhov and Maupassant, and in tones used by William Trevor and Alice Munro.

Significantly different was, at the time, the reaction of readers to Hong Kingston's book. Many of them were confused by her floating of very different and unfamiliar genres with what was supposed to be a personal autobiographical account. Hong Kingston (1982) replied to her critics in a piece that she called "Cultural miss-readings by American reviewers" where she expressed her frustration that even those who praised her book could not see beyond their own stereotyped thinking. This included what she called the painful "exotic-inscrutable-mysterious-oriental reviewing," according to which everything unfamiliar to an established pattern of remembering and identity appeared to be "obscure" and reinforcing the feeling that, as one critic wrote, "East is East and West is West and never the twain shall meet" (quoted in Ling, 2009, p. 84).

There is no doubt that reading Hong Kingston's memoirs is not always easy. At times, I found it reminiscent of my struggle to understand the Canadian Vietnamese stories, which, too, never lost for me a certain enigmatic quality. Hong Kingston's stories often make one wonder, who is speaking. Who is the remembering I? Are we listening to a narrator who is a young girl, her mother, the author, or all of them? Some may even hear the voices—Chinese voices, that is—of those who told many of these stories before. Readers might feel confused by the continuous blurring of borderlines considered canonical in the Western culture of memory and life writing; among these is the borderline separating the personal from the collective. This is related to the expectation that autobiographical narratives are to be accurate and reliable accounts of individual experiences, clearly distinguished from folk narratives, fairy tales, myths, epic poems, and other social discourse forms. This borderline partly coincides with the one assumed to distinguish fact and fiction, the real and the imagined.[8] All these distinctions entail a complex cultural system not only of narrative but also of ethical and other philosophical conventions negotiating the meanings of "fact" and "fiction" under changeable circumstances (cf. Brockmeier, 2013a).

In addition, Hong Kingston's memoir draws on many resources of the English and Chinese languages. Sometimes her English reads like a literal translation of a Chinese epic poem, at other times, the protagonists from Chinese stories and myths speak with a strong American accent. Here and there we are addressed by a voice that ironically or, perhaps, even sarcastically performs a parody of what a "Westerner" imagines to be Chinese American lingo (again, I see Nhi Vu smiling while she performs for me how it sounds when a Vietnamese native speaker ironically imitates an English accent).

Finally, there is no stable distinction between the male and the female. For this reason, the book was read as advancing feminist discussions in the 1970s. In fact, even if most of its fury and bitterness is articulated vis-à-vis the history of oppression and disrespect for girls and women in China, it undeniably also takes a critical stance toward America, especially its racism and class distinctions. *The Woman Warrior* makes it clear that her author also remembers the long history of economic exploitation of and discrimination against Asian immigrants. "I've learned exactly," she asserts, "who the enemy are. I easily recognize them—business-suited in their modern American executive guise, each boss two feet taller than I am and impossible to meet eye to eye" (Hong Kingston, 1989, p. 48).

Although eventually successfully established in the American reality, Hong Kingston has not forgotten what "the Laws" meant in the everyday life of her community. "The Laws" were special legal restrictions limiting the civil rights of Asian immigrants in the United States, forcing them, among other things, to live in segregated ghettos, the infamous Chinatowns, at the end of the 19th and the beginning of the 20th century. Her memoir is about a childhood determined as much by Chinese and American memory traditions as by experiences linked to race, class, and gender. And what is more, it shows that in her autobiographical process the two traditions are indissolubly intertwined.

Obviously, personal anger is one of the driving forces behind this autobiographical quest—which is quite different from McEwan's portrait of

Perowne, which was driven by anxiety and a sense of threat and insecurity. A sense of anger also seems to have motivated the desire to identify with the half-mythical figure of the woman warrior. However, Hong Kingston writes that the weapon for the autobiographer is not "the sword of the swordswoman" but the act of remembrance of events that for a long time were not allowed to be remembered, let alone reported. "The idioms for revenge are 'report a crime' and 'report to five families.' The reporting is the vengeance—not the beheading, not the gutting, but the words" (Hong Kingston, 1989, p. 53).

Remembering no-name woman

An intriguing example of the power attributed to the autobiographical process—the "true weapon of the woman warrior"—is the story of "no-name woman." Do not tell anyone you had an aunt, said her mother, before going on to recount to her daughter the gruesome tale of Maxine's aunt's illegitimate pregnancy. An unacceptable offence in a patriarchal society, it causes the village to ostracize and terrorize the aunt, who eventually kills herself by jumping into the family well. In order to punish her even after her death and, at the same time, out of shame, neither her story nor her name is ever mentioned again. Even Maxine, the girl, does not dare ask or talk about her aunt, though this nameless woman hovers as an unspeakable memory, a permanent "absent presence," as Helena Grice (2002, p. 52) puts it, through her life.

To wrap a story in the paradoxical dictum "don't tell" is a widespread figure of speech (Cheung, 1988). But it is, after all, a telling rhetorical move. Yet, there also are more radical practices of memory denial, such as rigorous ritual silencing. Not only in the Chinese tradition does it constitute an important part of the collective remembering and forgetting of ethnic communities (Anderson, 2006; Halbwachs, 1992). I think, however, that Assmann (1992) has a point when he underlines that the social practice of "structural amnesia" is less a concern of communities but of authority, control, and power. Assmann describes it as the "alliance of power and forgetting" (1992, p. 71). Sider and Smith (1997) view it in terms of historical strategies that aim to silence certain events and their "histories" in the shadow of other events and their "histories." The Romans, for instance, introduced the practice of erasing the memory of a traitor or an emperor who fell in disgrace after his death and was officially "damned," the so-called *damnatio memoriae* or condemnation of memory. The name, images, and every trace of life and deeds of the person who must not be remembered were expunged from sight, in whatever form these writings, representations, and mementos were previously exposed to the public.

Yet oppression typically entails resistance and subversion, and this is also true for the dialectic of social remembering and forgetting. An exclusionary framing of public memory can provoke unintended acts of remembrance, collective and individual, and endow them with uncontrolled subversive power. This, indeed, is what Hong Kingston is interested in. Why, she wonders, does she only many years later talk and write about her memory of the story her mother told her about her aunt? Why was she silent for so long? Apparently, she concludes, the emotional texture of her autobiographical process has changed; now, however, the affective tenor is radically different: "My aunt haunts me—her ghost drawn to me because now, after fifty years of neglect, I alone devote pages of paper to her" (Hong Kingston, 1989, p. 16). A belated sense of horror and ire has her writing down her memories of this forbidden Chinese story in English. Searching for words for the unspeakable, she begins with naming the nameless, using the possibilities of English to turn no name woman into a proper name: No Name Woman. At a single blow her aunt is given an existence. She is remembered and her suicide reported as an act of revenge against patriarchal brutality. Leaving the realm of ghosts and shadows, she, too, transforms into a woman warrior. Her story becomes that of an avenger, of an ally in the same rebellious spirit of the autobiographer.

In a number of ways, I read this episode as highly characteristic of Hong Kingston's methods of creatively engaging in the autobiographical process. For one, it demonstrates how a terse narrative, once told by Brave Orchid to warn her daughter to obey the rules of tradition, is recalled and reinterpreted decades later and, in the light of the remembering subject's changed self-understanding, acquires new meanings and feelings. Hong Kingston leaves no doubt that there is no way to retrieve and reinstantiate any of the original or historical events. This is not one of the intentions driving her autobiographical enterprise. Her memories—many of which are, as we have seen, memories of stories she heard and whose traces she followed—are prompted by a sense of resistance and subversion. These are ideas that work for her in her present American life, the life of an adult woman and writer, which she is leading at the time of writing her memoir. Her entire project of remembrance-reimagining, as Shu-ching Chen (2000) stated, is rooted in her real-life predicament in which she finds herself unable to formulate an Asian American identity for the lack of appropriate narrative models.

Ghosts and selves

The amalgamation of various traditions of memory carried out in this memoir is, not least, a linguistic event. It takes place on a number of levels and by multiple means, ranging from naming (that is, identifying, foregrounding, individualizing) to the blending of various genres, as well as stylistic, rhetorical, and narrative forms. The blending effect is heightened by the intermingling of narrative points of view and voices from diverse traditions. Consider an example that seems to be only about semantics, that is, about words, but opens a much wider narrative space: Hong Kingston's use of the word *ghost*. Ghosts, as the title of the book already suggests, pervade the entire memoir. They are everywhere, and recognizing, labeling, and exorcizing them turn out to be essential mnemonic practices. Often the word ghost translates as the Mandarin *gwei*. But *gwei*, as Ling and Chu (1998) noted, has a broader spectrum of meanings than its common English translation, reaching from "demon" and "specter" to "barbarian" and "foreign devil." It can have a polite or insulting tone, it can be playful or serious, a precise reference or a metaphor.

But Hong Kingston's use of ghost is not merely about the various meanings of a word in Mandarin and English. The various Chinese *gweis* come with extended narrative entourages. They appear in ever changing guises. Establishing mysterious connections among the manifold occasions of their appearance, they come into sight in a variety of situations in the life of the little and the adult Maxine as well as in the lives of the other characters of her memoir. One effect of this is that the autobiographical process turns into a, at least for a Western reader, strangely animated and spirited enterprise of which the narrator herself seems to have only little control. Ling and Chu (1998) remark that Hong-Kingston's stories have a "fluid quality," as if "the text itself flows across the boundaries that separate genres, languages, and cultures" (p. 445).

We can suppose that Hong Kingston was well aware of how novel her understanding of the autobiographical process must have been for her readers. Drawing knowledgeably on both English and Chinese resources as well as on personal and collective memories (including oral traditions of folk and mythical storytelling, and literary, imagistic, filmic, and musical traditions), she even created her own tropes, such as the Mandarin ghosts. Surely she also was conscious of the difficulties that her break with traditional genre rules, both in the field of life-writing and autobiographical remembering, created for a mainstream audience. Take her use of the pronoun "I." At first sight an unimposing grammatical device, the English pronoun "I" brings with it an array of far-ranging assumptions about identity, subjectivity, and the self. On a theoretical, especially, linguistic and philosophical level these assumptions have been extensively investigated (e.g., Mühlhäusler & Harré, 1990). In traditional autobiographical narrative they are, however, rarely addressed. When it comes to concepts such as I, self, and identity, autobiographical discourse "tends to promote an illusion of disarming simplicity," as Eakin (1999, p. ix) has it. This illusion is commonly shored up by a straight representational understanding of the pronoun "I." Although, as Mühlhäusler and Harré (1990) argued, it first and foremost serves a grammatical function, this is mostly overlooked in favor of a naïve-realist interpretation that conceives of the first-person pronoun as a substantial autobiographical self. In most autobiographical narratives the "I-figure," Eakin (1999) observes, appears to turn into a real entity, a buddy like you and me. The use of the first person, which, significantly enough, is capitalized in English, compounds a unified and autonomous sense of being "in full command of our knowledge of our selves and stories." Eakin goes on to say that the use of the "I" not only "conveniently bridges the gaps between who we were once and who we are today, but it tends as well to make our sense of self in any present moment seem more unified and organized than it possibly could be" (1999, p. ix).

In contrast, Hong Kingston's "I" baffled and provoked audiences because it defied the commonsense assumption of a stable and sovereign self. Both for the adult autobiographer and her childhood self, the "I" is a force driven by diverse, indeed, conflicting interpretations, feelings, and desires. More than this, whenever there is an "I" there is a particular point of view upon the world that is built into the cultural grammar of the English language and that does not exist, in this way, in Chinese. Of course, Hong Kingston is not the only one doubting that the pronoun "I" is the straightforward expression of a solid and sovereign self. The South African writer Antjie Krog, pondering about the reason why she uses the I-word, finds that the English "I" is amazingly malleable. It allows her, as she puts it, to forge a new "I" that "allows many breathing spaces around the facts" (Krog, 2005, p. 103). Another reason is that she uses the "I" as if she is applying a mask to her face. This mask permits her to take a stance that she otherwise would never take. "Many of the things said by the "I," I would never say" (Krog, 2005, p. 103). To me, it seems that Krog, too, articulates some of Hong Kingston's motives. In distributing the narrator's and her—the author's—own point of view over multiple positions, some factual some fictional, Hong Kingston unfolds an idea of autobiographical subjectivity that, at the time, was so radically new that it left, understandably, many of her readers puzzled.

Even today we may feel a sense of bewilderment if we try to understand how the "I" of the *Woman Warrior* emerges as the focal point of an autobiographical synthesis that is neither exclusively Western nor Eastern, neither male nor female, neither factual nor fictive, but incorporates all of this into one seamless narrative. What this synthesis puts forward is a hybrid identity that tries to realize what, perhaps optimistically, has been characterized as "a model of transcultural identity" (Davis, 2005, p. 48). From a narrative perspective, it spans a continuum of stories that, despite all ruptures, reaches from Brave Orchid's initial admonition "You must not tell ..." to the intercultural and intergenerational vision of the auto-biographer: "Here is a story my mother told me, not when I was young, but recently, when I told her I also talk story. The beginning is hers, the ending, mine" (Hong Kingston, 1989, p. 206).

The classical Lockeian model of autobiographical integrity was based on the idea of an autonomous and sovereign self, the modern Western idea of individual subjectivity. Against this backdrop, Hong Kingston appears as an autobiographer grappling with challenges of remembering that reflect culturally very different conditions. Often, these conditions are labeled as a "culture of memory." In order to avoid a semblance of homogeneity that often is associated with the concept of "culture," I have preferred to speak of a cultural economy of remembering and forgetting, a notion that resonates better with a dynamic constellation of material and intellectual practices, technologies, and objects of remembering and forgetting, as well as concepts, rules, and values regulating this dynamic. Many aspects of Hong Kingston's cultural economy of remembering are different from John Locke's (and again there is a difference between the economy of remembering of little Maxine, the one protagonist, and the adult writer Hong Kingston, the other protagonist of *The Woman Warrior*). In fact, despite the thousand-year-old bats and ghosts that fly through this book, its primary reality is the present in which it is written—somewhere toward the end of the 20th century. That is, its reality is that of the fleeting, multiethnic, and multicultural life worlds of modern and postmodern societies, and the different kinds of self-experience that these life worlds entail. This experience comes in tandem with that of growing fragmentation, inequality, social tensions, and conflicts.

Even within the Western tradition these have been new experiences. Mark Freeman and I have argued that many personal experiences of the postmodern world can no longer be emplotted within traditional narrative genres of autobiography, such as the *Bildungsroman*, adventure story, life as process of self-finding, redemption plot, and so on (Freeman & Brockmeier, 2001). As we move into the heart of the postmodern condition, the challenge of achieving some measure of narrative integrity may, in fact, become intensified. *The Woman Warrior*, as Chen (2000) remarked, is a case in point of experiences in search of narrative models that live up to the cultural intricacy of these experiences. The ongoing creation of new autobiographical genres also might speak to this; recall that, according to Smith and Watson (2010), there are about 60 different genres, and the count goes on. How, "in the face of so voluminous a library of possible narratives," Freeman and I wondered, "is one to determine how best to tell one's story?" (2001, p. 92).

However, as my reading of Hong Kingston's memoir—as well as the case studies presented in the previous chapters—have indicated, there is more to the autobiographical process than the question of how best to tell one's story. My argument in this chapter has been that the Western cultures of autobiography are historically developed economies of remembering in which the autobiographical process is a form of life in Wittgenstein's sense. It is a process of self-localization in a cultural world of which autobiographical practices have become an essential part. In such a world, the act of writing one's own personal memories into a huge intertext, the symbolic space of cultural memory, is not simply what we commonly call a symbolic act. It is an inherent part of everyone's everyday life, something that has become intrinsic to the human condition. To put the same point another way, in the Western world, the autobiographical process has become one of the basic forms of life.

To bind oneself into a cultural world is one thing; the other is how the cultural world is bound into the microcosm of one's personal memories. This move is also carried out in *The Woman Warrior*. It demonstrates how it is that collective memories and, more generally, visions from what Taylor (2003) has dubbed the social imaginary—which in Hong Kingston's California encompasses "Chinese" and "American" memories that go far beyond the lived experiences of one individual—can be lodged in the autobiographical memories of that very individual. This also holds for the lacunae of past experience, the memories that seem to be forgotten and blacked out by the power of collective condemnation. Such memories of absence may be dormant until circumstances wake and again draw them into the dynamic of an individual's autobiographical arena. As the story of the No Name Woman reveals, in this process of reinterpretation, re-evaluation, and recomposition, the rememberer eventually manages to undo the *damnatio memoriae* that for many years weighed on her community and herself.

Instead of confining her autobiographical process to her own experiences, the narrator comes to view them within frameworks of cultural memories that embrace the wider ethnic community of her childhood. That is, individual memories are taken to be collective memories. At the same time, the narrator accommodates the Western tradition of auto-biographical narrative, transforming collective memories into personal events, into stories that were told to her by her mother and other members of her childhood world and have now become part of her own autobiographical experience. These are the stories from the hot and steamy laundry in Stockton, Confucius's wondrous cinema, and secretive whispers in the kitchen. At these sites of memory, all of which are linked to particular ghost stories and to the presence of *gweis*, the distinction between the social and the individual blurs once more. And so does the line, whoever once drew it, between the microcosm of individual experiences and the macrocosm of collective memories.

CHAPTER 8

Dissolving the Time of Memory

The Autobiographical Process as Temporal
Self-localization

IN WHICH DIRECTION FLOWS THE TIME OF MEMORY?

All remembering is about time. In Greek antiquity, only the gods need not remember because they do not know time. Theirs is a world of timeless eternity. Humans who have finite lives need to remember because they forget. Even Odysseus, a hero but not a god, forgets and must remember; in fact, he is remembering all the time, as we know in much detail from the great memory book of antiquity, the *Odyssey*. Yet the human condition is not solely characterized by remembering, forgetting, and temporality but by various types of these. This chapter is concerned with the temporal dimension of the autobiographical process, which I have called autobiographical time (Brockmeier, 2000b). I want to elaborate on the idea of autobiographical time by, first, putting it into a larger cultural and intellectual context and, second, taking a closer look at its narrative dynamic. So far I have explored the narrative dynamic of the autobiographical process as one of interpretive meaning-making; now I extend this focus to the nexus of remembering, narrative, and time.

To point out why this route covers new ground, let me start by briefly reviewing the traditional Western way of understanding the relationship between memory and time—that is, I start at the beginning, with Odysseus. When the Greek warrior sets sail to return to his home island of Ithaca after the destruction of Troy, many dangerous years are in the offing. Yet at the same time as he embarks on an uncertain future, he travels back in time, to his own past time, his childhood and his former life. Why has the story of this journey caught the imagination of countless generations of listeners and readers? I believe that much of the fascination of Homer's epic poem stems from the intertwining of future and past, from its conjuring up the idea of simultaneously moving forward and backward in time. The story of Odysseus is at the same time a story about anticipation and hindsight, fusing an outer and forward voyage with an inner and backward voyage. There are the wind and the waves that bring the ship of the hero to Ithaca, but there also is a vision of the past and the power of nostalgia that equally drive the journey.

Remembering is traveling in time, or so it is said. Ever since Odysseus's departure from the Trojan shores into a future guided by his longing for the past, remembering has been associated with a journey in time—an inner journey, a journey to the origin, a journey that leads from one time to another. This, again, is a different metaphorical and narrative field from that of the archive. But what kind of time travel is meant when we speak of this memory journey? Which direction do we travel and in which direction do we cross time when we remember? The traditional view of memory and time provides us with several answers that all come down to one basic scenario, whether metaphorical, narrative, or conceptual. In this scenario experiences (and often even emotions) from the past move, or are moved, to the present. At times we talk about them as something that is "brought back" to the present, or even "brought back to life." Accordingly, memories are *re*called, *re*trieved, or *re*membered; they *re*turned from the past to the present. And although this movement can be slow or quick, direct or hindered, immediate or distorted, voluntary or involuntary, it has, at any rate, a clear direction. We would not say that in remembering we bring the present to the past. Or would we?

Perhaps we could say that in remembering we go back to some earlier event or experience, and in this sense indeed move from the present to the past. *Oh bring me back to the sweetness of past time* is the name for happiness of the Proustian nostalgic, another hero of memory travels, who wants to go back in time. However, for the true nostalgic, the desired state of remembering can only be found, not searched for. A true memory is always *mémoire involontaire*, involuntary memory, triggered by a chance sensory cue that provokes a chain of sometimes overwhelming reminiscences of what before was seen as an irretrievable past. But what bliss, once this chain has started to unfurl!

Yet we also go back to the past when we remember intentionally, that is, when we consciously search or look for something particular. For instance, when we go into the underworld, as happens to Odysseus on his wanderings, or climb down into the pit of the memory archive, like Hegel, or dig something up in an archeological excavation, like Freud, or trace back neuronal activities to the hippocampus, like the neuroscientist. Then we patently reverse the direction and envision ourselves moving from the present to the past, turning around, as it were, the flow of time. Still, we do so in order to ultimately bring back the past to the present, to retrieve or recall precedent experience.

Both the forward and the backward view of the direction of remembering share two assumptions. One is that memory is an archive in which the past is stored; the other is the idea of time as a flow, river, or arrow—to mention just a few metaphorical expressions in this semantic field. Both ideas are deeply rooted in Western cultural history. From Aristotle's theory of nature and Christian teleology of history and salvation to the philosophy of Enlightenment and Newton's physics, time has been imagined as something that has a number of given qualities: it is continuous (ongoing and without interruption or stops), linear (straightforward and without deviation), homogenous (identical with itself in all its manifestations), and directional (moving toward what we call future).[1] In the Western tradition, these features are generally summarized as chronological, which is to say that time is measurable or, as Aristotle called it, countable (Coope, 2005).

This idea of time has been fundamental for the understanding of human memory. However remembering is conceived, it is commonly viewed as taking place against a fixed background of time. When remembering occurs involuntarily—as in the Proustian way—it more or less follows the flow of time; if it is voluntarily—as in the Homeric way—the idea is that in the act of remembering we hold on to or even reverse this flow, but only to bring a memory to the here and now. If the memory cannot be recovered, it will be forgotten and abandoned to the flux of time. In Odysseus's world, this flux is symbolized by the river Lethe, the river of forgetfulness.

Reading the memory journey of the *Odyssey* in this light, I was struck that the same assumptions about time and memory underlying the millennia-old Homeric epics are also widespread in modern discourses on memory and remembering. They are not only shared by modern common sense but also by the scientific study of human memory. Contemporary cognitive psychology generally ascertains that there is an objective trajectory of time, embodied by the cognizing mind or brain, which is continuous, homogenous, and directional. This trajectory forms a fixed temporal background, in synchrony with the Newtonian universe, against which cognitive processes of human timing ("processing of temporal information") are pictured (e.g., Beike, Lampinen, & Behrend, 2004; Block &

Zakay, 2001; Brown & Chater, 2001). This is the standard view. It also applies when time is seen as a knowledge, sometimes called "temporal knowledge," which is taken to be a component of one's autobiographical "self-knowledge" (e.g., Skowronski, Walker, & Betz, 2004). And it holds for approaches that conceive of the human sense of time as not merely bound to one chronology but to multiple chronological scales along which time is experienced and remembered (e.g., Friedman, 2001; 2004). Finally, since Piaget, the idea of a fixed background of objective time has been the basic assumption for developmental-psychological research on the child's emerging cognitive sense of time (Moore & Lemmon, 2001; Piaget 1969).

Turning to neuroscience, we encounter the same idea of time. Indeed, it is constitutive of the neuroscientific model of the brain's backward and forward time travels, a model that has become widespread in discussions about the neuronal basis of human time experience. Time travel has for long been a subject of religion, literature, and film, especially of science fiction, and—in the wake of Einstein's general relativity theory—of theoretical physics and philosophy of science (Nahin, 2001). Tulving, as we recall from Chapter 2, introduced into neuroscience the idea of remembering as mental time travel, an idea which was subsequently taken up by many researchers (e.g., Bar, 2011a; Nyberg, Kim, Habib, Levine, & Tulving, 2010; Suddendorf & Corbalis, 2007). Tulving claimed that episodic memory, the vivid recollection of events and their associated contextual details, affords humans the ability to engage in fictive time travel (Tulving, 2002c; 2005). Postulating "hypothetical mechanisms of memory" that allow us to mentally move backward in time as well as into the future, he has dubbed this assumed capacity "chronosthesia" and suggested that it singles out humans as the only species constantly aware of past, present, and future. According to this view, when we mentally shift back to the past and forward to the future we always move "in time." In fact, as the assumption goes, only because there is a fixed background—the universal Newtonian trajectory—can we tell whether we are in the present, the past, or the future.

Now, the argument I have put forward so far is that, although the traditional model of memory and remembering still dominates many quarters of academic memory discourse, new developments have radically undermined its presuppositions and encouraged us to conceive of remembering and forgetting in a different light. In the previous chapters, I have shown how one of the emerging new options, the narrative alternative, permits us to understand the complex dynamic of the autobiographical process in a way that reaches far beyond the conceptual imagination of the archival tradition. In further exploring the implications and consequences of this vision in terms of time and temporality, I want to point out that there are essential aspects of the autobiographical process that run counter to the trajectories of continuous, chronological, and homogenous time. If we examine these aspects up close, as we will do in a moment, these trajectories appear as an arbitrary imposition from the outside, as normative principles that do not have much in common with either the narrative or the temporal dynamic of the autobiographical process. My project, yet again, is to propose that the narrative alternative permits us a more appropriate, sensitive, and richly textured understanding of the narrative fabric of autobiographical time.

IN THE MODERNIST LABORATORY OF MEMORY AND TIME

In tracing a continuity in the Western vision of time from Aristotle to Newton and contemporary memory sciences, we should not forget that there is more than one tradition. In Chapter 2, drawing on McTaggart's thesis of the "unreality of time," I discussed a nonontological approach to memory that aims to identify the status of a memory through its temporal status, not through its "nature." I then went on to suggest, building on thoughts by Heidegger and Ricoeur, a narrative-hermeneutical perspective of time experience that enables us to understand autobiographical memories as the outcome of interpretive temporalization. What connects McTaggart, Heidegger, and Ricoeur is that they all are philosophers whose works have to be viewed against the backdrop of the modernist revolution in our understanding of time and memory at the beginning of the 20th century.

But the modernist revolution not only affected visions of memory and time; these visions were at its very heart. Einstein's general and special relativity theory was only one, even if arguably the most famous, of the cataclysmic changes of modernism. Other facets are associated with figures like Picasso, Proust, Woolf, Gropius, Eisenstein, Benjamin, Bergson, Man Ray, and Freud, to mention a few names from a long list. This list comprises writers, architects, film directors, painters, photographers, philosophers, sociologists, anthropologists, and cultural theorists. Obviously, the scope of the often-described intellectual and cultural rupture of modernism was broader than its articulation in theoretical physics. When the Newtonian idea of time as a fixed background began to lose its hitherto semblance of naturalness, new spaces for imagination opened up, setting the scene for the emergence of likewise revolutionary prospects of personal, individual, and autobiographical time. What makes these prospects particularly interesting for my line of argument is that they entwined the individual and social dimension of time and memory, akin to the entanglement of individual and cultural memory treated in the last chapter. To understand these amazing scenarios of time better, some historical context is helpful. This context makes the narrative alternative that I am advancing appear not quite so outlandish as it might seem if its only point of reference were the memory sciences.

The first steps in this new direction were taken in the experiments of literary modernism in the decades around the turn of the 20th century. The multitemporal visions brought up in the narrative laboratories of modernist life-writing mentioned earlier, were about settings of memory and time quite different than the movements from the past to the present and from the present to the past depicted at the beginning of this chapter. Many modern writers came to realize that their autobiographical experience of time did not have much in common with the epic tale of Odysseus's memory travels and, probably closer to home, the intelligibly ordered story time of 19th-century realist novels. Irrespective of differences in their styles, worldviews, and personalities, writers such as Proust, Woolf, Joyce, Mann, and Kafka all questioned, in one way or another, time and memory as continuous, homogenous, and directional. They ignored, if not rejected, the grids of chronological temporality as modeled on Newton and those of narrativity as modeled on Aristotle. In her diary, Virginia Woolf notes Thomas Hardy's remark that modern literature renders time in its own way: "'They've changed everything now,' he said. 'We used to think there was a beginning, and a middle and an end. We believed in the Aristotelian theory. Now one of those stories came to an end with a woman going out of the room'" (Woolf, 1954, p. 93).

One reason for the modernists' skepticism of objective or absolute time was, perhaps paradoxically, its very success. As the world was increasingly colonized by the clock and its measurement regime, the Newtonian manifolds got tighter and tighter. Their grids grew closer and extended to more areas of life and imagination, not only in terms of geographic and economic expansion, but also in terms of the extended time scales made apparent by the theories of evolution, geology, and astrophysics. These macro time scales were complemented by the micro scales of sub-atomic particles established by the discoveries of quantum physics. At the same time, technological innovations, including the automobile and the airplane, provided unprecedented standards of speed, offering new experiences of space and time. All of a sudden, enormous distances could be traversed in so short a time as was unimaginable previously. Telegraph, telephone, and radio made possible a disjunction of spatial and temporal distance that came close to the fantastic, which, on a pragmatic level, contributed to further standardization of the many different local times that until then existed side by side.

Various interests intersected in this development. From the point of view of power, control, and economic progress, the diversity of local cultural times had been for long a serious problem. It prompted the urge to homogenize time, turning local times into one abstract and universal time, comparable to the formation of one abstract and universal space—a process described in great detail by Stephen Kern (1983) in his magisterial study, *The Culture of Time and Space 1880–1918*, from which I draw in various parts of this section. Yet the tendency to standardize time also had technological and military reasons. Further, it found support in scientific advances and, even more, in positivist philosophy of science according to which the progress of science consists of the discovery of universal laws and regularities that underlie superficial changes and subjective experiences. In the process, subjective experience became more and more obsolete.

The universalist approach, as we saw above, was not entirely new. Objectivist and absolutist views had been dominating philosophy since Plato and Aristotle. Powerfully reinvigorated in modern times not only by positivist empiricism from Hume to Mill, but also by Kant, Hegel, Marx, they dominated most of 19th-century philosophical thinking. A comparable orientation confirmed many 19th-century historians in their conviction that there is one overarching historical process, encompassing the apparent variegation of local developments. In taking this point of view, history radically broke with the previously held proposition that there are multiple histories revolving around diverse local centers of event (cf. Koselleck, 2004). The new unified "universal history" unfolds along a continuum of a singular and linear time, substituting what earlier epochs had considered the many times of many different developments. Where there were *storiae*, histories and stories, now there was just one *storia*, one history and one story.

This trend, however, was not without contradictions and, particularly in modernist quarters, did not remain unchallenged. One modernist response to the standardization, mechanization, and collectivizing of public time was to emphasize the contrast with private and subjective temporality, with phenomenological and "inner time." Kern maintains that before the late 19th century no one within the Western tradition systematically questioned the homogeneity of time, with the possible exception of Laurence Sterne, who explored a sort of private time in *Tristram Shandy*. "The evidence for it," as Kern explains this exclusion, "are written on the faces of the millions of clocks and watches manufactured every year" (1983, p. 11). With the advent of modernism a counter-movement emerged that viewed this "evidence" with second thoughts. The thrust of many intellectual and cultural productions was to affirm the reality of subjective or personal time against that of objective or public time, which meant to present its nature as heterogeneous rather than homogeneous, fluid rather than atomistic, and reversible rather than irreversible.

It is striking in what a short historical span personal and autobiographical experience of time became a preeminent theme in contemporary novels, dramas, poems, and life-writings. Through newly developed narrative techniques such as "interior monologue"—a term that covers various forms of free direct discourse of which "stream of consciousness" became a particularly striking example—many authors began to explore the spontaneous, nonlinear, and discontinuous ramifications of their own time experience. McEwan's rendering of Henry Perowne's autobiographical process is part of this tradition. In this way, writers became even more aware of what Virginia Woolf called in *Orlando* the "extraordinary discrepancy between time on the clock and time in the mind" (2006, p. 72).

Philosophically, Woolf could draw, or at least could have drawn, on Henri Bergson's rejection of objectivist and absolutist accounts of time. This was, however, only one of a number of similar options within her reach (cf. Banfield, 2003). Like many thinkers in those years, Bergson (1946; 1990) was especially concerned with the subjective experience of time, putting forward arguments for its irrefutable reality. His case was the personalized meaning of the flux of time, *durée*. For Bergson, the experience of remembering was a special form of time experience that did not have much to do with the storing and retrieving of knowledge, let alone information. He rather conceived of time as a form of social engagement, as an activity on which our sense of *durée* depends. For the French philosopher, this sense was distorted by the categorical distinction of past, present, and future that he saw as artificially superimposed on the essentially fluid nature of time.

Bergson's was an influential philosophical voice in the choir of novelists, physicists, psychologists, and social scientists of the day who investigated the ways in which "individuals create as many different times as there are life styles, reference systems, and social forms," as Kern put it (1983, p. 15). With this formulation Kern alludes to a remark by Einstein contrasting Newtonian mechanics, which only permitted one clock, with relativity theory, according to which "we can very well imagine as many clocks as we like" (Einstein & Infeld, 1966, p. 181).

There is indeed much to be said for viewing such philosophical, literary, and scientific statements and the attention they drew to the subjective and intersubjective reality of time as a reaction to the historical trend of standardization and homogenization of time. This view also encompasses the work of Halbwachs and the origin of the modern study of collective memory. Halbwachs (1992) took Bergson's analysis of the subjective experience of time as a starting point to examine the difference and the relationship between subjective and objective or public (or social) apprehensions of the past. However, these "apprehensions" were not only reactions to material changes in the Western cultural economy of time and memory; they also were explorative interventions, put forth by the protagonists of a new culture of conceptual and artistic experimentation with time and time experience. They did not only mirror societal, technological, and scientific advances but were inherent to what Kern calls "a cultural revolution of the broadest scope," a revolution that involved "essential structures of human experience and basic forms of human expression" (1983, p. 6).

One of the most spectacular features of this revolution of human experience comes to the fore when we consider that almost all innovative works of the modernist period were created in big cities, at a time when the great majority of people even in industrialized countries lived in the countryside or in villages and small towns. The huge urban agglomerations that came into existence in Western Europe and North America in the late 19th century were themselves a product of the dynamic of modernism, and so were their cascading consequences. Life in the city became the focal point of new experiences that accumulated to form a novel quality, the metropolis. The modern metropolis set up the terrain for forms of life and time unparalleled in history. A picture often used to capture the new quality of time experience was that of a kaleidoscope of different times, reflecting a unique conflation (and dissolution) of processes of innovation and acceleration. Cities exploded in size, fueled by an exponential increase of industrialization, division and productivity of labor, commerce, and traffic, with all these developments overreaching and accelerating one another. City dwellers were witnessing a breathtaking expansion of transport and information systems, boosted by new technologies of communication via post, telephone, wireless telegraph, radio, phonograph, and cinema. Newspapers turned into media empires, providing an endless flow of information from around the world to stunned audiences who grew in the tens of millions.

Emblematically, in the prewar Europe depicted by Proust's *Recherche*, the car replaces the carriage and the aircraft ousts the balloon. Bear in mind that all of this means the loss of a familiar and beloved past that the protagonist of Proust's novel sets out to oppose with the power of remembrance, that is, with his individual reminiscence. To a significant degree, this power is due to a narratively induced new sense of time. This time, Proust's autobiographical time, is patently nonchronological and nonsequential, a time of memory that, whatever else it may be, undoubtedly is without speed and acceleration, vertigo and exhilaration.

At the turn from the 19th to the 20th century, sociologist and social philosopher Georg Simmel (1903) wrote an essay, "The metropolis and mental life," in which he considered the impact of the new social, technological, and institutional realities of the big city upon the mind of its inhabitants.[2] Simmel described the urban mentality as the result of a fundamentally altered way of life of which continuous change is a constant feature. A metropolitan existence means the permanent transformation of individual consciousness, as a rule and not as an exception. In Simmel's analysis, metropolitan life has irreversibly broken with the steady and even-paced sense of time of premodern small town and country people, creating "psychological conditions" of "permanent change," a "restless tempo of social life," and the "rapid compressing of ever shifting images" (Simmel, 1971, p. 326). All of this, Simmel suggests, intensifies the temporal flow of perception, imagination, and emotion characteristic of metropolitan time consciousness.

The second main feature of the metropolitan time experience examined by Simmel is the simultaneous occurrence and experience of different events and temporal processes. Simultaneity is a key category not just of literary and artistic modernism but of modernity altogether. Helga Nowotny (1994) distinguished between the emergence and the discovery of simultaneity. The emergence of simultaneity was prepared for in a long-term historical process in which it is at first connected with the spatial extension of state control, from modern nation-states to the territorial expansion of European colonialism; then with the economic expansion, the internationalization and globalization of the markets; and finally with the expansion of technologies, especially with those of communication (Nowotny, 1994, pp. 22–23). For Nowotny, all these processes create new forms of overlapping time experience. All of this once more increased exponentially with the digital revolution. Simultaneity translates into a universal present, as theorists of the digital age maintain: "Suddenly, the faded and fading past of old school friends, former lovers and all that could and should have been forgotten are returned to a single connected present via Google, Flickr, Ebay, YouTube, and Facebook" (Hoskins, 2013b).

But the interplay among parallel developments in the social, economic, and technological spheres that accelerate each other, including the way they are experienced (by means of new communication media), became an ubiquitous phenomenon even earlier. It is perceived and reflected upon, praised and complained about in all cultural milieus at the beginning of the last century. In 1916, the writer and arts critic Theodor Däubler declared "simultaneity" a key term of modernist aesthetics. Simultaneity, he wrote, was the quintessential "modern phenomenon" (quoted in Anz, 1994, p. 113). The sum of sensations and impressions being perceived and conceived by the modern subject engendered a "simultaneistic elasticity" (p. 113), as Däubler appreciatively recognized. He saw it even affecting the dynamic of modernist literature and arts itself, pointing out how the pressure of innovation and competition within the "cultural system" propelled the continuous emergence of new trends. Often these trends were hybrids in which the avant-garde was overlapping and intermingling with older forms, present-day innovations piggybacking on historical phenomena, European traditions appropriating non-European traditions, and so forth. Däubler came to no longer view the many different styles and trends of his time according to the model of diachronic succession but as "synchronic coexisting, as plural simultaneity of the disparate" (p. 113).

Literary modernism's sensitivity for time and time experience speaks directly to my inquiry because it engendered new narrative forms and techniques that made it possible to give shape not only to a new sense of personal and subjective time, but also to unprecedented polychronic scenarios. Both the concern with subjective time and different but simultaneously existing orders of time are central to the autobiographical process. Modernism played a crucial role in its genesis and thus the emergence of a culture of autobiography. It developed and tried out sophisticated scenarios of autobiographical time, and it disseminated them. Despite its avant-garde edge, these developments were not limited to the literary, artistic, and intellectual domain.[3] Modernism, the cultural expression and realization of modern metropolitan life, was much more than an event for the cultural elites. It also was more than the emergence of a new vocabulary, a vision, and a "mental life," to use Simmel's terms. With modernism, an array of new forms of life emerged, in tandem with new forms and practices to remember and reflect on them.

Memory's own time

In emphasizing the modernist background of complex autobiographical time scenarios, I am not saying that ideas of subjective time and multitemporality were unknown in earlier Western life-writing, and that

autobiographical narratives had simply followed the trajectory of linear and chronological time. Already Odysseus's mnemonic flashbacks
mingled present, past, and future in a way that laid out a simultaneous
moving forward and backward in time. In as far as Homer's epics can be
viewed as the beginning of written European literature, they also are the
beginning of nonlinear narrating. Only very few genres—such as folktales and fairytales—follow exclusively linear sequences of action and
narration. Epics tend to begin in the middle of things and then relate
earlier events through explanatory flashbacks, while novels likewise
strategically use flashforwards, as Genette observed in his study of how
narrative reshuffles chronological time (1988, p. 279).

Yet the narrative and imaginary horizon of modernism reaches much
further, outlining not only nonlinear and nonchronological subjective
experience but also intricately composed polychronic trajectories. At the
same time, modernist texts afford new possibilities for exploring the narrative fabric of autobiographical time; they represent, as Herman (2011c) has
shown, advanced temporal scenarios even by today's standards of literary
time experience. More than this, modernist and postmodernist narrative
texts not only represent, reflect, and explore temporal scenarios, they also
are lived time practices "to address "real-world crisis through . . . narrative
engagement," says Jesse Matz (2011, p. 275)—and we may add, they also
are lived practices to address real-life crises. In his assessment, Matz draws
on a narratological tradition of time theory that also includes Peter Brooks,
who called plot, the narrative configuration of time, the "product of our
refusal to allow temporality to be meaningless, our stubborn insistence on
making meaning in the world and in our lives" (1984, p. 323).

It is no coincidence that Proust's (1983) *Recherche*, an emblematic modernist text, has been already mentioned a few times. Drawing its readers
into an enormous autobiographical process and its endless interpretations, it also provides them with extended meditations on the phenomenology of subjective and objective time. A self-portrait of a mind in search
of memory experiences, it invokes a unique time zone. Yet it also exposes a
more general, historical sense of time, modernist time. That the *Recherche*
encapsulates an entire culture is indeed the central argument of Jean-Yves
Tadié's (2000) monumental Proust biography. The bond between the cultural economy of remembering at large and the work is Proust's life. While
his novel becomes his life, his life becomes his novel, as Tadié's (p. xvii)
sees it. It is worth considering more carefully how Proust's novel is tied
into the overarching cultural changes because it gives us a more decen-
tered perspective on his practice of self-temporalization. I use the term
temporalization to bring into focus that autobiographical time—our

main subject here—is the outcome of a process of meaning-making, of that kind of meaning formation, to be more precise, that occurs in the autobiographical process.

The volumes of the *Recherche* open one of the aforementioned modernist laboratories for experimentation on memory and time; they present a site of production for a new description of the relations among remembering, imagining, and narrating. Proust was not simply a writer who dedicated his entire life to his writing, which is, of course, what many writers do and most aspire to. He was existentially entangled with language and autobiographical remembering, a connection he saw at the heart of what it means to live a life and to find meaning in living a life. Writing appeared to be the royal route to escape what troubled him most, the experience of transience, of time passing by. And it was particularly autobiographical narrative that promised him a mode to hold onto the passing moment, a way to lastingly recover "lost time."

But it was not just any time he wanted to recover. He was after something he considered the "essences" of lost time, by which he meant the sensuous experience of lived life in its fullness. Proust was fascinated by autobiographical reminiscing because he had come to believe that in this way he could not only recall past memories, even after a long period of forgetting, but directly access their "essences" and thereby truly transform time lost into "time gained." The question of how such a transformation can happen is the central theme of the *Recherche*.

What makes this endeavour additionally challenging is that there is, for Proust, only one particular kind of memory that allows him to regain time lost in the fullest sense: *mémoirés involontaire*. Proust's narrative and psychological investigation of involuntary memory have made him famous far beyond the literary world. "No single work of literature," writes Schacter (1996, p. 26) in his discussion of the phenomenon of involuntary recollection, "is more closely associated with human memory than Marcel Proust's *À la recherche du temps perdu*". Proust's faith and hope in involuntary memories is closely linked to his conviction that our mnemonic life eludes the laws and categories of common or public time. Differently put, he insists that memory has its own time. Besides its narrative and psychological aspect, this view, as noted before, also has a philosophical dimension, and this is ultimately what brings Proust to leave the familiar terrain of Newtonian time. A human being, he writes,

> ... is that ageless creature who has the faculty of becoming many years younger in a few seconds, and who, surrounded by the walls of the time through which he has lived, floats within them as in a pool the surface-level

of which is constantly changing so as to bring him within range now of one epoch, now of another. (1983, vol. 3, p. 627)

Understandably, faced with this Proustian scenario of simultaneity, experimental psychologists have sensed serious problems with the traditional notion of memory. And they are not alone. Landy wonders whether Proust's involuntary memories are proper memories at all; for when—according to Proust—"an odor, texture or sound returns us to a former state, we are not dragging into the light a set of impressions that have long since departed but, instead, summoning up a part of us that is still very much present within our mind" (2004, p. 110). Yet, there is another way to think about Proust's "pool of time," and that is to view it as an analogy of our simultaneous existence in different temporalities, with remembering, viewed as a constant oscillation back and forth in time, as the central mode of creating and mediating this simultaneity.

The pool of time may have been an original trope, as certainly was much of the narrative repertoire Proust employed to articulate the sudden time shifts between various pasts and presents. But, as already emphasized, the phenomenon he aimed to capture was anything but new, nor was the awareness of it. Other writers, philosophers, and scientists had already described the simultaneity of multiple temporalities in which human beings live. Everyone probably has experienced it in one way or another, even if this experience was not necessarily consciously searched for and reflected upon. Here, however, we find one of the reasons Proust's meandering explorations of the weave of memory and time were so spectacular: because its narrator intentionally seeks the experience of involuntary remembering. For it is this experience that allows him to float in the pool of time by being simultaneously in touch with different epochs of his life, epochs that by common standards might be separated from each other by years and decades. For the French writer, the multiple temporality of memories, in all their nonlinear and achronological randomness, represents most authentically the very time of human memory, indeed, of our life.

Involuntary memories blend past and present in an inextricable manner, bringing to the fore what is common to both and, in this way, fusing the "essences" of the past with the "essences" of the present. Roger Shattuck (1962) described this perspective as "binocular" and "stereoscopic": It captures past and present, the experience of then and the experience of now, and simultaneously brings both into one focus. This stereoscopic focus necessarily must be out of time, thus creating a situation of timelessness.[4] For this reason, Genevieve Lloyd concluded that "Proust's 'involuntary' memory goes beyond the mere co-presence of memory and perception to assert a daring assimilation—a certain identity even—of memory and perception, of past and present. ... In involuntary memory the past is restored in the fullness of its reality, while yet it is grasped in a present perception" (1993, p. 129).

Being in search, then, not so much of "lost time" but of this kind of experience, both the narrator and the author of the *Recherche* have come to retire into the elusive realm of involuntary memories, with almost complete disregard for what they perceive as the external, mechanical, and mindless time of clocks and calendars. As a consequence, as the novel progresses, the more their lives revolve around these memory experiences and the quest for them, Proust's involuntary memories gradually become more voluntary, Shattuck (1962) observed. What came, for example, as an entirely unexpected surprise at the beginning of the narrative—the childhood memories triggered by the taste of tea and the *petites madeleines*—has become the experience of a clearly voluntary recollection in the last volume *Time Regained*, where Marcel, at a gathering of old friends he has not seen for a long time, tries hard to recall his memories of them in order to trace their former identities.

The problem with experiences of this kind remains, however, that they cannot be completely planned for and arranged. They may or may not happen. But when they materialize, all of a sudden, evoked by the smell of flowers, the sound of a violin, the taste of a cake, they give way to incomparably privileged sensations, to *moments bienheureux*, blissful moments. Moments of stunning emotions, they release streams of associations that conjure a sense of fullness and immediacy in which the distinction between past and present dissolves, indeed, the idea of time does as well.

There is a second aspect to Proust's investigation of memory and time that is similarly important if one wants to examine their interwovenness: both appear as narrative phenomena. And they are not just narrative in the sense one would expect in the work of a narrative artist. The assumption is much stronger, echoing what I called, in Chapter 4, the strong narrative thesis. For Proust, autobiographical remembering and time *only* take on a gestalt in narrative form. His claim comes very close to the argument at the center of this book, namely, that both remembering and time, as well as their fusion in autobiographical time, only become intelligible insofar as they exist in linguistic form. They are exclusively thinkable and imaginable as autobiographical discourse and narrative time. This makes Proust's observations and reflections supremely appropriate for playing through the notion of narrative temporalization that I have proposed. To do so, my next step is to consider how narrative temporalization relates to and differs from that view of time I have referred to as Newtonian. In the concluding part of the chapter, I return to the Proustian articulation of autobiographical time, comparing it to that of another modernist writer, Walter Benjamin.

THE NEWTONIAN VIEW AND THE NARRATIVE VIEW

Fundamental dimensions of human existence, memory and time are highly contested areas of investigation and contemplation. Two views are particularly relevant here; by now, we are familiar with both: the Newtonian view and the narrative view. The ontological assumption underlying the Newtonian view is that time is an objective and absolute system—in Newton's words, "without relation to anything external"—a fixed background against which all events in the universe are spatiotemporally localized.[5]

Because all knowledge is perspectival, the Newtonian view does not preclude that time appears in various and changing subjective versions: in human experience, memory, and narrative. Nor does it rule out that time is perceived and reflected upon in phenomenological, cultural, and historical terms. But whatever the specific interrelationship between mind and time, the basic supposition is that ultimately it can be represented in terms of an underlying Newtonian trajectory—in the same fashion as, in classical narratology, the "discourse time" of narrated and narratable events and experience can be mapped along the linear and homogenous trajectory of "story time."[6]

The narrative view, in contrast, draws on a meaning-based ontology. The primary level of temporal reality here is constituted by the relations and interactions among human agents. Because it thus does not depend on the fixed background of a space-time manifold, it is an independent ontology. It claims that our ideas and concepts of time are neither universally given entities nor epistemological preconditions of experience; rather, they are outcomes of symbolic constructions. That is to say, all patterns or orders of time are cultural and historical constructions, created by human beings. Their purpose is to help organize our societal life and make sense of our existence. And as human meaning formations are amazingly variegated, so are our constructions of time.

On a cultural level, this view corresponds to Einstein's argument that time is a framework relative to local reference systems. In his *Special Theory of Relativity*, Einstein claimed that time appears slowed down in a system moving away at constant speed—a phenomenon unimaginable within Newton's absolute manifolds of time and space. The *General Theory of Relativity* of 1916 extended the framework to accelerated bodies and their gravitational fields. Because all bodies and all matter in the universe engender gravitational fields, and because every gravitational field constitutes a system of time, every body has its own time. Hence the universe can be imagined as populated by an infinite number of clocks, each representing an independent temporal system. The cultural analogue to this polychronic universe needs, however, a qualification. In the realm of human matters we also may say, with Einstein, that we can imagine as many clocks as we like, but this is so because it is we who make them, whereas we obviously do not make gravitational fields of matter. It is human beings who create the powerfields of culture and define the scope of their temporal models. In this process of meaning-making or temporalization, humans use all kinds of material and symbolic aids, from the movement of the stars and self-made timepieces to social rituals, mathematical algorithms, and mythological and historical narratives.

From this assumption follows the main point of the narrative view. The more complex human temporal constructions become—for example, when they go beyond basic representations of duration, chronology, speed, and frequency, and when they comprise simultaneous combinations of different times and time orders, including times of possible, "subjunctive" worlds, as typically is the case in autobiographical narratives and other life stories—the more they create scenarios like those with which Proust is concerned. That is, the more we deal with human temporalities (and only these are the subject of Proust's contemplations) the more the construction site is language, and in particular the language of narrative.[7]

Narrative discourse is our most advanced way to shape complex temporal experiences, including remembering. All natural languages provide a broad spectrum of semantic and grammatical resources and, on an overarching and integrative level, narrative forms and models by which humans temporalize themselves, that is, by which they localize their being in a self-woven symbolic web of temporality. In telling stories about ourselves—and this is the type of discourse in which I am first of all interested—we not only give meaning to experiences present and past, as well as question given meanings and reflect about possible new and future meanings, we also unfold, explicitly or implicitly, temporal scenarios. More than just aligning events and experiences in time, these scenarios define and evoke "time" and its meaning in the first place —for example, by configuring an experience as past or present, or as a mix of both, or as simultaneous with another experience, or as relating otherwise to other events. This is what I call temporalization.

To consider time as a relational construct rather than an absolute given was first proposed by Gottfried Wilhelm Leibniz toward the end of the 17th century. A contemporary of Newton, Leibniz challenged the absolutist philosophy of time of his English colleague, suggesting instead to refer to time as the way in which nonsimultaneous events relate to each other.[8] Viewed philosophically, a relational mode of self-localization is also implied in Proust's pool of time, whose surface level, in floating up or down, connects distant epochs of time "in a few seconds." Even in this scenario, temporal structures appear not as a fixed background measure of narrative (as the Newtonian would claim), nor as an epistemic condition of the possibility for narrative experience (as the Kantian might put it), but as a consequence of narrative acts of meaning, of narrative temporalization. In this sense, a substantial portion of our time constructions can be understood as a result or effect, indeed, as the side effect of meaning constructions, with narrative as our most powerful "anthropomorphic operator of time" (Brockmeier, 1996).

All theories, in the strong sense of the word, try to recast different and opposing theories in their own terms. While the Newtonian view incorporates the narrative view as a subjective or phenomenological version of a universalist given, the narrative view frames the Newtonian view as a particular cultural-historical conception that emerged in the 17th and 18th centuries and was itself replaced at the beginning of the 20th century. John Bender and David Wellbery (1991) have described the difference between the Newtonian and the post-Newtonian modern and modernist conceptions of time in terms of two distinct "chronotypes." *Chronotype* is a variation on the term *chronotope* that was introduced into narrative theory by Bakhtin (1981). Bakhtin borrowed the term from Einstein's physics to portray the fusion of temporal and spatial structures that characterizes space-time formations in specific narrative genres, such as the romance, the folktale, and the picaresque novel. Bender and Wellbery have slightly shifted the scope of the concept to focus on comprehensive cultural conceptions of temporality: "Bakhtin's term," they state, "is suggestive because it points to the diversity of prototypical cultural forms within which time assumes significance" (1991, p. 3).

Yet even if we agree with Bender and Wellbery's argument that the post-Newtonian chronotype tends toward a more constructionist, pragmatist, and contingent point of view—an argument elaborated in detail by Rorty (1989)—and that the new chronotype thus encompasses "the drive to comprehend temporal construction as a function of narrative formation" (Bender & Wellbery 1991, p. 3), this still does not explain how exactly autobiographical temporalization can be seen as a "function of narrative formation." Why does narrative play such a pivotal role in our understanding of the temporal dynamic of remembering and forgetting?

Temporal self-localization

Let me offer two reasons. The first emerged with the historical development, beginning in the 18th century and culminating with modernism, in which narrative evolved as the royal road to autobiographical remembering. Countless autobiographical authors—writing for literary and personal motives, published and unpublished, famous and unknown—have dedicated themselves to examining their own practices of remembering and forgetting; and among these practices, again, narrative has proven to be essential. I mentioned Nalbantian's (2003) point that the meticulous accounts of memory phenomena given from Rousseau to Octavio Paz offer a spectrum of narrative test cases for the functions of human memory that is as broad and differentiated as human memory itself.[9] For many autobiographical writers, this dedication to remembering has even turned into an obsession, an all-consuming way of life, which fits in well with the Western culture of self and autobiography as outlined in the last chapter. Autobiographers, as the anthropologist would say, live permanently in the field, blurring the limits between object and subject of observation, third- and first-person perspective, teller and told, the fictive and the factual. Their field notes and research reports have yielded numerous thick descriptions, undercover investigations that often extend over years, decades, and sometimes over entire lives.

Viewing autobiographical narrative not only as a form of representation but as a practice of investigation affords "unparalleled access to the mind and experience and memories of their subjects," as Saunders (2008, p. 323) writes. For Saunders, autobiographical writing displays much more than how rememberers individually construct and reconstruct themselves, although this individualist focus was long the hallmark of academic studies. It also demonstrates how this concern is propelled, guided, and constrained by cultural imperatives. These imperatives, as Saunders (2008) proposes, make the genres of life-writing routes into culture and cultural constructions of memory.

Once more, Marcel Proust is an exemplary figure. Between 1909 and the time of his death in 1922 he continuously worked on the *Recherche*. The result was a 3,200-page version published in seven volumes. Although not strictly autobiographical in terms of genre and plot, this unparalleled endeavor of self-examination attributes to its protagonist personal experiences, concerns, and micropsychological observations that undoubtedly originated in the life of its author—even if the relations among Proust the person, the publicly performing writer, the narrator, and the protagonist of the *Recherche* are anything but clear and mimetic (cf. Landy, 2004). Still, as we know from Proust's biographers Carter (2000), Painter (1977), and Tadié (2000), much of his life happened analogously to his work: as something that only gradually took shape and brought out its themes, motifs, and goals, most of which never found any definitive closure.

A case in point is Proust's fascination with the multiple times of memory and the remembering self. In Proust's narrative universe, this oscillating multiplicity is crucial to the entire process of narrative identity formation. It is, for example, a vital concern of the novel's protagonist, the younger Marcel, and its narrator, Marcel at the time of the story's telling, for the continuous shifts in the pool of time are closely related to the remembered simultaneity of the "innumerable 'selves' that compose our personality" (Proust, 1983, vol. 3, p. 437). Thus it makes no difference whether one self becomes another self after a lapse of years in the putatively natural sequence of time, or whether one self changes at any given moment into another, for both changes expose the same blend of "the incompatible persons, malicious, sensitive, refined, caddish, disinterested, ambitious which one can be, in turn, every day of one's life" (p. 657).

On a narrative level, this becomes manifest by Proust's permanent use of anachronisms, which defies reckoning by any common time order. If one would review it with a timepiece in hand, as Hans Robert Jauss (1986, p. 139) remarked, one could believe that the narrator continuously turns the hand of his clock back and forth, so that his protagonist simultaneously dines with his lover and plays ball with his nanny. Hence even the concept of a natural flow of time, as suggested by Bergson, reveals little about the shifting simultaneity of different experiences, heterogeneous temporal states, and, in fact, different "selves" of the experiencing or reminiscing narrator. Often, Proust writes, we simply forget how many of our different "selves" there are.

> There were some of these "selves" which I had not encountered for a long time past. For instance (I had not remembered that it was the day on which the barber called) the "self" that I was when I was having my haircut. I had forgotten this "self," and his arrival made me burst into tears as, at a funeral, does the appearance of an old retired servant who has not forgotten the deceased. (1983, vol. 3, p. 437)

Eventually, the assumption of a given time within which we are to localize ourselves appears itself as an attempt to cope with our fundamentally unstable and relational identity or, more precisely, as an effect of our narrative strategies to make sense of our fluid forms of life.

In terms of autobiographical memory, Proust arguably brought to its fullest expression the age-old saying that the remembered self is unavoidably intermingled with the remembering self. Since the *Recherche*, the narrative and temporal nexus of these two "selves" has become an almost natural concern at the heart of innumerable writers; it also has become an established topic in the world of letters (cf., e.g., Bruner, 1994; Eakin, 1999; Olney, 1998). This is not to say that all shared Proust's version of this nexus. But the French writer has sensitized us to read much of 20th-century autobiographical literature through this lens. This literature either explicitly deals with the lives and minds of the writers themselves, with their selves in time (that is, in various times), or it indirectly draws on and exploits the dramas of their lives. If we want to know what it means to look at one's own existence and the existence of others from a first-person point of view, clearly autobiographical literature is a privileged site for investigations of this sort.

Autobiographical writers, as Ender (2005) remarks, are writers who have "a vocation for remembrance" and are highly aware of its "subtle complexities"; they know from their own work, "that memories are constructions, that they are dependent on mood and context, and above all that there is no ready-made template to be found somewhere in the brain that reproduces an initial impress or trace" (p. 5). Many writers have emphasized what seems to be true for all autobiographical remembrance, that processes of autobiographical temporalization include the simultaneous configuration of scenarios and selves in very different times, and that these "times" are inextricably tied to the narrative reality of the stories in which they gain their meaning.

The point I drive home from these observations adds to an argument made earlier in this book: both the articulation and study of the autobiographical process, as we encounter them in many works of self-writing, allow for insights that no cognitive and neuroscientific memory research can provide. We have to consider them as indispensable complements for an understanding of the autobiographical process as a form of life.

This leads to the second reason why narrative plays such a crucial role for our understanding of the temporal dynamic of remembering and forgetting: because this dynamic, as we recognize yet again, is itself fused with that of the narrative process. We are not only talking about the narrative representation or reflection of a prior entity "time" or "remembered time" or, on a different level, about distinct cognitive memory systems responsible of mental time travels. Rather, the focus once more is on narrative as carrying out a process of meaning-making, this time of temporal self-localization. This implies that there is no autobiographical temporalization "in itself," independent of narrative.[10] I take as also significant for autobiographical temporalization what Bruner said about human life in general, namely, that to look at it "as if it were independent of the autobiographical text that constructs it is a futile a quest for reality as the physicist's search for a Nature that is independent of the theories that lead him to measure one rather than another phenomenon" (1993, p. 55).

The narrative experiments we observe in the autobiographical literature invite us to inquire how modern individuals try to localize themselves in a modernist version of Heraclitian fleetingness, a world that—in contrast with the Newtonian world and its fixed spatiotemporal background—does not provide any temporal, let alone existential, stability. Moreover, these experiments invite us to examine how people engage in interpreting and making sense of themselves in continuously changing time frames and how they employ, in the process, the narrative models, genres, and strategies of temporalization offered to them by the cultural world in which they live. From this perspective, the autobiographical process offers an intriguing venue for the study of our attempts to make sense of temporal experiences that are part and parcel of our modern and postmodern reality.

REMEMBERING, TIME, AND INTENTIONALITY

Returning to the multiple temporality of the autobiographical process, let me summarize my point. Drawing on the narrative view, I have argued that our ideas of time are side effects of our meaning constructions, rather than their ontological (or epistemological or narrative) preconditions. How and whether we qualify, in the autobiographical process, experiences, emotions, hopes, and fantasies in terms of the Newtonian trajectory of past, present, and future (or combinations of these), depends on the special features of the process of meaning formation in which they play a role. Clocks, calendars, and other forms of societal time regulation are extremely useful when we organize our everyday life; yet as soon as it comes to the autobiographical process, Virginia Woolf is right: such devices, as sophisticated as they may be, are of no great help. Reading them has to be replaced with the effort to understand the meanings of our narrative time scenarios. These meanings relate to the time of clocks like the meanings of our lives relate to the chronologies listed in a curriculum vitae.

To take a closer look at such meaning-based temporalization, I want to distinguish two sides of this dialectical process. On the one hand, there is, as noted before, the cultural and historical world with its specific semantic and grammatical resources, as well as its discursive orders, concepts, and narrative models of time and memory. On the other hand, there is the individual as a subject of intentionality, a person with a social life, emotions, motives, and desires that, embedded in this social life, is the agentive force in these meaning constructions, including their temporalizations. Without recognizing the subject's intentional attitude toward his or her present, past, and future, or the personal significance of specific memories, we cannot comprehend the concrete temporal scenarios that emerge in any autobiographical discourse. We cannot even comprehend whether a certain experience or mental state is interpreted as related to the present, the future, or the past.

Resonating with this view is a renewed focus in narrative theory on the role of intentionality in discourse and narrative understanding. This interest is inspired by research in several areas about the human tendency "to read for intention" (Herman, 2008) or, differently put, to reach for meaning (Brockmeier, 2009). For Bruner, this is one of narrative's central psychological features: "narrative deals with the vicissitudes of intention" (1986, p. 17). In making sense of characters' actions and reflections in a story—and this, again, is true for literary and everyday stories—we try to understand their intentions, read their minds, interpret the landscape of consciousness in which they move (as, most likely, did the narrator who told the story). Almost unavoidably, we try to figure out what that narrator or author might have had in mind, what could possibly be his or her intentions (as, again, that very narrator or author might do in view of the readers of or listeners to the story). For Herman, storytelling, stories, and storyworlds are "irreducibly grounded in intentional systems," while "intentional systems are grounded in storytelling practices" (2008, pp. 240–241). Drawing on this hermeneutic rationale, we can view autobiographical narrative as, to use Herman's terms, a "primary resource" for (re)constructing psychological states and, more generally, states of consciousness, "thanks to which circumstances, participants, actions, and intentional states of various kinds can be connected together" (p. 241).

Now, within the Proustian universe of discourse, I want to highlight one element of such a connection: the narrator's (and, in this case, also the author's) intentional stance toward time and remembering. Consider, once again, Proust's picture of the pool of time and his idea of human life as encompassing at any given moment a multitude of different epochs. We understood this as essentially suggesting the simultaneity of experiential states and temporalities that, in traditional chronological terms, would be conceived of as situated at distinct past and present moments in time. Can we discern a profile of intentionality behind this vision of autobiographical time? Let me take this picture as the starting point in attempting to indicate an answer. Of course, this can only be a short hint, for the entire *Recherche* is nothing else but an extended project of temporalization.

Time is the great theme of Proust's work, explored by philosophers like Ricoeur (1985), critics like Jauss (1986), narratologists like Genette (1980; 1988), and writers like Beckett (1957). The entire existence of Marcel, which also is the name of the *Recherche's* protagonist, is a search for lost time. The sphere of time is the domain of the origin of art ("time regained" is the very material of artistic beauty) and its foremost subject of reflection. Furthermore, it is supposed to define the form of the work as well as its overall composition (at the end of his search, after Marcel has undergone a series of experiences in the resuscitation of time lost, he resolves to write a book that will have "the shape of time," the book the reader just finished). A concern with time even insinuates itself into the style. Think of Proust's notorious syntax as a form of reminiscing that assumes a timeless or multitemporal universe of discourse, with meandering sentences whose epic dependent clauses are like mnemonic search movements, determined at the onset but then all of a sudden hesitating, moving back and forth, to the side and ahead and returning again, as if they had forgotten something and came back for it.

Remembering the lost future

What I am most interested in, however, lies on a more elemental psychological or, perhaps, more existential plane. Is there a distinctive quality of Proust's overall attitude to time and memory, an intentional stance that shapes not only the experiences he wants to remember and the stories he tells about them, but also his temporalization of certain events as memories and of others as immediate experiences in the here and now? With this question in mind, I want to compare, in the final pages of this chapter, Proust's writing with that of another autobiographical writer, Walter Benjamin. This comparison is far from random. Benjamin was an early admirer of Proust; he was not only an addicted reader, as he called himself, but also a translator, commentator, and sympathetic philosophical critic of Proust's work. Benjamin's own autobiographical prose, first of all the collection of short pieces of his *Berlin Childhood around 1900*, reveals many features reminiscent of Proust—the bittersweet memories of the beloved mother, the noises from the courtyard and thus from a foreign world, and the places whose magic caught the boy and never left him. Not least, there is what Peter Szondi describes as the key experience of Proust's work and his idea of remembering: "that almost everything childhood was can be withheld from a person for years, suddenly to be offered him anew as if by chance" (2006, p. 10). Further, at the level of theoretical reflection, Benjamin comes close to Proust's vision of the simultaneity of multiple times in the autobiographical process, for example, when he ventures the idea that a remembered event is infinite, because as a memory it is a key to everything that happened before and after it (Benjamin, 1968).

Nevertheless, Szondi suggests in his analysis of the relationship between Proust's and Benjamin's work that little ultimately is gained by such comparisons. In fact, it would be difficult to refute the objection that such similarities only reflect that both writers tackle typical auto-biographical raw material situated in the same fin-de-siècle epoch (cf. Martens, 2011), material whose presence in their lives they attempt to trace in many-layered tableaus of time and remembrance. Yet can we even be sure, Szondi asks, that

> Proust and Benjamin really share the same theme? Does their search for "lost time" arise from the same motive? Or is the common element merely an appearance that should be pointed out because it could obscure the fact that the intentions of the two works are not only not related but are in fact totally opposed. (2006, p. 11)

To understand Szondi's suspicion regarding the different intentions embodied by the two works, we first have to follow his reading of Proust's novel. It tracks the meaning of Proust's search for time past as evolving out of two main emotions, a painful one and a happy one. Both run through the entire *Recherche*. The inexplicable feeling of happiness seizes the hero first when, with the madeleine dunked in tea, the whole world of his childhood reappears. Whereas the other feeling, that of consternation, takes hold with the recognition that there is one, existentially threatening dimension where he does not stand outside of linear and chronological time but is subject to its law. The high point of Marcel's autobiographical undertaking is at the end of the book when he recognizes that these two feelings of happiness and terror are intrinsically connected. "That," writes Szondi, "which underlies the feeling of happiness in the one case liberates him from the terror of the other" (p. 12).

It is remarkable to see that this point is illustrated by a passage from the *Recherche* in which Marcel, in describing his feelings of happiness and his memories of them, also reflects on their temporal status. The experience of the simultaneity of different times coincides with the liberating emotional experience of breaking free from the sway of temporality itself.

> I caught an inkling of this ... when I compared these various happy impressions with one another and found that they had this in common—namely, that I experienced them simultaneously in the present moment and in some distant past, which the sound of the spoon against the plate ..., or the peculiar savor of the madeleine even went so far as to make coincide with the present, leaving me uncertain in which period I was. (Proust, 1983, vol. 2, p. 995)

For Proust, this sense of "identities between the present and the past," is triggered, as we saw, by an involuntary memory. This experience allows him to escape from the threat that the idea of the irreversible flow of time exerts on him and, instead, to "live and enjoy the essence of things ... entirely outside of time" (p. 995). For Benjamin, both time and remembering have a different meaning. The intentional stance behind his autobiographical *Berlin Childhood* can be readily perceived, and again I follow Szondi, from scenes that present moments of departure, emerging, and first times. Consider the scene when Benjamin recalls his walks as a boy to the *Tiergarten*, to the "the strangest part of the park," where he feels drawn not to the statues of the royals but to their pedestals, the place of a first time sensation: "Here, in fact, or not far away, must have lain the couch of that Ariadne in whose proximity I first experienced what only later I had a word for: love" (Benjamin, 2006, p. 54).

Like the *Tiergarten* memory, there are many experiences in which Benjamin detects signs of his later life, early traces of things to come that are irrevocably gone once those things have come: "I can dream of the way I once learned to walk. But that doesn't help. I now know how to walk; there is no more learning to walk" (p. 142). Such observations and memories—which do not limit themselves to personal concerns but include historical and social matters—are not so much about the past as about a perspective in which present and future are brought together, where the premonition of the child and the knowledge of the adult are merged. What Benjamin is interested in, as Szondi concludes, is not the past in itself but the invocation of those aspects of his childhood "in which a token (*Vorklang*) of the future lies hidden" (2006, p. 21).

Proust's search for time lost is driven by his desire to defend himself from the imposition of chronological temporality. The real goal of his absorption of all times past and present in the simultaneity of the autobiographical process is to escape from the present and, perhaps even more, from the future, with all its uncertainties and threats, of which the ultimate one is death. For Benjamin, in contrast, the future is precisely what matters most and what he even seeks in the past.

> Almost every place that his memory wishes to rediscover bears "traces of what was to come," as he puts it at one point in *Berlin Childhood*. And it is no accident that his memory encounters a personage from his childhood "in his capacity as a seer prophesying the future." Proust listens attentively for the echo of the past; Benjamin listens for the first notes of a future which has meanwhile become the past. Unlike Proust, Benjamin does not want to free himself from temporality; he does not wish to see things in their ahistorical essence. He strives instead for historical experience and knowledge. Nevertheless, he is sent back into the past, a past however, which is open, not completed, and which promises the future. Benjamin's tense is not the perfect, but the future perfect in the fullness of its paradox: being future and past at the same time. (Szondi, 2006, p. 19)

Benjamin's autobiographical quest for time gone by, for lost time, is, in sum, a quest for the lost future. This future never became real; it only emerged briefly in moments of promise and *Vorklang* in the past. We must keep in mind that even this past only emerges in hindsight, in the act of remembrance that takes place in the here and now as the invocation of a utopia that never came true. The here and now, that is Benjamin writing his memories in the 1930s, trying—in vain, as we know—to escape from fascism, a man haunted and hounded without any hope either for his own future as a writer and philosopher or for the future of humanity. Without being aware of this historical context, this cultural constellation of "intentionality" (of which the individual intentional stance of the author is only one instance), the temporalization of Benjamin's autobiographical scenarios remains unintelligible. And so it does for Proust's elegiac visions of a past that he tries to evoke as a timeless present.

This difference between their ideas of time and remembering is also responsible for what Szondi (2006) calls the formal difference between Proust's and Benjamin's narrative works, the "gulf which separates the three-thousand-page novel from the collection of brief prose pieces" (p. 21). But despite their different formal shape, both texts resonate with the case I make in this book: that the emerging scenarios of autobiographical time are more adequately understood as results and side effects of narrative worldmaking than as mnemonic representations of "the" past in "the" present. The temporal scenarios of the autobiographical process do not unfold a "time of memory" that is to be found, along a Newtonian trajectory, somewhere in the past. Nor can they be reduced to or projected onto such an ontological model of time. Rather, if we closely investigate such scenarios of remembering and time they prove to be inextricably interwoven with their very narrative fabric, a fabric whose understanding, as both Proust and Benjamin suggest, necessarily reaches beyond mere narrative analysis.

CHAPTER 9

Beyond Time

The Autobiographical Process as Search Movement

Austerlitz, the last book of W. G. Sebald, is one of the most stunning explorations of human remembering and time ever conceived. It continues the narrative efforts outlined in the previous chapter to understand autobiographical time in a way that radically differs from the itineraries of Odysseus. Although the modernists tried to temporalize their being in the world in new and unheard-of literary forms, Sebald's *Austerlitz* is a work that transcends time and temporalization as meaningful dimensions of self-understanding and world-understanding altogether. On Austerlitz's sea chart the island of Ithaca has disappeared.

The book was written at the end of the 20th century, a century that started with the modernist revolution and its challenge of long-established ideas of identity, remembering, and time, to which the last chapter was dedicated. Often described as perplexing and disturbing, many see their difficulties with Sebald's book reflecting an all but easy literary style. No doubt, *Austerlitz* demands a serious reader who follows attentively an ever meandering syntax without clear paragraph structure, a peculiar mixture of the narrative voices of the protagonist and the narrator, several layers of free indirect thought and discourse, and wide-ranging associative chains that encompass accounts of very specific details. All this may or may not contribute to a labyrinthine plot, if we can call it a plot at all. But my sense is that this book has left many puzzled not only because of its demanding narrative composition but also, more importantly, because it suggests a postarchival vision of the autobiographical process that goes even beyond the modernist imagination.

Among the numerous studies of this book, there is no agreement as to what makes this vision so perplexing. Many would concur that Sebald's writing can be seen in line with modernist experimentation with time and memory. *Austerlitz*, however, lacks the literary playfulness and lightness that was part of the experiments of Proust, Joyce, Woolf, and Kafka. What characterizes Sebald's universe of discourse, both linguistically and emotionally, is a tone of inconsolable disarray. A sense of existential urgency sets the scene.

Even if one situates Sebald's writing in a post- or late-modernist cultural context—after all, it takes place nearly a century after Proust's and Benjamin's celebration of "metropolitan mental life"—this does not necessarily place it in opposition to the early modernist repertoire of styles and narrative practices. In what follows, I read Sebald's portrait of Jacques Austerlitz, the enigmatic protagonist of the book, as a study in the overlapping border zones of autobiographical process, narrative, and time. What complicates this study is that Sebald, although following in the footsteps of the modernists, radicalizes their views and narrative techniques to the point where all three—remembering, narrative, and autobiographical time—lose their traditional meaning.

By this I do not claim to reconstruct Sebald's views and thoughts on time and remembering as general theoretical pronouncements. My goal here is different. I want to stake out the narrative-psychological scope of the notion of autobiographical process and explore its constructive and imaginative reach from various points of view: in Chapter 6, it was that of identity formation, in Chapter 7, it was a cultural perspective, and in the previous and the present chapters, it is time, autobiographical time, that is.

AUSTERLITZ'S TIME

Remembering is the subject, method, and aim of Sebald's writing. In fact, it may be said that his books have created a new genre of memory writing. Though not easily read, as already noted, they have been highly celebrated on the literary and intellectual stage both in North America and Europe, with *Austerlitz* triggering the most enthusiastic though not unperturbed reactions. The book is a haunting account of Austerlitz's search for his lost memory. In an article entitled "In a no man's land of memories and loss," Michiko Kakutani (2001) writes that in reading Sebald "we are transported to a memoryscape—a twilight, fogbound world of half-remembered images and ghosts that is reminiscent at once of Ingmar Bergman's *Wild*

Strawberries, Kafka's troubling fables of guilt and apprehension and, of course, Proust's *Remembrance of Things Past*." Kakutani goes on to observe that the story of Austerlitz slowly "assumes the shape of an autobiography" or, at least, shows "the resonant texture of a memoir." What appears so foreign, even exotic to many is a view of remembering that has little to do with the spatial visions that we met earlier in the archival tradition of memory. Whereas the idea of memory as such, and of remembering as relating past and present, was, as we saw, still shared by modernist writers, Sebald gives a different outline of remembering, one that emerges as an undirected, speculative, and ever-ongoing search movement—a diffuse activity that has lost any ability to anchor one's personal identity in one's lived past.

I believe there are at least three different reasons why one can feel at a loss with Austerlitz. First, as a work about human remembering, it revolves around the account of an individual, Austerlitz, who has forfeited crucial childhood memories and begins, at one point of his life, an increasingly desperate search of his lost memory, indeed, his identity. So far this resembles a quite traditional quest. But what does autobiographical identity mean if an important portion of one's personal past is beyond the reach of any autobiographical remembering? The book recounts an inquiry into the meaning of memory lost that extends over some 30 years. Yet the chronological time frame does not really matter, for it becomes obvious that such an inquiry, even if it were successful and not hampered by various difficulties, cannot but be a never-ending enterprise because there is no moment in time in which we can claim to have fully recalled and exhaustively interpreted an experience that we believe to have had in the past.

Second, *Austerlitz* also is bewildering as a work about human temporality and, specifically, autobiographical time. It not only rejects the idea that our minds reliably distinguish what is past and what is present, what is a memory of a past experience and what is a present imagination of a past experience, let alone a memory of a past imagination. It also defies any notion of chronology, sequentiality, and directedness within the realm of human time experience. Instead, it discloses scenarios of temporalization that ultimately dissolve the Newtonian trajectory of time altogether. At several points, the book makes this case explicitly, as when Austerlitz remembers a visit to the Royal Observatory in Greenwich and its collection of chronometers, regulators, and other time measuring devices:

> Time . . . was by far the most artificial of all our inventions, and in being bound
> to the planet turning on its axis was no less arbitrary than would be, say, a

calculation based on the growth of trees or the duration required for a piece of limestone to disintegrate … If Newton thought, said Austerlitz, pointing through the window and down to the curve of the water around the Isle of the Dogs glistering in the last of the daylight, if Newton really thought that time was a river like the Thames, then where is its source and into what sea does it finally flow? Every river, as we know, must have banks on its sides, so where, seen in those terms, where are the banks of time? … Why does time stand still and motionless in one place, and rush headlong by in another? Could we not claim … that time itself has been nonconcurrent and nonsimultaneous over the centuries and the millennia? (p. 100)[1]

The River Thames, the growth of trees, and the duration for a piece of limestone to disintegrate are just a few of the metaphorical, allegorical, and symbolic references to phenomena of nature that flank Austerlitz's ongoing dispute with the Newtonian model of time. A further rhetorical topos used not without an ironic slant is the weather, which serves to describe temporal experiences that escape the model of clock and calendar time:

> … And is not human life in many parts on the earth governed to this day less by time than by the weather, and thus by an unquantifiable dimension which disregards linear regularity, does not progress constantly forward but moves in eddies, is marked by episodes of congestion and irruption, recurs in ever-changing form, and evolves in no one knows what direction? (pp. 100–101)

Emphasizing that he can demonstrate through his own life how questionable the idea of linear and directed time is, Austerlitz goes on in a more personal tone, linking these general reflections with his personal sense of autobiographical time:

> A clock has always struck me as something ridiculous, a thoroughly mendacious object, perhaps because I have always resisted the power of time out of some internal compulsion … in the hope, as I now think … that time will not pass away, has not passed away, that I can turn back and go behind it, and there I shall find everything as it once was, or more precisely I shall find that all moments of time have co-existed simultaneously, in which case none of what history tells us would be true, past events have yet occurred but are waiting to do so at the moment when we think of them … (p. 101)

At stake, then, is a far-ranging philosophical issue, generalizing a personal experience of simultaneity that we already encountered in Proust's

Recherche. For Amir Eshel (2003), the "poetic eruption" in the passage just quoted describes a most personal, indeed, highly emotional concern, as it did for Proust's protagonist. Intimately linked to his own sense of time, Austerlitz puts forward an idea of time as a mode of simultaneously coexisting moments and episodes from very different periods of clock and calendar time, moments that include present experiences and memories from the past, yet also from the future. And as it is for Proust, this view is also central to Sebald's writing about remembering and time as a whole. But insofar as the meaning of this view is concerned, Sebald takes it one step further. His consequences are, in Eshel's words, a "poetics of suspension" that not only suspends notions of chronology and succession, but also of comprehension and closure (2003, pp. 74–75).

And there is a third reason *Austerlitz* is perplexing: as a work of narrative. Probing an extreme life experience, it employs correspondingly challenging narrative resources. It incorporates nonlinguistic elements such as pictures, photographs, bills, prints, travel tickets, and other documents, all of them uncaptioned, which are turned into constitutive components of the narrative text. Several authors have identified here a novel and unique narrative technique, or a set of techniques, which are linked to Sebald's central concern with remembering and autobiographical time (e.g., Harris, 2001; Kilbourn, 2004; Weber, 2003). The plot—again, if we can call it a plot—consists of a series of conversations between two men, Austerlitz and a nearly anonymous narrator.

Sebald was a writer, scholar, and intellectual who himself also can be located at a juncture among literature, science, and philosophical reflection. Combining psychological and historical investigation with an interest in the idiosyncrasies of narrative self-examination, he seems especially to have been attracted by eccentric and mysterious exemplars of narrative self-exploration. Although the book industry has labeled his works as fiction, Sebald himself simply called them texts or prose (Sebald, 1993). For the character of Austerlitz he drew on several authentic historical biographies, among them one of a close colleague who taught history of architecture, and fused them (cf. Sebald, 2001b).

The three books Sebald published in the 1990s (*Vertigo*, *The Emigrants*, and *The Rings of Saturn*) can be seen as leading up to *Austerlitz*. All four books are presented as recollections and observations made by a narrator who travels around parts of Europe, but also (in *The Emigrants*) to America. Yet the travelogue and the reportage blend with the description of dreams, the essay with storytelling, and historical and philosophical reflections with autobiographical and biographical accounts. Sebald's writing not simply undermines traditional boundaries between genres and styles; it does not just play with them, offering artful riddles or puzzles, or a new variation of them—such as a "semi-documentary," "authentically fictionalized," or "semi-fictional" novel, as critics have labeled it. It rather explicitly refuses the distinction between fiction and nonfiction, or, as Samuel Pane remarks, it "seems to occupy an undefined (indefinable) space vis-à-vis travel writing, history, fiction, non-fiction, and autobiography" (2005, p. 37). We also could say that Sebald rejects playing by the rules of these language games, in contrast with most of the criticism on his books. His rejection regards all registers of the traditional labeling vocabulary: "My medium is prose, not the novel," he remarked (1993, p. 49).

Take the character and identity of Austerlitz as a case in point. The prose of *Austerlitz* intermingles fact (or apparent fact), recollection (or apparent recollection), and fiction (or apparent fiction), making all of them indistinguishable. What interests me here is not the challenge this prose poses for the critical, narratological, and epistemological reflection of these borderlines, but something else: in blurring the lines between the documentary and the fictional, Sebald seems to come close to the dynamic of autobiographical remembering and forgetting. What is needed, he ponders, to trace this dynamic and "to overcome the dissociative relationship to the past, is the organization, in an at least halfway discursive form, of what unobservedly occurs as remembrance (*Eingedenken*) in one's memory and what is understandable for no one" (Sebald, 1990, p. 121).

Susan Sontag (2000), in her essay on Sebald, reminds us that fiction and factuality have never been really opposed, as might have fiction and truth. A founding claim of the modern novel, she argues, is that it is a true story. "What makes a work fiction is not that the story is untrue—it may well be true, in part or in whole—but it's use, or extension, of a variety of devices (including false or forged documents) which produce what literary theorists call 'the effect of the real.' Sebald's fictions—and their accompanying visual illustration—carry the effect of the real to an extreme" (p. 3).

But the narrative evocation of the effect of the real is only one aspect, and I am not sure if it is a particularly specific one, of Sebald's writing. More significant is the analysis and deconstruction of what may be called the reality effect of remembering. Moreover, what makes Sebald's undertaking really special is that it sleuths the reality effect of the autobiographical process *without* using the traditional repertoire of archival models of memory. Austerlitz is a case study in the mind and life of a person for whom both the Newtonian time of clock and calendar and the idea of the memory storage have lost their binding power in his efforts at self-understanding. Who, then, is Austerlitz, this mysterious wanderer between the ruins of memory and time?

Autobiographical search movements

Jacques Austerlitz is a British historian of architecture who, in spite of many forebodings, discovers only late in his life his true origin and the terrible events of his childhood. Realizing that both his official identity as well as his own idea of himself was based, for most of his life, on an autobiographical void, a narrative lacuna, he faces dramatic psychological and psychiatric consequences. At least on one level one can read the life story of Austerlitz as illness report: as an account of a traumatic experience (Garloff, 2006), an account in which photography figures as a particular locus of trauma (Panc, 2005). This account is comprised of the entire range of common symptoms: from anxiety attacks and lingering bouts of sadness and social isolation to drastic forms of posttraumatic desperation, derealization, depersonalization, and the impossibility to temporally localize the traumatic experience. Finally, there is stupor, collapse, and suicide. Austerlitz tells the narrator about most of this during their sporadic encounters. The men meet at various places in several European countries over a period of 30 years. The book consists of a report of these conversations provided by the narrator and completed by other materials, written after Austerlitz had died and bequeathed a collection of black and white photographs to the narrator.

As with all protagonists in Sebald's books, not only is Austerlitz's past enigmatic, it somehow remains so despite all his efforts to recall and despite the ongoing investigations of the narrator. There also is a penetrating air of melancholy, a sense of "a mind in mourning," as Sontag (2000) entitled her essay. "The Anatomist of Melancholy" is the title of a collection of essays on Sebald, edited by Rüdiger Görner (2003). J. M. Coetzee speaks of Sebald's "lugubrious prose" (2002, p. 25). Less enigmatic, however, is the basis of this melancholy. Austerlitz's remembering monologues may be melancholic, they even may be atrabilious, but they also are reflexive and analytic. They are propelled by an investigative curiosity. They decisively exceed the primarily private and aesthetic tenor of modernist melancholia and Weltschmerz.

All of Sebald's protagonists are marked by the burden of a past that is both individual and historical. For all of them the trouble with their memories, or the loss of them, is part of a troubled cultural memory. For all of them, these individual and collective memories are those of a catastrophe, something that has happened in the gray zone between language and beyond what language can reach. Time and again, the reader learns that it is the catastrophe of modern European history, a history of war, violence, displacement, and destruction, of which the Holocaust is the ultimate manifestation (c.f. Dreyfus & Wolff, 2012). It is this ever present chasm in the continuum of historical remembrance that robs these characters of their personal sense of continuity. "Internally," as J. M. Coetzee observes, "they are wracked by a conflict between a self-protective urge to block off a painful past and a blind gripping for something, they do not know what, that has been lost" (2002, p.25).

What has been lost for Austerlitz, the reader finds out only after a few hundred pages, and only when Austerlitz himself has learned—after many years of searching and wandering around the places and spaces of that ineffable personal catastrophe—about his past and its entanglement with history. At first, the narrator's conversations with Austerlitz are concerned with the buildings at and in which they meet: the Palace of Justice in Brussels, the French Bibliothèque National, big railway stations such as Antwerp Centraal and London's Liverpool Street Station. Yet in Austerlitz's historical descriptions and interpretations of their architecture it becomes increasingly clear that they are not just about the meaning of architectural space but about a larger and deeper space of meaning. Many of the aesthetic and historical observations seem to be triggered by a search for autobiographical traces and clues. Often the starting point is the architecture historian's sharp eye for the sign quality of the material world, an uncanny sense that perceives its signs as strangely reminiscent of his own past.

Austerlitz's monologues realize autobiographical search movements, albeit wary movements. But what is searched for in the silent spaces of halls, staircases, domes, and urban landscapes? Like Austerlitz himself, we are not really sure about this. Surrounded by thingness, at times one might sense mnemonic reverberations, moments of empathy and affinities echoing personal memories. But whether they are real or imagined, they remain ineffable. But then, how do we know about their existence? Austerlitz speaks of "incomprehensible feelings" weighing on him for days, keeping him thinking, "like a madman, that there were mysterious signs and portents all around me here; how it even seemed to me as if the silent façades of the buildings knew something ominous about me" (Sebald, 2001a, p. 216). This, too, may explain why a large part of the book consists of detailed descriptions and interpretations of spaces, urban designs, and other examples of architecture. The bewildered reader wonders about their meaning until it becomes obvious that their invisible vanishing point is that of an autobiographical perspective. Although we find ourselves here in a nonverbal or preverbal territory of experience, it is not an overtly psychoanalytic or otherwise individual-psychological notion of memory that Sebald suggests, as Kilbourn (2004) points out in examining the architectural metaphors in *Austerlitz*. Sebald's preoccupation with architecture affords him an ample reservoir of metaphors, allegories, and symbols for memory as a cultural and historical phenomenon. This does not override every psychological concept of memory but rather shows its "irreducibly metaphorical or tropological nature" (Kilbourn, 2004, p.140).

The more Austerlitz's autobiographical perspective takes shape, the more imaginary stories shine through the detailed portrayals of, for instance, railway stations. Monuments of mobility but also of migration and flight, stations are associated with the stories of countless refugees, deportees, and emigrants in the 20th century, not to mention with Austerlitz's own personal past. As he will learn (and along with him the narrator and the reader) in the course of the book, his Czech-Jewish mother managed to save him as a boy of four and a half from a Prague occupied by German troops by including him in one of the so-called Kindertransports to England. His Kindertransport arrives at London's Liverpool Street Station where he is greeted by his new foster parents. Growing up in Wales under a new name, in a new family, with a new identity, and in a new language, he is never told about his previous past or the fate of his family. In fact, nothing is even mentioned to him. Whether it is despite or because of this, he begins to suffer from recurrent bouts of anxiety and dread.

When he, years later, eventually finds out about these events, the search for what he believes are submerged memories becomes the primary purpose of his life—a quest for something of which he only senses a vague outline. His efforts to fill this void, and to reconstruct how his family was destroyed along the shattered lines of European history, a history that Austerlitz captures first and foremost through its likewise mute architectural ciphers, lead him to Prague. When he detects that his mother was deported from Prague to the concentration camp Theresienstadt and from there farther to the east to her death, he decides to visit the town of Theresienstadt or Terezín, near Prague. I would like to offer a reading of this visit in which I examine what I take to be a key feature of Sebald's account of his protagonist's autobiographical process prompted by this visit to Terezín: its nonchronological, nonsequential, and nondirectional understanding of autobiographical time.

REMEMBERING THERESIENSTADT

The point of departure of my reading is Prague. Prague is the city where Austerlitz lived as a child, from where his mother was deported, and from where, about 50 years later, he sets off to trace her. He travels first by train and then on foot to Terezín, passing the lowlands at the confluence of the rivers Eger and Elbe. What he first encounters are the brick walls of the outer fortification of Theresienstadt that, surprisingly low, rise from a broad moat. Built in the 18th and 19th centuries as part of an Austrian fortress, the walls now are dilapidated and overgrown. Arriving in the inner city, the most striking aspect of Terezín, although it has been for many years an ordinary town again, is its emptiness. Wherever Austerlitz walks, he meets no people in the streets. Not a single curtain moves behind the blank windows of the houses.

As already mentioned, it is a peculiar characteristic of Sebald's books that they contain visual representations of documents and pictures, most of them photographs. Rarely do they just illustrate the text; mostly they continue, complement, and expand the narrative. Often they go beyond the written word, break it and, invoking what cannot be said otherwise, invite the reader to further interpretation and investigation. They establish a new kind of interpretive remembering, whose reference is not an original experience but the consciousness that such "authentic event" is irrevocably lost. In this sense, Richard Crownshaw (2004) has described photography in *Austerlitz* as a sort of "postmemory," using a concept introduced into the study of intergenerational memory by Marianne Hirsch (2001). There is, for example, a snapshot of what might have been one of Austerlitz's first sights of Theresienstadt on his arrival, the view of the outer fortifications of the old town. The picture inserted in the text shows how shrubs and bushes have covered the former grass-grown ramparts, giving the impression that the town is not so much a fortified monument of history but one half-hidden and sunk into the marshy ground of a floodplain, as if nature is in the middle of undoing the work of civilization.

In another grainy photograph we view one of the empty streets of Terezín lined with the dark façades of what might have been former garrison buildings. The entrance of the house closest to the viewer has been bricked up and another door barricaded. It features an old sign on which we read in large letters the word IDEAL. What does it mean? Is it the sign of a former shop? Or the name of a person or a good that once was sold here? Or does it mark a meeting place? And what kind of meetings? But then, we recall another hint shortly before, almost escaping our attention, when Austerlitz was musing over the oppressive sense of abandonment in the fortified town laid out to a strictly geometrical grid, an allusion that brought up, for a second, the ideal Sun State of Renaissance philosopher Campanella. From there the chain continues, suggesting a historical continuum of modern-time social and urbanistic utopias from its beginning to 20th-century Theresienstadt.

Looking closer at this photograph, we notice that, in contrast to all other pictures from this journey, the shot with the IDEAL sign is organized by a classic central perspective, featuring an empty street that runs into an imaginary vanishing point. As if walking toward this imaginary vanishing point, Austerlitz continues along the street. The closed gates and doors, an element which Austerlitz previously noticed only incidentally, come back to his mind. Are we mistaken in understanding it metaphorically as the closed gates and doors of his journey of remembrance, of remembering Theresienstadt how it "really" was?

> What I found most uncanny of all, however, were the gates and doorways of Terezín, all of them obstructing access to a darkness never yet penetrated, a darkness in which I thought, said Austerlitz, there was no movement at all apart from the whitewash peeling off the walls and the spiders spinning their threads, scuttling on crooked legs across the floorboards, or hanging expectantly in their webs. (p. 190)

As there already is a dream quality to his acts of remembering, or non-remembering, it needs only a minor metonymical shift to continue with the memory of a "real" dream.

> Not long ago, on the verge of waking from sleep, I found myself looking into the interior of one of these Terezín barracks. It was filled from floor to ceiling with layer upon layer of the cobwebs woven by those ingenious creatures. I still remember how, in my half-conscious state, I tried to hold fast to my powdery gray dream image, which sometimes quivered in a slight breath of air, and to discover what I concealed, but it only dissolved all the more and was overlaid by the memory [of the walk through the town]. (pp. 190–194)

Note that this description of a dream and the awakening from it captures an autobiographical memory in a strict sense. It is a twofold act of recall: a rememberer ("I still remember") recalls how he remembered a dream ("I tried to hold fast to my . . . dream image"). But this is only one element of the intricate time construction unfolding in this narrative passage; the more we become aware of it, the more it turns into a powerful allegory of the weave of remembering and time itself.

Like a metaphor, an allegory is figurative language, language that has a nonliteral meaning, but it extends beyond the format of a metaphor to that of a story. Given that I have put much emphasis on the narrative nature of our understanding of time, let me unravel this allegorical story. Right now we are in Terezín, at least, in terms of what narrative theorists would call story time. But that is not our only time. Austerlitz just talked about a dream he had at some time after his visit in Terezín, that is, from the point of view of Terezín plot time, a dream he will have in the future—a flashforward. In this dream he tries to find a clue of what happened in Terezín, that is, in the Theresienstadt of the past ("looking into the interior of one of these Terezín barracks"), a past long ago before his visit to Terezín. We, the readers, learn about this dream only on the basis of another flashforward: because Austerlitz will tell, even later, the narrator about all this, then, however, in autobiographical hindsight. Again later, after Austerlitz's death, the narrator will write down, also in retrospect, the entire story, the story we are reading now.

Returning to Terezín story time, Austerlitz finds himself on his walk through the town, by accident, outside of the so-called Ghetto Museum. Here he will spend the rest of the day immersed in plans, graphs, compilations, and pictures of the annihilation system of Theresienstadt. And he looks at things, a huge array of things that although he names them remain nameless.

> I understood it all now, yet I did not understand it, for every detail that was revealed to me as I went through the museum from room to room and back again, ignorant as I feared I had been through my own fault, far exceeded my comprehension. I saw pictures of luggage brought to Terezín by the internees from Prague and Pilsen, Würzburg and Vienna, Kufstein und Karlsbad and countless other places; the items such as handbags, belt buckles, clothes brushes, and combs which they had made in the various workshops ... I saw balance sheets, registers of the dead, lists of every imaginable kind, and endless rows of numbers and figures. ... (p. 199)

The signs of the past are mute, and the stories behind them remain forever untold. But could it be that their unrealized meanings, their openness to the narrative imagination are what make them loom so powerfully in the present? For Austerlitz they are mementos without any historical patina, signs of a timeless present.

When he leaves the museum and boards the bus back to Prague, the journey to Terezín reaches its last phase. This journey has finally demonstrated to Austerlitz that it is impossible to impose any temporal directedness or chronological hierarchy, indeed, any sense of external temporal order on the various layers of his memories, images, ideas, historical and personal reflections, and their ongoing interpretations—the uninterrupted steam of consciousness that went on during the entire visit.

Sebald's suggestive picture for this is the bus ride back to Prague, which Austerlitz recalls as

> ... going steadily downhill, particularly, when we reached the suburbs of Prague and it seemed as if we were descending a kind of ramp into a labyrinth through which we moved very slowly, now this way and now that, until I had lost all sense of direction. (p. 201)

If we conceive of Austerlitz's visit to Terezín as a memory journey—obviously quite a different one from that of Odysseus—the bus ride comes close to the simile of a movement that is all but localizable on a chronological and homogeneous trajectory, be it one of geography, remembering, or temporality.

NARRATED TIME AND NARRATING TIME

In Chapter 5, I referred to the two concepts of *fabula* and *sjuzhet* first introduced by the Russian formalists to distinguish the elemental sequential succession of events in a story, the fabula, from their particular narrative composition and presentation, the sjuzhet. Much discussed in the history of narratology, and for some time now substituted by the concepts *story* and *discourse,* this distinction establishes a juxtaposition of two spheres or orders of narrative. Correspondingly, two temporal orders are differentiated, *story time* and *discourse time.* Even if narratologists in the tradition of Genette (1980) have added a third order called *narration* to capture the production and communication of narrative, they, too, go along with the basic distinction between a sphere of chronological story time and a less restricted sphere of discourse time (though Genette, as noted, granted the possibility of "achronic" or temporally "undatable" narrative structures). These two temporal orders, as Fludernik (2003) ascertains, represent the two major levels of analysis on which temporality has been treated in narrative studies.

The idea of this binary opposition of two time spheres enshrined in story and discourse implies that whatever becomes the subject of narratological investigation is predicated on a concept of chronology. "It is assumed," writes Fludernik, "that the *story* level of a narrative, i.e. the sequence of events reconstructed from the surface level of the linguistic medium, can be viewed as a chronological order, whereas on the discourse level (the sequence of words on the page that constitute the text) several reshufflings take place to produce a number of *anachronies,* as Genette calls them (flashbacks and flashforwards)" (2003, p. 118).

But even Genette's (1980) anachronies presuppose a frame of reference that allows us to determine what is forward and what is backward in time and thus retains the underlying idea of time as chronological, sequential, and homogeneous. And this also holds true for the other aspects of Genette's concept of the temporal "order" of a narrative, as well as for things like narrative "speed" or "duration" and "frequency" (which are Genette's major subcategories of what he refers to as "tense" or narrative temporality). Despite its complicated conceptual apparatus, Genette's basic assumption of what makes up narrative time is soundly grounded in a traditional Newtonian ontology.

The question is, however, whether this model of narrative time is universally applicable to all forms and practices of narrative, including the narrative forms of the autobiographical process at issue here. As Fludernik elucidates, we are "tempted to see time as an objective, measurable and unambiguous category that can be pictured as a dotted line progressing from past to future" (2003, p. 119). Accordingly, as she goes on to write, "[T]emporality is conceptualized on the story level in the common-sense 'objective' manner that we all take for granted. On the discourse level, with the reading and viewing of narrative discourse, however, a cognitive order of temporality is instituted which is based, not on sequentiality or chronology, but on holistic structures of narrative comprehension" (p. 119). But can we be so sure that all narrative, including nonliterary forms and practices, can be modeled on Newtonian time, as Fludernik (and Genette) seem to suggest? Moreover, is not discourse time, even if it is viewed as nonsequential and nonchronological, per definition always conceived of as against the background (or underground) of story time's chronology and sequentiality?[2]

I suspect that it is especially difficult, if not impossible, to make use of this model of narrative time in the understanding of texts like *Austerlitz* that seek to enact the textual fabric and the temporal dynamics of an autobiographical process. These dynamics, I have suggested, evade models of chronology, linearity, and homogeneity—and we see why Sebald must be viewed in a tradition that also includes Virginia Woolf's and other modernists' astonishment about the discrepancy between time on the clock and time in the mind.

Notwithstanding the limits of the traditional narrative time model, I want to offer a short analysis of the different story time levels of the Terezín episode. I do this for two reasons. One is to understand better the multitemporal scenarios underlying Austerlitz's memory of his Terezín visit. Again, as in the passage from McEwan's *Saturday* examined in Chapter 5, what we view here is a time horizon that clearly stretches beyond the autobiographical to the historical. In this case the otherwise problematic concepts are helpful. The second reason is because I want to use this analysis as a point of departure for supporting my argument that the reality effect engendered by this sort of autobiographical narrative is actually not based on the representation of a realist time line, the putative given order of story time; on the contrary, it offers a point of view from which all supposedly given chronological levels of autobiographical time disintegrate. They collapse, we might say, into one temporal space. This dissolving of time—time according to the Newtonian trajectory—goes further than what Fludernik, drawing on Genette (1980), has called the narrative "reshuffling" within the expressive order of discourse time (2003, p. 118). Rather, it is a dissolving of the kind we saw allegorically displayed in Austerlitz's bus ride back to Prague at the end of the Terezín episode.

Yet before we reach the end, let us look again at the beginning—Austerlitz approaching Terezín through the marshy ground of a floodplain. What he first spots is the half-sunk fortress that seems to be disappearing into natural temporality, or timelessness, out of which it once emerged. Human civilization as part of natural history: this is the first level of time evoked in this episode. But civilization soon becomes more specified. It was in modern times that Theresienstadt was founded, with the spirit of rationalism and enlightenment leaving its mark on the checkerboard pattern of its design. The story of all of this is told by Austerlitz in passing, as part of his ongoing observations that do not claim the spotlight but contribute to an omnipresent sense of historical temporality. Further layers or aspects of historical time become visible as this narrative universe unfolds, indicated, for example, by the references to Campanella and the history of social utopias. In this key, the fortress town embodies several distinct strata of this history, reaching to 20th century catastrophes and the deserted streets of the "ordinary town." Such is the historically saturated temporal terrain on which we follow Austerlitz on his uncanny stroll, a stroll that, by the way, on a mere plot level does not take longer than one day.

But analysis of the common fabric of time, remembering, and narrative does not stop here. So far we have only reviewed the domain of what sometimes is referred to as narrated time or *erzählte Zeit*, to use the terms of Günter Müller (1968). This is the time or the times that unfold in the story told, the time the narrative is about. Different from this is the time in which the narrative is told, *narrative time* or *narrating time* or *Erzählzeit*, as Müller called it (what Genette dubbed *narration*). This is the time in which the narration takes place. Just as the narrated time of the Terezín episode comprises various individual and historical time levels so, too, does the time in which the narration takes place set up a multilevel scenario. In our case, this includes at least three different planes. First, there is the time in which Austerlitz tells the narrator about his memories from his Terezín visit; second, the time in which the narrator reports his memories of the conversations with Austerlitz and the story he learned therein; and third, the time in which we, the readers, read and try to understand the story.

As the scenarios of narrated time and narrative time are intermingled in a number of ways, they conjure up a dense universe of temporal discourse. To sort it out requires quite an analytical effort. Still, it might be surprising that we, as ordinary readers, do not become aware of this temporal complexity. Why is that so? There is an easy answer and a difficult answer. The easy one: because a good narrative does not need a narratologist and memory researcher to be read and understood. And the complicated one: typically, the narrative flow would keep us interested not in its temporal organization but in its content, its meaning construction. This is the dimension where things happen, the things that keep us reading and listening and engaged in stories. But a close tracing of the various movements of meaning that go on in the narrative stream of action and consciousness reveals, as we see, a continuous moving back and forth, an oscillating among all planes.[3]

"I work using the system of bricolage, in Lévi-Strauss's sense," Sebald comments, referring to the French anthropologist's work, *The Savage Mind*; "it is a form of savage work, of pre-rational thought, in which one nuzzles in findings until they somehow make sense" (1993, p. 51; my translation). The term bricolage is indeed helpful to describe not only how much of Sebald's memory combinatorics is based on a kind of "metonymic mnemonics," as Anne Fuchs (2004, pp. 59–62) has shown. It also captures his entire mnemotic style that is both post-Newtonian and, in his own understanding, pre-Newtonian. It seems that Eshel has this in mind when he speaks of *Austerlitz's* "unstable temporality that shifts between different layers of the past and different aspects of the present" (2003, p. 92). In my view, it might, however, be more appropriate to conceive of it in a Proustian sense as the simultaneous presence of all these different temporal strata and moments, avoiding any echo of a hierarchical model of different times. To picture such a temporality we need concepts different from story and discourse time, which are based on assumptions of chronology and hence miss the mark of the atemporal simultaneity that defines this space of meaning.

I believe that this post-Newtonian (or, for Sebald, pre-Newtonian) space of meaning comes closest to the temporal reality of the autobiographical process. Walter Benjamin has described such spatial simultaneity or copresence, the *Nebeneinander* of moments and events that appear to the modern eye as chronologically distinct, as a fundamental feature of human imagination. This feature is integral to the narrative weave of remembering and autobiographical time that we find in *Austerlitz*. Its hallmark is what Benjamin called the timeless *now*, the moment in which present experiences, mental representations (*Vorstellungen*), and memories become indistinguishable.[4]

THE TIMELESS NOW

To flesh out Benjamin's timeless now, I once again return to the Terezín episode, focusing on the narrative configuration of spatial simultaneity in close up and slow motion, so to speak. So far I only briefly touched on a scene in which Austerlitz walking through the empty streets of the town observes the window display of the only shop in this haunting place. The shop with the name *Antikos Bazar* exerts such power on him that it is a long time before he can tear himself away from staring, his face pressed against the window, at the hundreds of different objects, "as if one of them or their relationship with each other must provide an unequivocal answer to the many questions I found it impossible to ask in my mind" (p. 195).

> What was the meaning of the festive white lace tablecloth hanging over the back of the ottoman, and the armchair with its worn brocade cover? What secret lay behind the three brass mortars of different sizes, which had about them the suggestion of an oracular utterance, or the cut-glass bowls, ceramic vases, and earthenware jugs, the tin advertising sign bearing the words *Theresienstädter Wasser*, the little box of seashells, the miniature barrel organ, the globe-shaped paperweights with wonderful marine flowers swaying inside their glassy spheres.... (pp. 195–196)

The list of ornaments, utensils, and other objects Austerlitz notices and meticulously describes goes on and on, and the longer it gets the more it becomes an endless accumulation of finds that stands for a likewise endless accumulation of signs. But what they signify is lost—a universe of mementos, of memory objects that have been forgotten and now are mute. We only can suspect the dramas of life of which they were a part. Last things, perhaps, which were at one point irrevocably separated from their owners who may have loved them until their final moment. Now having lost their stories and, in a sense, their histories, they have become a silent assembly of signs of what is absent. Undecipherable signs. Brought together in a strange spatial simultaneity, it seems as if they were for a second, for a *timeless now*, awoken through Austerlitz's glance. It is this glance that makes the stories behind these mementos appear as untold.

Ultimately, then, this scene is not primarily about the universe of untold stories but about Austerlitz's autobiographical glance, which turns out to be the affective vanishing point, the emotional center of gravity of this scene. It connects the objects with life, with *a* life, Austerlitz's life. For his life is as unknown and its story is as untold as the stories of the objects in the shop. Now they appear as mementos of his own lost memory.

This is Austerlitz's dilemma: the present cannot be informed by memories of the past that have disappeared beyond recovery. Yet at the same time, there are countless material traces of the past, physical mementos, that swarm through every aspect of the present. Past and present grow into each other almost organically, and it is this grown *Nebeneinander* or simultaneity that is captured in one of the most emblematic visual metaphors of the book inserted in the text at this point. In a photograph of one of the windows of the *Antikos Bazar* we see branches of storefront trees mirrored in the window as if they were literally reaching into the display mingling with the objects. We pause and think about whether this optical reflection means something, and then realize that this also is the very moment in which Austerlitz (or Sebald?) must have taken the shot. Indeed, when we look carefully at the next photo on the opposing page showing another window of the shop we recognize the faint image of the photographer himself, his barely perceptible reflections on the window pane.

Could it be the silhouette of Austerlitz (or Sebald)? A frozen *hic et nunc* of Austerlitz's memory, simultaneously held onto with the objects displayed in the window? Becoming aware that we are looking at the display through the silhouette of the photographer, we, the readers and viewers of the book, enter the scene. And we do so—from the point of view of the photographer—at one point in the future, peering through this window, as well as through the lens of the camera that pretends to hold onto this moment, at the mementos in the *Antikos Bazar*.

The entire scene encapsulates what I conceive of as the dissolving of the temporal grid behind the distinctions of past, present, and future. While the scene operates, in filmic terms, like a zoom and, in rhetorical terms, like a metaphor, it is immediately followed in the book by an allegory that captures this timeless now from a still different angle. Austerlitz has just left the museum and again finds himself in the deserted town square. Suddenly the situation in Theresienstadt in December 1942 comes to him, a time when his mother must have arrived there. About sixty thousand people were squeezed together in the ghetto, a built-up area of one square kilometer at the most. It seems to him that all these people were still living in the buildings and basements and attics, as if they were incessantly all over the place, looking out of the windows and moving through the streets, "and even, a silent assembly, filling the entire space occupied by the air, hatched with gray as it was by the fine rain" (p. 200). Imagining a vast number of people actively going about their business crammed into such a small ghetto once more intensifies the idea of timeless, spatial simultaneity that emerged in the scene in front of the *Antikos Bazar*.

The co presence of different mental states, including memories, dream scenes, and mental images, mingling and mutually embedded, is widespread in 20th-century literature concerned with consciousness and the mind. Various literary theorists have shown that the presentation and creation of a character's states of mind is a crucial concern of the modern novel, and that narrative mind-presentation and mind-creation can get very complex (e.g., Herman, 2011c; Palmer, 2004; 2010; Zunshine, 2006). Decisive for the evocation and interpretation of this complexity are a number of narrative techniques and strategies that articulate and give existence to mental states that occur simultaneously. Not least, this includes memories, whether they are clear and vivid or vague and blurred to the point that it is not even clear that they are memories.

In Sebald's writing we find this simultaneous co-presence of different mental states and sensations with memories radicalized in a way that severs the linkage with any temporal system of reference. It even extends to the dead. Past and present, life and death, become to the same indistinguishable extent co-present as real and imagined memories.

> It does not seem to me, Austerlitz added, that we understand the laws governing the return of the past, but I feel more and more as if time did not exist at all, only various spaces interlocking according to the rules of a higher form of stereometry, between which the living and the dead can move back and forth as they like, and the longer I think about it the more it seems to me that we who are still alive are unreal in the eyes of the dead, that only occasionally, in certain lights and atmospheric conditions, do we appear in their field of vision. (p. 185)

The perspective of the dead does not represent the intrusion of the spectral or demonic but elaborates a mode of imagining that we have come across through the entire book. It gives shape to a further gestalt in which Austerlitz/Sebald repudiates the Newtonian vision of time and the idea of remembering as "the return of the past," a past which has be stored in the dark chambers of some memory archive.

In terms of narrative theory, this is the terrain of "fuzzy temporality," as Herman describes a category of narrative "that order[s] events in a fuzzy or indeterminate way as stories engaging in a 'polychronic' style of narration" (2002, p. 212). Further developing Genette's (1980) discussion of achronic or temporally undatable time, Herman proposes "polychronic" narrative as a "temporal sequencing that is strategically inexact, making it difficult or even impossible to assign narrated events a fixed or even fixable position along a timeline in the storyworld" (p. 212). Traditional narratology locates polychronic narration on the plane of discourse time; this is the place where "fuzzy temporality" may occur. Its status is that of a strategy or technique of narrative composition. But, as noted before, the basic assumption of narrative time in this conceptual frame is that discourse time only "reshuffles" the Newtonian story time that ultimately underlies all events and experiences. Sometimes, Newtonian story time is only a hypothetical abstract model, because in the narrative act story time and discourse time are always inextricably interconnected.

In contrast, I have suggested in my reading of *Austerlitz* that the Newtonian ontology fails to capture the temporal dynamics of the autobiographical process in which the "inside perspective" is pivotal. To use Herman's expression, the autobiographical process demands an understanding of polychronic temporality that also extends to story time, the temporality the narrative is about—if we then still want to use the terms discourse time and story time, with all their metaphysical implications, in exploring the autobiographical process. Austerlitz, for one, surely did not share this metaphysics.

I have called this chapter *Beyond Time*. But if we nevertheless want to talk about time in Sebald's *Austerlitz*, then we should talk in a strong and literal sense (albeit not Genettian sense) about *narrative* time, the time that is evoked in the process of narration. Eshel (2003, p. 91) remarks that Sebald's narratives do not simply count off times gone, but create their own mode of counting, of accounting for their own times. The argument I have put forward is that this kind of temporality is the outcome of a linguistic figuration, the result of a process of narrative temporalization. What marks Sebald's writing, to borrow again Eshel's words, is "the ways in which the effects of figuration themselves constitute the work's ultimate referent, that is, its unique 'time effects,' the way in which the text forms time and conditions the reading experience" (p. 91).[5]

We have seen how some of these narrative "time effects" are intermingled with what likewise can be called the narrative "memory effects" created in the autobiographical process. The picture that emerges from Sebald's dissection of Austerlitz's remembering does not presuppose or expose any order of time as a precondition of narrative and remembrance. Rather it reveals that "time" emerges as one possible result or effect, indeed, as a side effect of the narrative process of meaning construction and self-localization. Newtonian time may be, under certain circumstances, an important parameter for our autobiographical self-localization, especially, if this localization follows a perspective of retrospective teleology, as I have pointed out elsewhere (Brockmeier, 2001b). But it is neither a fundamental nor an a priori condition of it. Sebald's portrait of Austerlitz's autobiographical search movements makes the case that in the center of humans' concern with their identity is not an effort to account for our existence in terms of a chronological or sequential order of time and memories but the hermeneutic effort to make sense of, and give significance to, our being in the world—even if this world, as for Austerlitz, is no longer a place to be remembered.

CHAPTER 10
Reframing Memory

In much of Western history memory has been a concept with gravitas. It is one of those terms that appears both as common currency in our everyday life and, since Plato ennobled it metaphysically and modern academia scientifically, as a conceptual heavyweight. The starting point of this book was the observation that this gravitas is dissolving; in fact, memory has already lost a lot of its once substantial weight. What is left is a different term, an airy word that points to an amazing variety of diverse and fuzzy discourses—without, however, having entirely lost its former meanings. They continue to stay attached to it like old memories of which one has become fond.

Can we at least assume that all these different discourses have something in common? Even here, skepticism is part of the answer. We can say for sure that the search for a treasure at the end of the rainbow, for something that *in reality* corresponds to the vocabulary of memory as an archive of the past has resulted in the sobering recognition that there is no such thing as "memory." Nor is there a physical reality or capacity or a number of neuronal systems or mechanisms localized in the brain that could claim this term. The word memory is like the word time: there is no place, no spatiotemporal field, no *res extensa* that it can capture, although it has the flavor of it. We should keep in mind that most people, including most memory scientists and scholars, might still think of memory as something that has "a home, even if still a hidden one, in the brain" (Tulving, 2002b, p. 20).

One of the objectives with which I started my inquiry was to synthesize recent developments in various areas of memory studies that have contributed to the insight just summarized. At the same time, I tried to show that these developments have given way to radically novel perspectives on remembering that go far beyond the traditional storage idea and transcend the assumption of memory as something located in an isolated brain. These perspectives tend to reframe remembering and forgetting as social activities, as practices of persons who are steeped in cultural worlds abounding with mnemonic activities and artifacts, including an increasing portion of digital memory technologies. Moreover, moving beyond an archival model of memory might also afford new avenues for understanding, caring for, and treating those suffering from memory problems linked to dementia, a disease increasingly affecting large parts of the population. This shift in focus might lend support to what I have called a postautobiographical perspective of human identity which, conversely, sheds new light on conditions of persons with serious memory troubles (Brockmeier, 2014; Medved & Brockmeier, 2015).

This cultural paradigm shift in our understanding of memory and remembering outlined in the first chapters has been the backdrop for my exploration of an alternative, the "narrative alternative." I have presented it as one of a number of alternative perspectives and visions of memory, that is, of alternatives to the archival model. This exploration has concentrated on one specific area of memory research, the autobiographical process. What makes this domain of human remembering particularly fascinating is that it interlaces biological and psychological, individual and cultural, linguistic and imagistic aspects in a unique fashion. It also entwines individual with historical processes of temporalization, which, as I have suggested in the last two chapters, is a view that challenges the time-honored assumption of remembering as a movement in (Newtonian) time.

Within the autobiographical domain, I have further concentrated my investigations on the narrative fabric of the autobiographical process, using the linguistic and psychological dynamic of narrating as a model to re-describe what traditionally had been called autobiographical memory. One chief advantage of this approach is that it gives center stage to the interplay of cognitive-interpretive, social-communicative, and emotional-motivational aspects of remembering. Typically, these aspects are studied in isolation; a case in point is psychological and neuroscientific memory research (which, at any rate, has been overwhelmingly a cognitive enterprise). In contrast, the understanding of this interplay and the resulting synthesis of the various narrative and psychological components of the autobiographical process was the main concern of the case studies presented in the previous chapters. What they have shown is that this synthesis is at the heart of the meaning formation that takes place in the autobiographical process.

Closely linked to this proposition, another objective of this book has been to bring into sharper relief that remembering is one of those multilayered phenomena whose assumed material reality cannot be distinguished from our views and thoughts about it. This has led to the outline of a de-substantialized and de-ontologized notion of memory that shifts the focus of attention from the single organ, the brain, to the biological–social–cultural lives of people, to individuals, that is, who remember and forget in the midst of a cultural and historical world. A consequence of this shift is an important qualification to the concept of personal identity, which results from the limits of its traditionally autobiographical and self-centered grounding. Vis-à-vis the experiences of individuals with atypical developments (like Fragile X), injuries (like neurotraumas), and diseases (like Alzheimer's), it appears that the autobiographical and narrative anchoring of identity, based on individual remembering and language, is too narrow a defining criterion of identity. In contrast, the cultural, intersubjective, and embodied understanding of identity that I have proposed is not predicated on its autobiographical and narrative dimensions—albeit neither does it exclude them as a possibility, a component of self-construction.

Now, in this last chapter, I want to drive home these points integrating them into a larger picture that takes on a slightly philosophical framework. Because I have used philosophical categories such as *epistemic, ontological, post-positivist, post-metaphysic,* and *res extensa* in various chapters, this framework is also meant to draw together the philosophical lines of sight underlying the previous studies and discussions. In order to avoid making this too categorical and theoretical an enterprise, my arguments are arranged around an artwork, a sculpture or, more precisely, an installation. Created by a contemporary European artist, Anselm Kiefer, it tackles exactly the dilemma that has been made visible by the quotation marks that I sometimes have put around the word "memory." These quotation marks are the marks of a concept that gives form to something that, as I have argued, does not exist along spatiotemporal dimensions but nevertheless is deeply moored in our cultural economy of remembering. Shaped by a long history, it is continuously reinforced by the way we talk, think, imagine, feel, and act. In this way, it has taken on a derivative, metaphorical, and narrative existence—a tropical gestalt that is emblematically embodied in the vision of the mnemonic storage and its many variants. An omnipresent example of this discourse, mentioned in many chapters, is the set of archival concepts encapsulating the *encoding, storing* (or *retaining* or *maintaining*), and *retrieval* of memories.

To deal with this dilemma I have used two vocabularies, two perspectives, two epistemological trajectories. On the one hand, I have referred to the phenomenon I am interested in with traditional terms such as autobiographical memory, sometimes with, sometimes without, quotation marks. On the other hand, I have used terms more appropriate to my investigative lenses such as autobiographical process, remembering, and mnemonic practice. In fact, the further along we have progressed in the book, the more the *memory* vocabulary has shifted to a *remembering* vocabulary. Sometimes, however, I have used both vocabularies as if they were interchangeable. But are they not supposed to exclude each other? Was the autobiographical process not meant to reframe the idea of autobiographical memory? To offer a kind of counter-trope to the master-trope of the archive, still dominant in many areas of memory research as well as in everyday discourse? How can these opposing vocabularies coexist?

Before I take a look at Anselm Kiefer's installation—which I view as a possible answer to this question—let me outline how Richard Rorty formulated the problem. Rorty (1989) has contended that arguments against the use of a familiar and venerable vocabulary unavoidably run into trouble because they cannot but be couched in the same vocabulary against which they are directed. It is a contradiction in itself to use a concept in order to reject the same concept. The coherent and meaningful use of a concept implies that it makes sense within a given vocabulary and its particular framework of meaning. For Rorty, we cannot simply reject and replace terms from an old vocabulary or even reject or replace the entire vocabulary itself but have to demonstrate that a better, more appropriate vocabulary for the description of a problem is available or, at least, can be imagined. Many important intellectual and scientific debates, Rorty adds, are not primarily an examination of the pros and cons of a thesis; usually they are,

> ... implicitly or explicitly, a contest between an entrenched vocabulary which has become a nuisance and a half-formed new vocabulary which vaguely promises great things. The latter "method" ... is to redescribe lots and lots of things in new ways, until you have created a pattern of linguistic behavior which will tempt the rising generation to adopt it, thereby causing them to look for appropriate new forms of nonlinguistic behavior, for example, the adoption of new scientific equipment or new social institutions. ... This sort of [method] works holistically and pragmatically. It says things like "try thinking of it this way"—or more specifically, "try to ignore the apparently futile traditional questions by substituting the following new and possibly interesting questions." (1989, p. 9)

What Rorty points out is a strategy of suggestion. It advocates that we might want to stop doing certain things the old way and do something else. But it does not put forward this suggestion on the basis of what he calls an "antecedent criteria common to the old and the new language games" (p. 9); which means, applied to our issue of memory, it does not argue, say, for a "better" archive or a neuroscientifically updated notion of memory as a neuronal, molecular, or system-based storehouse. Rather, it tries to make the vocabulary it favors look convincing by showing how it may be used to re-describe the involute processes of remembering and forgetting in a more comprehensive and sensitive way, that is, in a way that brings into prominence the narrative and cultural dynamic of the autobiographical process.

Kiefer's installation, to which I turn now, also offers a reframing of the idea of memory, although, as a work of art, it does so in an altogether different manner. Still we can view it as an attempt to capture both the dilemma of "memory"—an entity that does not exist but still haunts us—and the "method" of reframing old things by re-describing them in new ways.

CHRONOS'S ARCHIVE

I am not sure whether visitors to Berlin's Museum for Contemporary Art are aware that its main hall once was the home base of the first steam locomotives in that part of the world. The museum still carries the name of its earlier purpose *Hamburger Bahnhof*, Hamburg station, conjuring up the mid-19th century, when it was erected as the Berlin terminus of the Berlin–Hamburg railroad line, one of the first stations of the rail system. On a sunny day when the light shines through the old iron-framed roof windows of the hall it falls on the place where the passengers boarded their cars. There are photographs on which the trains look like dark and ponderous iron figures and it becomes clear why people called these vehicles *Eisenbahn*, iron train. In fact, Eisenbahn became the German word both for railroad and train.

When it was decided to put a sculpture by Anselm Kiefer on this very spot, stories of Eisenbahn, steam engines, and the people who left from here for Hamburg might not have played a role. What certainly mattered was the solid foundation. Iron is heavy stuff, one of the early steam locomotives might have weighed more than a thousand tons and Kiefer's imposing installation I imagine is not much lighter. It is made out of lead and steel, an ensemble of shelves filled with larger-than-life books or, perhaps, files or other documents: a massive archive whose sheer lead-heaviness seems to turn it into an indestructible monument. A statement of resistance against the flux of time. There is an almost archaic feel to its metallic physicality, an air of Stonehenge or Egyptian grave chamber. Anyone who approaches it cannot help but feel small.

But there also is a more concrete historical memory to which the sculpture makes reference. Called *Volkszählung* (Census)—see Figure 10.1—it was created 1991 in the aftermath of a controversial census, opposed and boycotted by civil rights groups and protest movements, in what then was West Germany. Yet this is only one of the connections to the outside world this compact block of an archive suggests. Lead, its main material, is another one. Kiefer has produced many artworks out of lead, which today are in museums all over the world. Lead, he says, is a material considered to be eternal and in full force, but in reality is soft and malleable. Lead is always about heaviness and lightness at the same time, about fixity and movement. As an artist with a profound historical

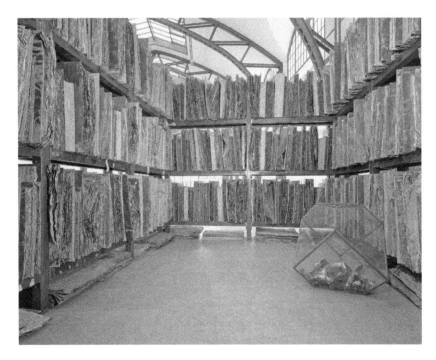

Figure 10.1: Anselm Kiefer: *Volkszählung* (Census), 1990
Nationalgalerie Berlin—Museum für Gegenwart (Museum for Contemporary Art), Hamburger Bahnhof, SMB. © Bildagentur für Kunst, Kultur und Geschichte (bpk), Berlin. Photograph: Jens Ziehe. With kind permission of Anselm Kiefer and Galerie Thaddaeus Ropac, Salzburg and Paris.

consciousness—many of his works revolve around the Holocaust, violence, and destruction, meditating on those events against a wider historical and cultural backdrop—Kiefer knows about lead's mythical aura and the long tradition of powerful qualities attributed to it. Since Antiquity, lead was associated with Saturn, the god and the planet, and, therefore, with time, transience, death, and melancholia—the Saturnine temperament.

Saturn is the Roman version of the Greek god Kronos, the father of Zeus. Kronos is a Titan, the first generation of gods, and thus close to another Titan, Mnemosyne, the goddess of memory, time, and language. We encountered her earlier, taking a closer look at Plato's conceptualization of memory. Mnemosyne, an important figure of reference for Plato, seems also to be an influential player in the background of Kiefer's art of lead: she is the mother of the Muses, of the arts. And like the arts, the origins of the metal lead reach back to prehistorical and mythical epochs. We know that it has been extracted from ores for at least 10,000 years. Alchemists and astrologers considered it to be the "basest" of the traditional seven metals.

At the same time, there is a strong affinity to another central mythical figure, Chronos, Father Time. Chronos is an ambivalent character, a father who also represents death and decay. Countless representations show Chronos as a skeletal figure. In fact, lead is a highly poisonous metal; its history is a long history of murder, disease, and dying that culminates in modern times. Especially in England, lead is linked to a century-long tradition of poisoning the general populace; one reason for this was that wine and cider were drunk out of pewter goblets containing lead. In the figure of Chronos, the ancient myth joined both the timelessness of gods like Kronos and the limited lifetime of humans, a time passing and irreversibly running out. It might have been also for this reason that, in the realm of human time, life needed something to hold on to—a stable archive, perhaps, or the never-ending narratives of myth.

Kiefer's Berlin version of Chronos's archive is arranged as a square of steel shelves with lead books and documents that opens to a walk-in space. Entering this space one encounters a strange geometric body, a polyhedron. Its most famous representation in the history of art is on a Renaissance engraving, Albrecht Dürer's *Melencolia I*. So is it the Saturnine temperament that one finds, according to Kiefer, in the very center of the archive? Is it the sense of human life's fugacity that erects the archive as a fortress against the flux of time?

If one stops to listen to visitors who explore this inner space, one overhears a variety of associations attributed to the installation. Obviously there is the library, the archive, and the storeroom. But one also hears talk of a castle, stronghold, studio, prison, and watchtower. I remember a woman who extensively photographed the installation and carefully drew a site plan. It's like an archeological finding, she said, something mysterious from a time long ago but still, you don't know why, it's very familiar.

This feeling of familiarity and strangeness is enhanced by the fact that the archive, despite the countless documents that seem to have been collected in it, does not give visitors any information about their content and function. Although it offers some hints. This is one: All books and documents are seeded with peas, peas and again peas. Peas? I once showed them to a friend who looked at me in disbelief: What peas? I only see bullets here, lead bullets all over the place. Whatever it is, one could think there is one of these little round pieces of lead for each of the millions of people who were to be counted in that contentious census from which the installation got its name. Counting peas is, in American parlance, counting beans. Counting people is the literal meaning of the German word for census, *Volkszählung*.

It is, however, not only the bewildering reductionism of the equation of one person = one pea that seems to be a concern here, but also the permanence and timeless solidity that the institution of an archive promises—at least, at first sight. For on closer inspection this promise becomes dubious. We notice that some of the books have opened and their lead pages separated and rumpled to the point of being unusable. You look at them and expect them to continue disintegrating before your eyes. And then there is the even more disturbing fact that none of these monstrous documents are actually readable. To begin with, who would be able to take them off the shelf? As it looks, not even a couple of strong persons would be able to lift one of these massive blocks of lead. In fact, they were placed there by a heavy-duty crane.

Do we have to conclude that what we see are the relics from previous epochs? A storage technology that went out of use, to the point that nobody knows to decipher its code anymore, or to access its writing at all? Who then will ever remember those millions of individuals archived here? Who recounts the stories of their lives that are attested to only by silent peas, mysterious peas of lead? After all, the installation might be not so much about an archive but about how even the heaviest and "basest" of all archives lost its struggle against oblivion. The entries it was supposed to store have become illegible, they have faded away despite and because of the lead that was meant to bestow on them a timeless present.

The longer we walk around the installation, the more it turns into an enigmatic fossil. A memento mori from an era whose messages have become unintelligible as time has gone by. Who knows, after all, whether they were ever *meant* to be messages? We certainly can say that the meanings we now associate with these books would not arise if there were letters and texts to be read on their pages.

So is this another of Kiefer's infamous works on human failure in the face of history, scrutinizing memory as a case in point? Or is it about the failure of the idea that there is an unfailing memory? Is it about the end of the age-old utopia that there can be an archive that is not part of the flow of time against which it was erected? And this despite an attempt to make use of a metal that the alchemists considered the most robust because it was the least human of all matter?

Yet, whatever else it is, the installation is first of all a work of art. And it is the notorious hallmark of artworks that their meanings only can be fathomed in processes of interpretation that themselves are not free from history. This is where narrative comes in: as the attempt to find a story that allows us to make sense of an object, an experience, a memory. If things and processes gain a certain degree of entanglement and, especially, temporal complexity, understanding their meaning unavoidably takes on the form of a story—which is a claim I discussed earlier in terms of the strong narrative thesis.

Sometimes this story remains enigmatic, as might, after all, Kiefer's sculpture, notwithstanding all our efforts to make sense of it. Sometimes the story branches into multiple stories, encompassing more than one or even two vocabularies that open up a variety of perspectives. This multiperspectivism—as we saw in studying narrative scenarios by McEwan, Hong Kingston, Proust, Benjamin, Sebald, and other writers, as well as stories from everyday contexts—is crucial to humans' unique imaginative capacities. So if we read Kiefer's memory installation in a narrative mode, we simultaneously deal with stories about the Hamburger Bahnhof, myths about Chronos, fairytales about alchemists, legends about the history of lead, anthropological field reports, historical accounts of a census, and reflections about the historical nature of our ideas of memory. They all charge the meaning of the artwork.

Surely this is not to say that all these stories ultimately condense to one comprehensive and final story. Even if sometimes there might be the narrative terra firma of an original and authentic *ur*-story, in being told and retold to others—and that is what stories are made for—it is continuously reinterpreted and adapted to new circumstances until the ur-story is irretrievably lost and forgotten. And all that remains are what in Kiefer's artistic language is symbolized by peas. But these peas can become seeds, the starting point of new narratives; they can provoke stories that capitalize on the resources of fiction and fantasy to reconstruct the meaning of things past. Perhaps these stories can even help us understand the people counted in that census, or at least those of them who opposed the census, like Kiefer.

MEMORY'S HISTORICAL ONTOLOGY

If I think of the scholars and scientists on whose work I have drawn to delve into the nexus of autobiographical remembering and narrative, I feel a sense of trepidation when it comes to my second main concern in this book, the outline of a de-substantialized and de-ontologized notion of remembering. I am afraid many will be reluctant to what they might call "forfeit" an ontological notion of memory, especially, if they conceive of it in terms of "social (or collective) memory," or "cultural memory," or "narrative memory." Although I understand and respect the reluctance, I do not share the misgivings, because to me my goal appears more as a constructive one: as an endeavor to make sense of remembering and forgetting as "colorful" activities, that is, as a complex of cultural inter-pretive practices, including artifacts, that reach far beyond the individual domain of consciousness (including the unconscious), or cognition, or neurocognition, which has traditionally be postulated as the privileged domain of "memory." Still, I am aware that the postarchival and post-ontological impetus of this project might encounter disagreement and incomprehension, possibly more so than my other main concern, advanc-ing the "narrative alternative." As I have been grappling with both con-cerns for some time, presenting and discussing them on many occasions and in various places, I want to anticipate, as a way of concluding, a few likely objections and, in trying to avoid possible misunderstandings, flesh out my de-ontologizing proposition in one important respect.

By suggesting that, in the wake of the cultural paradigm shift described in the first three chapters, the binding force of the archival notion of memory is about to disintegrate, I have in mind a particular conceptual architecture, a discursive blueprint. We might call it memory's historical ontology. Historical ontology is a term coined by Ian Hacking (2002) to describe the interplay between the concept of memory and its reality.[1] To view the ontology of something—the conception or perception of the particular kind of being that we ascribe to this something—as historical has two implications. The first is that objects of knowledge, ways of know-ing, and ways of being in the world are viewed as organized within larger cultural frameworks of a certain period (I described these frameworks in Chapter 3 as "epistemes"). The second implication is that they only can be understood within culture-specific semantics, the meaning systems of these frameworks.

I mentioned Foucault's argument that these frameworks and their dynamics are not merely conceptual or mental. Foucault's (1970) effort to tie together conceptual structures of knowledge and historical structures of power is linked to an investigation he called *archeology of knowledge*. The point of this archeology is not to study specific social or natural phenomena or statements, or to identify a problem, but to investigate how a particular phenomenon, statement, or problem has come into existence and how it may again cease to exist. How do concepts and discursive structures define ideas, assumptions, and views as *knowledge*? And how do they exclude other structures from being part of our knowledge, or at least what is considered knowledgeable, worthy, and possible to know?

Hacking draws on this Foucaultian linkage of knowledge, categories, and power when he argues that memory came into being as an epistemic subject in accordance with the 19th-century positivist agenda of the emerging memory sciences. This was the same agenda that set out to transform the "soul" into a subject of "positive" natural-science investigation. To drive home this point further, my argument has been that more than a century later the same epistemic subject "memory" is about to dissolve because the cultural imperatives that once brought it into existence have lost their hegemonic force. They are overridden by a number of new cultural, technological, political, and scientific developments (as summarized in Chapter 2).

To view the cultural frameworks of the notion and the reality of memory in the light of such a historical epistemology also stresses the second aspect foregrounded by the focus on memory's historical ontology. This is the inherently unstable order of such frameworks, an instability that defies all universalist claims. Viewed from a historical point of view, cultural frameworks appear to be continuously altering and, by extension, so do the subjects to which they give rise. We thus can take memory as one such subject, which reveals its truly cultural nature only if it is viewed as historical, be it from a large-scale perspective (for example, comparing modern and premodern ontologies of memory) or from a small-scale perspective (reviewing the quickly changing ideas of memory's reality in the last three decades of neuroscience).

PLANETS, GLOVES, AND MEMORIES

I have used Hacking's conception of historical ontology in my exploration of memory's ambivalent status because it was already put to a test in his own studies on the formation of memory as a scientific and epistemic subject. The upshot of his inquiries is that at stake is one of those conceptual entities that not only highlight, define, and represent, but also structure, evoke, and constitute the reality to which they refer. Building on Foucault, Hacking calls his approach dynamic nominalism. I touched on nominalist epistemologies earlier in this book, because they are influential in many of the new memory studies. Nominalists maintain that the concepts or *nomina* that we use to denote mnemonic processes and artifacts are tools of knowledge, reflection, and communication, rather than representations of real things, *realia*. But such an account, as Hacking states, can be static. By this he means the view that concepts—categories, classes, and taxonomies—are not only created by human beings (rather than found in nature), but that once in place these concepts are fixed and do not interact with what is classified and categorized. It is this interaction that makes nominalism dynamic. It would be preposterous, Hacking argues, to believe that the only thing material objects such as planets have in common is that we call them planets. Although the heavens may have looked different after we grouped the earth with the other planets and excluded the sun and the moon from this classification, the similarities and differences of the celestial bodies we call planets are real enough. And they also remain real enough when one day we do not call them planets anymore because life on planet earth has ceased to exist, together with our concept of planet.

This is not to say that there is only one episteme and one vocabulary by which we would describe our planets. Astronomers, astronauts, astrologists, air traffic navigators, astrophysicists, and poets all use different languages to speak about celestial bodies. It would be impossible to claim that there is just one timelessly adequate description of our planets, both in view of the history of science and in view of its future. This even holds true for the internal discourses of natural sciences, as Stephen Jay Gould (2003) has elucidated for his discipline, evolutionary biology. What we call a scientific statement, or finding, or explanation is rarely uncontested. It is a moving position in an ongoing debate. This, Gould claims, is integral to the very business of scientific research. He quotes Darwin, writing to a close colleague, "how odd it is that anyone should not see that all observation must be for or against some view if it is to be of any service" (quoted in Gould, 2003, p. 35). Rather than mirroring the world as it is (or as it is supposed to be), science means to be engaged in a never-ending debate among all kinds of people and among diverse theories and thoughts.

At this point, a further argument must be mentioned, put forward by Rorty (1990) to support the view of multiple simultaneous descriptions that exist at any given point in history. With this view, Rorty represents still another species of nominalism, slightly different from Hacking's dynamic and Foucault's discursive brand, one that could be called pragmatist. For the pragmatist, Rorty explains, "it is useless to ask whether one vocabulary rather than another is closer to reality. For different vocabularies serve different purposes, and there is no such thing as a purpose that is closer to reality than another purpose" (1990, p. 3).

So far I have considered planets and the like. However, there also are things that differ from planets and suns, as there are categories that differ from those of celestial bodies, and these things and categories are closer to our concerns here. The core categories used in these pages, indeed, do not refer in such a straightforward manner to phenomena of nature like celestial bodies. To explain what makes them different, I use two more of Hacking's examples, gloves and human beings. First gloves. Gloves are different because we manufacture them. "I know not which came first," Hacking writes, "the thought or the mitten, but they have evolved hand in hand. That the concept 'glove' fits gloves so well is no surprise; we made them that way" (2002, pp. 106–107). So far gloves. Now, second, human beings or persons. Persons are in a few important respects more like gloves than like planets, because "The category and the people in it emerged hand in hand" (p. 107). Hacking speaks of a mutual process of "making up people," a process that involves human beings on the one hand and, on the other, the historical category of a person as a politically, legally, philosophically, and psychologically defined modern individual.

> We think of many kinds of people as objects of scientific inquiry. Sometimes to control them, as prostitutes, sometimes to help them, as potential suicides . . .. Sometimes to change them for their own good and the good of the public, as the obese. . . . We think of these kinds of people as definite classes defined by definite properties. As we get to know more about these properties, we will be able to control, help, change, or emulate them better. But it's not quite like that. They are moving targets because our investigations interact with them, and change them. And since they are changed, they are not quite the same kind of people as before. The target has moved. (Hacking, 2006, p. 23)

Making the same point within the context of cultural psychology, Bruner (1996) has suggested that the concepts and narratives that humans use to make sense of the world around them reflect deeply the cultural world into which they are born. At the same time, every cultural world makes sure that we learn exactly those concepts and narratives that constitute this world and make us become its members. For Hacking, understanding the processes in which our investigation interacts with, and changes, the subject we want to explore involves us unavoidably in the business of nominalism:

> The claim of dynamic nominalism is not that there was a kind of person who came increasingly to be recognized by bureaucrats or by students of human nature, but rather that kind of a person came into being at the same time as the kind itself was being invented. In some cases, that is, our classifications and our classes conspire to emerge hand in hand, egging the other on. (2002, p. 106)

Whereas in the prototypical natural sciences our categories rarely change the way the world works, the matter is different when it comes to human beings. Prototypical human sciences are characterized by all kinds of interactions between concepts and systems of classification and the people they categorize and classify. By comparison with natural phenomena, psychological and social kinds are constituted by humans, value-laden, and uniquely reactive (cf. Martin & Sugerman, 2009).

In this respect, then, there is no way to escape the Foucaultian interplay between categories and the categorized reality. This interplay is particularly momentous—not least of all politically—in disciplines that investigate aspects of people and their lives in terms of psychic or mental diseases or disorders, categorized (at one time or today), for example, as posttraumatic stress disorder, hysteria, schizophrenia, obsessive-compulsive disorder, or dissociative identity disorder (or multiple personality disorder). Obviously, medicine, psychiatry, and psychology give wide room to such controversial categorical-physical interactions. This applies to the definition and constitution of diseases, symptoms, and treatments, as well as to apparently neutral methods or instruments like the clinical case report, which is widespread not only in psychiatry.

The case report, technically viewed, is "a foundational text that enables clinicians to depict, reason, and instruct others about a sick person's medical situation," as Brian Hurwitz (2006, p. 217) states. But the genre, Hurwitz argues, is anything but merely representational and depictive. In its long history it has accumulated many narrative and constructive elements, besides numbers, formulae, lab results, tracings, images, and the like. Transforming into a discursive performance, it reorganizes clinical data in a way that "collapses together the reference to a person, the medical abstraction of him or her, and his or her textual realization as a report," as Hurwitz (p. 217) goes on to describe the transformation carried out by the report. As a consequence, "the distinction between the person who is ill (the patient) and the medically construed picture of him or her is at times difficult to maintain" (p. 217). Elsewhere, Hurwitz drives this point about the case as a particular "epistemic genre" even further, suggesting that "the case is the contested and troubled ground where distinctions between person, patient, experience, symptom, subjectivity and objectivity jostle and intermingle" (2011, p. 55).

Clinical case reports belong to the category of concepts, instruments, and systems of classification that intervene into the reality they purport to represent and reflect. Hurwitz speaks of "hybrid" storied construals. Their history is as long as the history of medicine, and their history of being disputed is also that long. Which is understandable, because at stake are no neutral classifications but practices or "epistemic operations" that define and, in fact, constitute the space and direction of action. Jean-Paul Sartre once said that changes in such categories do change the ways of being that are open to individuals. With Foucault, Hacking, and Hurwitz, we may say that they also change the way individuals who fall under such categories are treated.[2] In the domain of the human sciences, new classifications of physical and mental disorders, new treatments, and institutions alter not only the space of talk, but indeed that of existence.

The same complex interaction characterizes the relationship between memory and our conceptualization of it. Both the emergence of the modern episteme of memory and the fading of this episteme are, as we have seen, a case in point. Let there be no mistake, like Hacking and his warrantors Foucault and Wittgenstein, I do not claim that concepts alone produce or engender reality, or that they alter or annihilate it. There is no direct way, as we have learned from Wittgenstein (2009), either from things to words or from words to things. To understand the meaning of a word or concept we need to understand the language games in which it is used, and to understand these language games we need to understand a culture.

When, in the course of history, a cultural world transforms and the meaning of a concept changes or disappears—something that, according to Hacking (1995), happened to the concept of the soul with the coming into being of the new sciences of memory and mind—this "disappearance" does not necessarily leave a void in the lives and experiences of the people, a void where there was something before. It would be absurd to maintain that the disintegration of the memory archive will create a lacuna where there was fullness. People will not stop doing what they call remembering and forgetting, basic practices of life and temporal self-localization that are essential to the human being in the world. They will not cease looking at photographs of their parents with babies on their laps, watching videos of their first steps, telling stories about first dates, and tracing back states of sadness and distress to sorrows from their early childhood days. They also will continue erecting memorials, celebrating remembrance days, and recalling other historical and personal anniversaries, as they will continue participating in political, religious, and many more ritualized memory ceremonies.

I have not concentrated on the specific content and the affective depth of such social and individual remembrance practices, but on trying out new ways of thinking about such practices—especially, practices carried out in the autobiographical process. My intention has been to take a closer look at the models, metaphors, and stories needed for such new thinking, in order to get a sense of how remembering and forgetting look if we drop the demand for framing them in an archivalist way. Yet this is a different thing than to drop or deny the existence or the demand for memories themselves.

REMEMBERING AND NARRATIVE: ENVISIONING THE CULTURAL INTERPLAY

How we can possibly picture a reframing of thinking, narrating, and remembering is the subject of an essay by Bruner (1987c), titled *Life as narrative*. Bruner takes on a notion as thorny as memory, namely, that of human life. His aim is to carve out the cultural-psychological dialectic of how we give meaning to our lives, a dialectic that comes close to the interplay between the notion and the reality of memory. Whenever we tell first-person life narratives, Bruner observes, we are guided by historically shaped cognitive and linguistic models and conventions. Yet at the same time, these narratives tend to become a shaping force themselves. They come to "achieve the power to structure perceptual experience, to organize memory, to segment and purpose-build the very 'events' of a life"; in the end, Bruner writes, "we become the autobiographical narratives by which we tell about our lives" (1987c, p. 15).

I take this to be an illuminative metaphor and model of the cultural interplay of narrative and remembering. It combines two principles. One, which leads back to Aristotle, is that art imitates life; the other, as stated by Oscar Wilde, is that life imitates art. Bruner proposes that an important way to characterize a culture is by the narrative models and prototypes it makes available for shaping the gestalt of a life, or in Hacking's sense, for making gloves and the concept of glove fit. Viewed in this way, cultural models of narrative turn out to be the central hinge between life and story. They make it appear, as Hyvärinen (2008, p. 264) has it, as a circle of mutual imitation.

In a study on the intergenerational handing-down of cultural conventions of autobiographical remembering in China and the United States, Qi Wang and I examined how narrative conceptions of self, life, and remembering constitute and support each other—which is, of course, undergirded by the fact that they all are bound into the same cultural economy of remembering (Wang & Brockmeier, 2002). We suggested that it is one of the central functions of a society's memory values to make sure that its hegemonic practices of autobiographical remembering and identity construction are transmitted from one generation to the next. Typically, this transmission is flanked by detailed ethical and educational agendas. Again, we were confirmed in assuming that narrative models and conventions are pivotal in this transmission and, what is more, that they also are instrumental in driving the circle of mutual imitation. They drive it to the point that our autobiographical narratives eventually affect not only the ways in which we understand but also live and remember our lives. Conflating cognition with social interaction, real-life with fiction, and account with fantasy, autobiographical narratives lay out a plurality of different life options. They realize, and often enough expand, the space of possibilities offered to each individual. They make us aware that our lives are possible lives, narrative gestalts of experience that never cease to be the subject of interpretation and reinterpretation.

There is, however, one aspect of Bruner's elegant metaphor that needs clarification. In his view, the interrelation between autobiographical memory and narrative identity works as a historical and cultural constant. The self-told life based on personal memories is seen as a universal feature of human existence, what varies culturally is the narrative form in which it is expressed. Those who are aware of the objections to the universalism of such a view, which generalizes a specific Western mode of autobiographical self-construction, will hesitate to take this outlook in this form. But imagine that Bruner, faced with these qualms, had taken the next step. And although Hyvärinen (2008) has expressed caution that Bruner's radical thesis of an intrinsic dialectic between narrative identity and culture has remained largely undeveloped in his later work, I do not see a reason why he would not have done so.

So imagine Bruner had viewed remembering practices as being subject to historical and cultural change in the same differentiated sense as the formation of our ideas of life and personal identity, then surely he would have found the same dynamic operative for the autobiographical process that he outlined for the relationship between living and narrating a life. Why, we wonder, can the new models, metaphors, and stories guiding the telling and interpretation of memories ultimately not achieve the same power to reframe and, eventually, reorganize the very processes of autobiographical remembering?

NOTES

CHAPTER 1

1. A collection of these artworks were on display in the exhibition *Brain Boxes & Boundless Books* at the Hackney Museum, London, in 2010.

2. Some variants and the advances of the systems model that reflect this awareness are discussed in more detail in Chapters 3, 5, and 6.

3. That memory is a set of processes organized around its central function, storage, is the key tenet of the chapter on memory in Eric R. Kandel's *Principles of Neural Science* since its first edition in 1981—to refer to only one, albeit arguably the most authoritative neuroscientific textbook (edited by Kandel with various coeditors; the latest version is by Kandel, Schwartz, Jessell, Siegelbaum, & Hudspeth, 2013). The formula "memory is the process by which...knowledge is encoded, stored, and later retrieved" (Schacter & Wagner, 2013, p. 1441–1460) has not changed since the third edition of 1991 (where it is found on p. 997). The storage function of memory is also pronounced as fundamental for the two dimensions along which it is commonly classified: "(1) the time course of storage and (2) the nature of the information stored" (Schacter & Wagner, 2013, p. 1442). What *has* changed over the last decades is how the storage is understood. Whereas in earlier editions of the *Principles of Neural Science* the information-processing orientation of cognitive psychology dominated, today it is neuroscience models, and accordingly "Storage refers to the neural mechanisms and sites by which memory is retained over time" (p. 1447). In terms of location, this means that "The storage of any item of knowledge is widely distributed among many brain regions" (p. 1446). On this view, the storage of memories ultimately takes place on the cellular level (cf. Kandel & Siegelbaum, 2013).

4. Historically, this premise emerged as part of experimental psychology's general orientation toward the individual, whether it be the individual's consciousness, behavior, mind, or brain. As Kurt Danziger (1990; 1997; 2008) has shown, this epistemic focus has reflected from early on "an essentially Cartesian metaphysics that prioritized the thinking individual's mind excerpted from any social and cultural entanglements" (2008, p. 10; cf. also Wilson, 1995). I discuss Danziger's analysis of the implications of this Cartesian metaphysics in Chapter 3.

5. Assmann (1992); Caruth (1995; 1996); Lambeck & Antze (1996a); Felman & Laub (1992), Hirsch (1997), Huyssen (1995), LaCapra (1994), Schacter (1995a), Terdiman (1993); Young (1993), and others.

6. The entire *Les Lieux de Mémoire* appeared in three volumes in 1996–1998 under the title *Realms of memory: Rethinking the French past* (Nora, 1996–1998).

7. To mention just 10 examples: Assmann, J. (1992, 2011); Danziger (2008); Eakin (2008); Erll & Nünning (2008); Etkind (2013); Farr (2012); Hunt (2010); Middleton & Brown (2005); Olick, Vinitzky-Seroussi, & Levy (2011); Radstone & Schwarz (2010).

CHAPTER 2

1. E.g., Brockmeier (2002a); Connerton (1989); Middleton & Brown (2005); Middleton & Edwards (1990a); Winter (2006), to mention a few. Not surprisingly, Barlett's *Remembering* (1932) and its constructive/reconstructive understanding of remembering as a social practice looms wide in these discussions, as do Halbwachs's, Vygotsky's, and Mead's social theories of remembering, all elaborated at about the same time (cf. Wagoner, 2012).
2. More precisely, the Internet as a memory technology has become cheap, for electronic communication hardware once was very expensive. Yet it has become cheap and accessible in a stunningly short period of time, a period that in part overlaps with what I have discussed under "memory boom." According to James Gleick (2011), the turning point was 1965 when Gordon Moor formulated "Moor's Law," which has become an important theoretical trajectory in information theory. Within information theory, the storage of information is called memory, and the processing of information or memory is called computing. Moor's Law stated that the price of electronic components would decrease and the production of these components would increase by a factor of one hundred every decade. These predictions, as Gleick (2011) points out, have proven to be amazingly accurate. Since 1965 the price of electronic equipment has decreased by a factor of a billion, nine powers of ten. The available amount of memory and computing has grown by the same factor, transforming not only the sheer quantity of information, but also its very nature. The flood of (ever cheaper) hardware has turned into a flood of memory.
3. It should be mentioned that the claim of a particularly social and interconnecting dimension of Internet technologies is not undisputed. For a different perspective see, for example, the work of Sherry Turkle (2011), which represents a growing body of "cyber-sceptic" literature. Contesting what she calls the "heroic narrative" of the Internet, Turkle argues that digital technologies originally meant to establish new and more socially engaging ways of communication and remembering have in reality pushed people closer to their individual computers and farther away from each other. From a more political point of view, a likewise ambivalent picture is drawn by Tim Wu (2010) who cautions that the Internet's potentially distributed and democratic structure (which has enabled many novel peer-to-peer or many-to-many user strategies that favor bottom-up social and political activities) is not immune to tendencies to take control of it and subdue it under political powers and economic interests of large corporations.
4. I examine the relationship between writing and memory in more detail in Chapter 3.
5. In addition to the literature already mentioned, there is a great deal of material to support this claim in Eakin (1999; 2008); Ender (2005); Herman (2011b); Nalbantian, Matthews, & McClelland (2011); and Olney (1998), among others.
6. In this section I draw on neuroscientific research by Addis, Wong, & Schacter (2007); Addis, Pan, Vu, Laiser, N., & Schacter (2009); Bar (2011a); Gazzaniga, Ivry, & Mangum (2009); Edelman (2004, 2006); Harris (2000); Prebble, Addis, & Tippett (2013); Schacter (1996; 2001); Schacter & Addis (2007); Schacter,

Addis, & Buckner (2008); Schacter, Addis, Hassabis, Martin, Spreng, & Szpunar (2012); Spreng, Mar, & Kim (2009); Suddendorf & Corbalis (2007); Suddendorf, Addis, & Corballis (2011); a number of chapters from Squire (2009); Szpunar (2010); Szpunar, Addis, McLelland, & Schacter (2013), and Szpunar, Chan, & McDermott (2009), if not otherwise specifically referenced. I concentrate on this focused selection of key publications because my intention is not to present a comprehensive research review but to stage an argument. This argument, however, is built on solid neuroscientific backing.

7. This does not exclude that there also are differences between neuronal activities associated with remembering and imagining future events (for a review of commonalities and differences, see Schacter et al., 2012; and Schacter, Benoit, De Brigard, & Szpunar, 2015).

8. Some neuroscientists believe they have identified brain areas that are specifically involved in the interpretive activities by which we are to distinguish perception, imagination, and episodic remembering. These areas, which include the anterior medial prefrontal cortex and the posterior cingulate, are thought to be particularly active in processes of self-reflection and thinking about one's own and others' mind. They also are seen as active when we try to understand a mental scene as a perception, an imagination, or a memory. Summarizing the research in this research field of "source monitoring," Fernyhough (2012) suggests that the process of "scene construction" is accompanied by activities in additional ("add-on") brain regions "where some of the effortful stitching-together of memories take place" (p. 156). "This extra activity," Fernyhough goes on to write, "is the basis for our knowing the difference between an event we actually experienced and one that we (for whatever reason) imagined" (p. 157). For Marcia Johnson and colleagues, this sense of "knowing" results from a neurophysiologically localizable act of attribution or interpretation that we make about a particular experience in order to get a sense of its status (Johnson, Raye, Mitchell, & Ankudowich, 2012).

9. What Hassabis and Mcguire (2007) call "scene construction" is described by Szpunar (2010), Schacter et al. (2012; 2014), and others as a process of "imaginatively simulating a hypothetical scenario" or "episodic simulation." It is believed that in this process a number of related neurocognitive activities are integrated, including some non-mnemonic ones, such as self-construction and autonoetic consciousness. Traditionally, the neurocognitive processes hypothesized to support these activities have been treated as distinct. After earlier reviews drew attention to the topic of "memory of the future" (e.g., Ingvar, 1984; Tulving 1985b) and, in 2001, the term "episodic future thought" was suggested (Atance & O'Neill, 2001), neuroscientists recently have started to consider mental functions associated with memory, imagination, and the anticipation or simulation of future scenarios as integrated within the same brain networks (e.g., Mullally & Maguire, 2014; Schacter et al., 2012; Szpunar, 2010).

Along these lines Buckner and Carroll (2007) have proposed "self-projection" as the central feature of these underlying neurocognitive activities, namely, as "the ability to consider alternatives to events in the immediate environment" (p. 49). This ability, they assume, is based on a shared network of associated brain regions that support diverse forms of self-projection. These include remembering the past, thinking about the future (prospection), conceiving the viewpoint of others (theory of mind), and navigation or "way finding" (Buckner, Andrews-Hanna, & Schacter, 2008; see also Spreng, Mar, & Kim, 2009). This brain network—the "constructive" or "prospective" or "proactive brain"—also underlies the projection of oneself into another time, place, or perspective and in this way the imaginative simulation of possible events in the past, present, or future. "Mental time travel" (Suddendorf, Addis, & Corballis, 2011; Suddendorf & Corballis, 2007) is another term meant to provide an overarching description of these different abilities from a neuroscientific point of view.

Buckner and Caroll (2007) argue that the flexibility of this underlying brain network might be its central adaptive function, "rather than the accuracy of the network to represent specific and exact configurations of past events" (p. 55). This is echoed by McDermott, Szpunar, & Arnold (2011) who view as the brain's main function its constructive nature that enables "one to piece together fragments from memory in the service of imagining potential future scenarios" (p. 89).

10. For more evidence supporting Tulving's view, see Svoboda, McKinnon, & Levine (2006). In some areas of the neurobiology of memory, concepts have emerged that seem to react to the mismatch between new findings and inadequate language to grasp them. Terms such as "memory consolidation" and "reconsolidation" are interesting examples (cf. Dudai, 2006). They aim to reflect "memories" as fleeting and unstable excitation patterns, rather than "information" "encoded" in some neuronal storage. The crucial question that comes with this take is, however, how to explain the possibility of more or less stable long-term memories (or neuronal circuits with long-term mnemonic functions) at all, wherever they may occur between the hippocampal region and the cerebral cortex. "Memory consolidation" hints at a possible answer. It is based on the presumption that some kind of consolidation process of exciting patterns may lead to a "gradual stabilization" over time—a "stabilization," though, that is based on ongoing change, because every time a neuronal "memory" pattern is accessed, it becomes unstable until it is "reconsolidated" again. What is meant by memory consolidation, then, is quite the contrary of an act of encoding and a subsequent process of storing of information, but, as Bontempi and Frankland assert, "a highly dynamic process that involves large-scale reorganization at both the synaptic and entire interconnected brain system levels" (2009, p. 733). The authors qualify this proposition, however, by saying that the "mechanisms underlying this reorganization are largely unknown" (Bontempi & Frankland, 2009, p. 733).

CHAPTER 3

1. The discussions on difference and relationship between metaphor and model are not especially relevant to the line of thought I am pursuing. If not otherwise specified, I use both terms in a nearly synonymous fashion, with *model* addressing more a conceptual element and *metaphor* more an imagistic element that extends to what is sometimes called metaphor's preconceptual grounding. Like icebergs, metaphors' visible, linguistically articulated shape is often only the smaller part of a much larger body, a pictorial region of meaning that is not verbally explicit but essential for the work of imagination. It is in this space, occupied by the iceberg's invisible underwater region, where metaphors can reach into the preconceptual and prelinguistic imagination.

2. E.g., Assmann, A. (2011); Carruthers (1990); Draaisma (2000); Hacking (1995); Rossi (1991); Yates (1966).

3. But do not modern brain imaging technologies finally permit us to view memory's "primary reality"—in the same way Harvey viewed the primary reality of the heart? Brain imaging technologies such as fMRI and MEG are the most powerful instruments of research at the brain's neuronal level. But they have not demonstrated in which part(s) of the brain memories are "stored," although there have been many claims to that. Rather, what they engender are computer-generated images representing, in fMRIs, the measurement of changes in blood flow in isolated regions of the brain and, in MEGs, tiny changes in the magnetic fields surrounding electrical signaling in the brain's neuronal circuits. These images, then, have been *interpreted* by making use of the familiar language of the archival memory tradition and its vocabulary of encoding, storing, and recalling.

CHAPTER 4

1. The question is asked by Trofimov in Act 2 of *The Cherry Orchard*. I quote from Tania Alexander's translation (Chekhov, 2007, p. 39).
2. For a more detailed discussion of these criticisms, especially Strawson's, see Eakin (2006; 2008); Hyvärinnen (2008); Meretoja (2013); and Ritivoi (2009).
3. This theme is developed throughout Benjamin's work, beginning with the early texts *On perception* (Benjamin, 1917/1996) and *On the programme of the coming philosophy* (Benjamin, 1918/1996). For a more detailed discussion see Caygill (1998).
4. "Experience," for Benjamin, is to be conceived "with regard to the individual, body and mind uniting person and their consciousness, rather than as systematic specification of knowledge" ["Erfahrung, so wie sie mit Bezug auf den individuellen leib-geistigen Menschen und dessen Bewusstsein und nicht vielmehr als systematische Spezifikation der Erkenntnis gefasst wird" (Benjamin, 1918/1991, p. 162)].
5. These discussions were been particularly lively in France in the second half of the 20th century where, as Meretoja (2014b) has shown, major theoretical and aesthetic movements—from structuralism to poststructuralism, existentialism to hermeneutics, and semiotics to narratology—involved not only philosophers and narrative scholars, but also many writers and artists debating the crucial role of storytelling for human experience and the entire human condition.
6. Implicitly, this is assumed by many authors; explicitly it is stated, for example, by Carr (1986) who maintains that "no elements enter our experience [...] unstoried or unnarrativized" (p. 68).
7. In recent years, Tomasello (2005; 2008), Nelson (1996; 2007a), and their collaborators as well as other researchers in the wake of Vygotsky (see, e.g., Wertsch, 2007, on Vygotsky's notion of semiotic mediation) have provided abundant material for such a reading of narrative as a complex semiotic system.
8. "Being that can be understood is language," is a much discussed remark by Hans-Georg Gadamer (2004, p. 474). In his commentary on this dictum, Richard Rorty (2004) points out that there is no way of getting behind language to experience the object as it is in itself. This is not because our experiential faculties are limited but because human experiences, even ineffable experiences, always take place within a symbolic space, that is, a culturally and historically mediated space in which language plays a pivotal role. Another hermeneutic philosopher, Emanuel Lévinas, relates Gadamer's statement to Martin Heidegger's notion of language as "the house of being." "There never was a moment," writes Lévinas, "meaning came to birth out of a meaningless being, outside of a historical position where language is spoken. And this is doubtless what is meant when we were taught that language is the house of being" (1987, p. 79).

9. There is, however, one important exception to this proviso, one area of human experience where I agree with Herman's view of narrative as a condition "for the having of an experience." This is constituted by narrative's capacity to deal with, evoke, and interpret complex temporal scenarios.

10. I draw here from material of the "National 9/11 memory consortium" gathered in the aftermath of the 2001 terrorist attacks on the World Trade Center in New York City and other places. I am grateful to William Hirst for being able to participate and access this material for an independent study on traumatic memory (Brockmeier, 2008b).

11. Not surprisingly, Fludernik has no difficulty fitting comprehensive processes of autobiographical remembering into her picture of the narrative mind. In her view, the purpose and function of storytelling is that of "a process that captures the narrator's past experience, reproduces it in a vivid manner, and then evaluates and resolves it in terms of the protagonist's reactions and of the narrator's often explicit linking of the meaning of this experience with the current discourse context" (Fludernik, 2003, p. 245).

12. This applies paradigmatically to the hermeneutics of historical stories, which, as Koselleck (2004) pointed out, remain open in the twofold sense in which neither narrative nor history ever reach a final endpoint. "The past," writes memory historian Matt Matsuda, "is not a truth upon which to build, but a truth sought, a re-memorializing over which to struggle. The fragmentary, disputatious, self-reflective nature of such a past makes a series of 'memories'—ever imperfect, imprecise, and charged with personal questions—the appropriate means for rendering the 'history' of the present" (1996, p. 15).

13. E.g., Brockmeier (2005); Bruner (1990a; 2001); Herman (2009b; 2012); Sarbin (2000).

14. See, e.g., the special volume of the journal *Style,* 45 (2) on "Social minds in criticism and fiction" with a target article by Palmer (2011) and critical comments by Herman (2011d) and myself (Brockmeier, 2011), among others.

15. How our understanding (and its changes) of mind and memory is embedded in historical traditions of narrative (and their changes) has been pointed out in great detail by Grafton, Most, & Settis (2010).

CHAPTER 5

1. My usage of the term "autobiographical process" draws on the one hand on a critical reading of Freud's interpretive approach to remembering and forgetting (Brockmeier, 1997) and on the other on the notion of meaning-construction developed in Bruner's narrative psychology (Brockmeier, 1999). As far as I can see, it was Bruner (1993) who first explicitly applied the term autobiographical process to describe the narrative fabric of identity and autobiographical remembering. I recall a seminar in 1992, in Turin, Italy, where he presented a draft of his 1993 paper. He pointed out that what he had previously called a "new look" (Bruner 1990b) at identity and autobiographical memory—which he linked to the project of a culture-based narrative psychology—had to break with the traditional notion of memory as prelinguistic storage of the past. When I asked him whether he could envision a completely new conceptual perspective for a different view of remembering and forgetting that might emerge with the idea of the "autobiographical process," he seemed skeptical, however. Referring to Vygotsky's point that thoughts are not independent from the language in which we conceive of them, he remarked that it ultimately depends on whether

we are able to overcome the deeply ingrained vocabulary of encoding, storing, and retrieving memories of the past, a vocabulary that has cemented the
traditional view.

2. To better understand the first-person perspective of a brain specialist, McEwan
not only did extensive literature studies in the field, but also spent two years
work-shadowing a neurosurgeon at London's National Hospital for Neurology
and Neurosurgery, which included attending his operation theater mornings.

3. "More than in any other novel of mine," McEwan remarks, "I've drawn on a
recognizable world to fill out the details" (Roberts, 2010, p. 146). By that he
means that "This book is going to be tied right into a world that is public, shared,
real. All the external events—the Iraq invasion and so on—are definable, clear,
checkable in your newspaper." (pp. 143–144)

4. The reader might think of Kafka's Josef K. who woke from troubled dreams, too.

5. James (1882) also speaks of a "field of consciousness" whose margins are indeterminate. "Inattentively realized as is the matter which the margin contains, it
is nevertheless there, and helps both to guide our behavior and to determine the
next movement of our attention. It lies around us like a 'magnetic field' inside of
which our center of energy turns like a compass needle as the present phase of
consciousness alters into its successor. Our whole past store of memories floats
beyond this margin, ready at a touch to come in...So vaguely drawn are the outlines between what is actual and what is only potential at any moment of our
conscious life, that it is always hard to say of certain mental elements whether
we are conscious of them or not" (p. 232).

6. To be sure, Nietzsche was not the only one who praised the advantages of forgetfulness on a philosophical, that is, for Nietzsche, existential level; ultimately,
his point was, forgetting makes us happier. But his arguments were particularly
influential. See Weinrich (2004, Chapters IV–VI) on other versions of this view.

7. The view of writing on which I draw here and in what follows is elaborated in
Olson (1994); Brockmeier (1998); Harris (2000); and Brockmeier & Olson
(2002; 2009).

8. I adapt at this point the common linguistic meaning of "model," referring to
the view I want to advance as the narrative enactment model or the narrative
model, in order to compare it with other theoretical models. Within the narrative model, however, I consider autobiographical narrative not as a model in
the strong sense or a representation of the autobiographical process but as its
enactment, for reasons pointed out in the last section.

9. Over the years, Tulving has more and more modified his theoretical views of
the episodic memory system and, by implication, of autobiographical memory (which he, for one, does not consider to be a memory system of its own).
In the theoretical reflections of some of his later papers, it is difficult to attribute any precise meaning to the concept of system—especially vis-à-vis new
neurobiological findings—except that it is a label introduced a few decades ago
to set apart the then new and rising neurocognitive approach from the then
established old-school cognitive approach of information processing (cf., e.g.,
Tulving, 2005, p. 9).

10. The idea that an original experience (the original experience of the burning airplane), once encoded and stored in memory, can survive an extended period of
time—unaltered like a photograph ("flashbulb memories")—is as old as the idea
of memory (see Chapter 3). In more recent times, it was shared not only by many
memory scientists, but also by Freud and his followers (cf. Bergstein, 2010).

Among its critics were Montaigne (1580/1993), Goethe (1830/1891), William James (1890/1981), and Ulric Neisser (1966), who ironically dubbed it the "reappearance hypothesis" (cf. Wertsch, 2011, p. 23). Still, it is astonishing that it has held sway not only over many autobiographers and life-writers, but also over so many psychological and neuroscientific memory researchers who have been searching for the physical trace of memory and (neuro-)cognitive mechanisms meant to underlie remembering. Steven Rose has tried to reconstruct how it was possible that a version of the reappearance hypothesis put forth by Karl Lashley, Donald Hebb, and others, in the 1940s and 1950s, postulating the permanence of discrete memory "engrams" or "traces" on the level of molecular processes (especially in synaptic junctions), could have "shaped all subsequent biochemical and physiological research in the field" (Rose, 2010, p. 203) for decades, despite contradictory and controversial experimental evidence. Dudai describes the long-held conviction "that the engram is indeed a lasting change induced by the learning experience, not much unlike inscriptions on wax tablets proposed by Plato" (2011, p. 30) as part of the zeitgeist in the neurobiology of memory. In fact, only recently the explicit and tacit influence of the engram hypothesis, especially its mechanistic assumptions, on the thinking of many biochemical and neurobiological memory researchers has lost ground, as neurophysiological memory researchers such as Steven Rose (2010, pp. 206–208), Yadin Dudai (2011), and Andreas Draguhn (2012; personal communication) have pointed out.

11. The study of the narrator, single and multiple, as well as his or her point of view, focalization, voice, and other narrative-constituting characteristics relative to a certain person (in fiction, usually a character) marks an extensive field of narratological scholarship (e.g., Genette, 1980; Phelan, 2005; Richardson, 2006). This might reflect the fact that "the history of narrative is peopled with an extraordinary variety of narrators" (Phelan & Booth, 2005, p. 389). These narrators, moreover, use an extraordinary variety of perspectival filters or "focalizations" to give shape to their narratives (Jahn, 2007) and, in this way, also to themselves. I only touch on those aspects in this field relevant for my discussion of the Perowne sequence.

12. I thank James Wertsch (2011) for his helpful comments on my previous and sketchier treatment of this issue, prompting me to the following excursion.

13. Cf. my account of the reconstructive, language-supported labor that comes with "remembering" a scene from a birthday dinner, in Chapter 2 (pp. 48–49, 54–55).

CHAPTER 6

1. For the record, this view is not uncontested; see, for example, Carr (1986, 1997). Polkinghorne (2004) has argued that Ricoeur's works on narrative identity can be read as an attempt to overcome the putative opposition of language/narrative versus life/identity. Overcoming an opposition is, however, not to ignore any difference, albeit only one of graduation within a continuum.

2. For a more extended discussion of this argument, see Ochs and Capps (2001); Georgakopoulou (2007); and, especially in clinical contexts, Hydén (2013); Hydén and Öruluv (2010).

3. In this respect, I build on a collection of earlier approaches to this issue that includes studies by Jerome Bruner, Donal Carbaugh, Mark Freeman, Rom Harré, Kristin Langellier, Jerome Sehulster, and myself, published in the volume *Narrative and Identity: Studies in Autobiography, Self and Culture* (Brockmeier &

Carbaugh, 2001b). The project—which ultimately led to this present book—aimed "to narrow the gap between the study of human identity, on the one hand, and narrative and cultural discourses on the other hand—a gap that in part coincides with the gap between psychology and the other human sciences" (Brockmeier & Carbaugh, 2001a, p. 3). The goal was— and still is —"to show that the focus on narrative is not only useful, but proves to be supremely productive for the exploration of autobiographical memory and identity" (Brockmeier & Carbaugh, 2001a, p. 3).

4. See Rudd (2009, p. 62), who outlines some background of this argument in terms of philosophical discussions on narrative and identity in the wake of MacInyre (2007).

5. See also Bamberg & Georgakopoulou (2008); De Fina & Georgakopoulou (2012); Mildorf (2010).

6. On this question, see also the discussion between Bamberg (2007, 2010) and Freeman (2007; 2010c).

7. I use here Muldroon's translation (Ricoeur, 1991c).

8. For an English translation of parts of the work on Antiquity see Misch (1950).

9. Smith and Watson (2010, Chapter 7) see the work of Gusdorf and other influential authors like Francis Hart (1970) and Karl Joachim Weintraub (1978) as marking a second wave of autobiographical theory and criticism that advocates the "transcendent model" of Western identity formation.

10. Besides psychology, this assumption runs in many variations through debates on self, identity, and self-knowledge in contemporary philosophy, irrespective of otherwise significant differences. For the hermeneutic and phenomenological tradition, see Ricoeur (1991a; 1991b; 1992) and Taylor (1989); for the analytic tradition, besides Strawson (2011) and Parfit (1984), see Cassam (1994) and Williams (2009).

It also is present in much of 20th-century autobiographical literature and life writing. Eakin (1999) claims that the majority of all autobiographies published at the end of the 20th century in English assume that the writer's main task is to autobiographically remember what happened in the past, as truly, honestly, and authentically as possible, and that an even larger portion of the public reception of autobiographical texts is dominated by these criteria. For Eakin (2014), one of the foremost experts of autobiographical literature, "telling the truth" of a life and its history is considered to be one of culturally normative basic rules of what he describes as the contemporary autobiographical "narrative identity system" (Eakin, 2014, pp. 22–23). This may explain why, as a consequence, questions of fact and fiction, truth and authenticity—the *bios* bias—have dominated debates, irrespective of the misgivings of Beckett and many other modernist and postmodernist writers and theorists.

11. Some brain scientists, such as Gazzaniga (1998; 2008), have gone so far as to neuroanatomically identify the left hemisphere as the site of a "narrator in the brain" specialized for interpreting our feelings, actions, and experiences in narrative.

12. In Chapter 5, discussing the relationship between narrative and experience, I already addressed the claim that there is a primordial pre-narrative level of "true" and "immediate" human experience that tends to be only falsified through narrative, in fact, through language in general (cf. pp. 105–109). Whereas this "anti-narrativist" argument is often presented, philosophically speaking, in epistemological form—narrative is a means to impose a secondary linguistic or conceptual order on reality—it also draws on a strong ontological premise: this is the assumption that there is a human reality "as such," free from any

linguistic and semiotic mediation, which is, like the epistemological argument, characteristic of the empiricist and positivist tradition (cf. Meretoja, 2014a).

13. This is in line with the main role assigned to narrative in academic memory research: that it serves as an instrument to gain information, as a means to an end. Narratives can be useful, for instance, when they are elicited in standardized protocols of autobiographical memory interviews where participants are asked to provide information about various life periods, such as in the wide-spread "Autobiographical Memory Interview" (Kopelman, Wilson, & Baddely, 1989; 1990). The stories elicited by these instruments are taken as unearthing information that affords researchers to assess what, how much, how vividly, or how "episodically" or "semantically" a person recalls.

14. Probably the most formalized version of the standard view is Martin Conway's "self memory system" (Conway & Pleydell-Pearce, 2000; Conway, 2005; Conway & Jobson, 2012).

15. I mentioned earlier the "engram assumption" that for long seemed to provide some neurophysiological support for this view. One of the perhaps best known formulations of the archival assumption in cognitive memory psychology is Brown & Kulik's (1977) theory of "flashbulb memories," which maintains that images of certain extraordinary events (such as the much-researched assassination of John F. Kennedy) are engraved in memory like unchangeable photographs ("flashbulb shots"). This vision is also echoed by influential conceptions of narrative in cognitive psychology such as Rumelhart's (1975) "story grammar" and Mandler's (1984) "schema theory." Additional theoretical background for these theories of narrative and memory is provided by the psycholinguist structuralism of the 1960s and 1970s. On this cognitivist account, stories emerge from deep structures of abstract, amodal knowledge (which may include linguistic information), stored in semantic memory combined with more recent imagistic or otherwise sensory information stored in episodic memory.

16. Among the few exceptions are the works of Katherine Nelson (e.g., 1996; 2007) and Robyn Fivush (e.g., 2009; 2011).

17. A comparable exclusion of individual subjectivity, intentionality, and agency— and thus of processes of individual remembering and forgetting—is implied in many definitions of *Social Memory Studies* (or *Collective* or *Cultural Memory Studies*). It seems as though the justified criticism of "the overriding individualism" (Olick, Vinitzky-Seroussi, & Levy, 2011, p. 45) of psychological memory research has brought a disregard, if not contempt, for the entire individual dimension of autobiographical remembering. For a critical discussion, see Kansteiner (2010) and Bietti (2011).

18. In the first years since its 2009 inception, the cross-disciplinary journal *Memory Studies* has become a productive site for the study of the nexus of individual and social/collective/cultural memory, not least by giving space to innovative approaches off the beaten track.

19. I owe special thanks to Lars-Christer Hydén, Elenor Antelius, and Linda Örulv from the Swedish Center for Dementia Research (CEDER) for hosting me and allowing me to use the material and the results of their investigations. For a more extended version of the interview with Oswald and Linda as an example of "narrative collaboration," see Hydén (2011; 2013; 2014).

20. In view of Oswald and Linda's story, I deviate here from Jakobson's (1981) order of the six language functions.

CHAPTER 7

1. I discussed this point in more detail in Chapter 3, drawing on Danziger's historical approach to memory.

2. The concepts of *social memory, collective memory,* and *cultural memory* are sometimes used distinctively, sometimes synonymously (cf., e.g., Erll & Nünning, 2008; Olick, Vinitzky-Seroussi, & Levy, 2011). Concentrating on the relationship between individual and social memory, I apply, for now, social and collective interchangeably, following the Halbwachs tradition (Namer, 2000). Whereas social memory is often contrasted with individual memory, cultural memory contrasts with biological memory and thus—emphasizing the semiotic, noetic, artistic, and technological traditions of social and societal life—suggests a slightly different focus than social memory. In this sense, I have used cultural memory in my own work as a notion encompassing both individual and social forms of memory. This marks a certain difference with Jan Assmann's (1992; 2006; 2011) important conception of "cultural memory," which distinguishes among three specific levels or kinds of memory—individual, communicative, and cultural—and thus continues *mutatis mutandis* the distinction between individual memory on the one side and social (that is, communicative and cultural) memory on the other.

3. Among the 91 papers included in *The Collective Memory Reader* (Olick, Vinitzky-Seroussi, & Levy, 2011), which are considered to be classics and landmark contributions defining the field of social memory studies, there are only two authored by psychologists, both from the first half of the last century—Sigmund Freud and Frederic Bartlett. The editors have justified their choice by referring to what they call the "predominant reductionism in contemporary psychology" (Olick, Vinitzky-Seroussi, & Levy, 2014, p. 134) vis-à-vis the social dimension of human remembering and forgetting, a reductionism that they see as grounded in the idea of an isolated individual and his or her likewise individually reified memory. As sociologists, they write, "we have indeed always begun from the assumption that it is individuality that is the special case requiring philosophical specification, not collectivity." Thus, "we believe—contrary, apparently, to many psychologists—that if there is such a thing as 'memory per se' it is to be found in society... [I]f anyone's enterprise needs an adjective, it is the psychologists who should employ the modifier 'individual' to refer to the special case they study, rather than sociologists who should be required to employ the seemingly metaphorical label 'collective' or 'social' (p. 135)." In view of the emergent field of cross-disciplinary memory studies where "much recent work has paid greater attention than heretofore to the complexities of social and cultural memory processes," Olick, Vinitzky-Seroussi, and Levy (2014, p. 136) have indicated they will extend their choice of relevant (psychological) approaches in future editions of *The Collective Memory Reader.*

4. In line with today's common usage I employ in the following the term Asian American without a hyphen.

5. Hawaii Senator Daniel K. Inouye, who published his *Journey to Washington.*

6. These were by Pardee Lowe and Jade Snow Wong, the latter was to become the most widely read piece of Asian American literature until the 1970s.

7. For example, by Daniel Inouye and Daisuke Kitagawa.

8. Whereas many literary critics read Hong Kingston's memoir as fiction, more politically and socially oriented commentators took it as nonfiction, as "nonfictional autobiography." In 1976, *The Woman Warrior* was awarded the National Book Critics Circle Award for Nonfiction.

CHAPTER 8

1. This does not exclude that there are other, derivative and phenomenological forms of time and temporality that manifest themselves, for example, in the circularity and repetitiveness of celestial movements, the ecclesiastical pattern of the church year (which symbolically represents, and recalls, the life course of Christ), and further societal cycles of temporal organization. There are many different forms of time coexisting under the overarching notion of a continuous and chronological world time—see, for example, Brockmeier (2008a), Koselleck (2004), Nowotny (1994), Young (1988).

2. Today, Simmel's analysis of the human existence under the condition of the metropolis is considered a prophetic anticipation of many developments to come (e.g., Weinstein & Weinstein, 1993). Julie Choi maintains that "Although Simmel's metropolis is based on his experience of Berlin at the turn of the last century, his discussion of the metropolis can be fruitfully extended backwards to the eighteenth-century experience of the rise of big cities" such as London (2006, p. 706). Choi notes that many novelists who were contemporaries of Simmel were engaged in similar projects as they took as their subject matter the mental life of individuals in the modern metropolis.

3. Kern (1983) conceives of modernism as a social and cultural movement that originated from the intersection of a number of diverse historical developments, all of which contributed to the pluralization of time. This pluralization was a general feature of many cultural domains in the decades around the turn of the century. Kern goes on to conclude that "the assault on a universal unchanging, and irreversible public time was the metaphysical foundation of a broad cultural challenge to traditional notions about the nature of the world and man's place in it" (p. 314).

4. Proust himself speaks of a "telescope pointed at time"—for example, in a letter from 1922: "The image (imperfect as it is) which seems to me best suited to convey the nature of that special sense is that of a telescope, a telescope pointed at time, for a telescope renders visible for us stars invisible to the naked eye, and I have tried to render visible to the consciousness unconscious phenomena, some of which, having been entirely forgotten, are situated in the past" (quoted in Shattuck, 1962, p. 46).

5. On this view, events are identified by reference to the places and times at which they occur. Taken together, all these possible places and times constitute an independent manifold of spatial locations and an independent manifold of temporal locations. In modern physics the two independent Newtonian manifolds of locations are replaced by what is called the Minkowski representation: a single manifold of locations, each of which is a place-at-a-moment. Against the independent background of this Minkowski space-time, all events have their places-at-times, constituting an absolute and fixed background of all events—including symbolic and imaginative events—in the universe. In this important respect, then, the Minkowski representation builds on traditional Newtonian metaphysics (cf. Harré, 1996), and because the ways in which it differs are not especially relevant to my line of argument, I continue using terms like the Newtonian view and Newtonian time.

6. Because it is sometimes difficult or impossible to infer story time from discourse time, Genette (1980) introduced "achronic" or temporally undatable structures, while keeping the fundamental distinction between the two orders of time in place. I return to this issue in the next chapter.

7. By human temporality I mean a temporality that is specific to and fundamental for the human being in the world. On a more general plane, this human-specific dimension of time (which includes phenomena discussed as social, cultural, historical, phenomenological, and noetic time) is to be distinguished from concepts of time that refer to biological and physical temporalities (cf. Fraser 1992; 1987, Chapter 3).

8. Leibniz's conception of relational time appears in various respects compatible with the narrative view outlined above (see, e.g., van Fraassen, 1991; Harré, 1996). I have further explored this perspective elsewhere (Brockmeier, 1995/2001; 1996).

9. Besides Nalbantian (2003), a number of authors have discussed aspects of this spectrum through the works of various life-writers; see, e.g., Eakin (1999); Ender (2005); Foster (1993); Nünning, Gymnich, & Sommer (2006); Lachmann (1997, 2008), Olney (1998).

10. This claim does not exclude that there is, on a psychological and philosophical plane, a sense of self and identity even without narrative and autobiographical self-reflection, indeed, without language and memory—as discussed in Chapter 6.

CHAPTER 9

1. All quotes from *Austerlitz* refer to Sebald (2001a).

2. The model of story time and discourse time can be, and has been, questioned in several ways (e.g., by Herrnstein Smith, 1981; Richardson, 1987; Shen, 2002). In particular, it is the concept of story time that appears to be problematic. Like *fabula* and *story*, the concept of story time has emerged out of the tradition of "narrative grammar" and the universalist higher-order grammars that preceded it (Herman, 1995). To my mind, the idea of story time raises two critical questions, one is narratological, the other is ontological. The narratological question challenges the assumption that all narrated and narratable events and experiences can be mapped along the linear and homogenous trajectory of story time. The ontological question challenges the assumption that there is a given ultimate temporal order in the world of human beings and experience, a natural order of clock and calendar time in the "common-sense 'objective' manner that we all take for granted," as Fludernik (2003, p. 119) put it. More precisely, the ontological question raises doubts as to whether this temporal order, reflected by the notion of story time, exists independent from our meaning constructions and the cultural-historical systems of signs, symbols, concepts, and other practices of temporalization. It thus also doubts that this temporal order can serve as a standard, a fixed background, against which these constructions and practices can be appropriately represented.

    The second, narratological question draws on the argument that the model of narrative underlying the notion of story time overprivileges the mimetic function of narrative, a function dominating the realist conventions of much of 19th-century literature. It misses, however, essential practices and techniques of 20th-century literary approaches to phenomena of consciousness, mind, and remembering (some of them addressed in the previous and the present chapters), as well as used in nonliterary and naturally occurring narrative discourse. It misses, in particular, forms of narrative, as of language use in general, dominated by the constructive and creative function of language, its potential to unfold its own realities, including its own temporalities, rather than only depict or reconstruct a nontextual reality and its putatively given (story) order of time. In contrast with the story time/discourse time distinction that originated in formalist and structuralist philosophies of language, the latter view is associated with the non- (or post-)structuralist philosophies of Wittgenstein, Derrida, Davidson, and Rorty.

3. In Chapter 5, I distinguish a number of such planes of meaning constitution in my analysis of McEwan's account of Henri Perowne's autobiographical process.

4. Benjamin's idea of the "the time of the now" is closely connected to what he called the *Jetzt der Erkennbarkeit*, the "now of knowability" or the "now of cognizability." This concept plays a major role in his reflections on time and, in particular, historical time, in his *On the Concept of History* (Benjamin, 1974, pp. 1237–1238) and his unfinished *The Arcades Project* (Benjamin, 1999). Benjamin's concept of the now aims at the moment of conflation of historical knowledge and individual knowledge. This moment, as he sees it, interrupts the historical continuum of time, because it extends the historical toward the individual. This also is the moment in which past and present experience are equally present (cf. Hamacher, 2002).

5. The term "time effects" is introduced and discussed in a study on Proust by Malcolm Bowie (1998).

CHAPTER 10

1. There are comparable concepts such as Taylor's (1989) "moral ontology", Rorty's (1979) "historicist pragmatism," Foucault's (1970) "episteme" or "discursive formation," and Koselleck's (2004) "historical semantics." Hacking's conceptualization of historical ontology is particularly apt for my discussion, not least, because it emerged from his reconstruction of the emergence of "memory" as a scientific subject in the 19th and 20th centuries (cf. Hacking, 1995; 1996a, 1996b), as discussed in Chapter 2.

2. For a collection of case studies with this focus see Donley & Buckley (2000).

REFERENCES

Aptelbaum, E. (2010). Halbwachs and the social properties of memory. In S. Radstone & B. Schwarz (Eds.), *Memory: Histories, theories, debates* (pp. 77–92). New York: Fordham University Press.

Addis, D. R., Pan, L., Vu, M. A., Laiser, N., & Schacter, D. L. (2009). Constructive episodic simulation of the future and the past: Distinct subsystems of a core brain network mediate imagining and remembering. *Neuropsychologia, 47,* 2222–2238.

Addis, D. R., Wong, A. T., & Schacter, D. L. (2007). Remembering the past and imagining the future: Common and distinct neuronal substrates during event construction and elaboration. *Neuropsychologia, 45,* 1363–1377.

Alber, J., & Fludernik, M. (Eds.) (2010). *Postclassical narratology.* Columbus, OH: Ohio State University Press.

Amsterdam, A. G., & Bruner, J. S. (2000). *Minding the law.* Cambridge, MA: Harvard University Press.

Anderson, B. R. (2006). *Imagined communities: Reflections on the origin and spread of nationalism* (1st ed. 1991). London & New York: Verso.

Andrews, M. (2007). *Shaping history: Narratives of political change.* Cambridge, UK: Cambridge University Press.

Andrews, M. (2007). Exploring cross-cultural boundaries. In D. Clandinin (Ed.), *Handbook of narrative inquiry: Mapping a methodology* (pp. 489–511). Thousand Oaks, CA: Sage Publications.

Andrews, M. (2013). Never the last word. In M. Andrews, C. Squire, & M. Tamboukou (Eds.), *Doing narrative research* (2nd ed.) (pp. 205–222). London: Sage.

Andrews, M. (2014). *Narrative imagination and everyday life.* Oxford & New York: Oxford University Press.

Andrews, M., Squire, C., & Tamboukou, M. (Eds.) (2013). *Doing narrative research* (2nd ed.). London: Sage.

Antze, P., & Lambek, M. (Eds.) (1996a). *Tense past: Cultural essays in trauma and memory.* New York: Routledge.

Antze, P., & Lambek, M. (Eds.) (1996b). Preface. P. Antze & M. Lambek (Eds.), *Tense past: Cultural essays in trauma and memory* (pp. vii–xxxviii). New York: Routledge.

Anz, T. (1994). Zeit und Beschleunigung in der literarischen Moderne [Time and acceleration in literary modernism]. In Sandbothe, M., & Zimmerli, W. C. (Eds.), *Zeit, Medien, Wahrnehmung* (pp. 111–220). Darmstadt, Germany: Wissenschaftliche Buchgesellschaft.

Appiah, K. A. (2005). *The ethics of identity.* Princeton, NJ: Princeton University Press.

Appiah, K. A. (2006). *Cosmopolitanism: Ethics in a world of strangers*. New York: Norton.

Arendt, H. (1998/1958). *The human condition*. Chicago, IL: University of Chicago Press.

Aristotle. (1971). *On Memory*. London: Duckworth.

Aristotle. (2004). *Metaphysics*. London: Penguin

Aristotle. (2013). *Poetics*. Oxford & New York: Oxford University Press.

Assmann, A. (2011). *Cultural memory and Western civilization: Functions, media, archives*. Cambridge, UK & New York: Cambridge University Press.

Assmann, A. & Conrad, P. (Eds.) (2010). Introduction. In A. Assmann & P. Conrad (Eds.), *Memory in a global age: Discourses, practices and trajectories* (pp. 1–15). Basingstoke, UK: Palgrave Macmillan.

Assmann, J. (1992). *Das kulturelle Gedächtnis: Schrift, Erinnerung und politische Identität in frühen Hochkulturen* [Cultural memory: Writing, remembering, and political identity in early civilizations]. Munich, Germany: Beck.

Assmann, J. (2006). *Religion and cultural memory*. Stanford, CA: Stanford University Press.

Assmann, J. (2008). Communicative and cultural memory. In A. Erll & A. Nünning (Eds.), *Cultural memory studies: An international and interdisciplinary handbook* (pp. 109–118). Berlin, Germany & New York: de Gruyter.

Assmann, J. (2011). *Cultural memory and early civilization: Writing, remembrance, and political imagination*. Cambridge, UK, & New York: Cambridge University Press.

Atance, C. M., & O'Neill, D. K. (2001). Episodic future thinking. *Trends in Cognitive Sciences, 5*, 533–539.

Athens, L. (1994). The self as soliloquy. *The Sociological Quarterly, 35*(3), 521–532.

Augustine. (1991). *Confessions*. Oxford: Oxford University Press.

Austin, J. L. (1962). *How to do things with words*. Oxford: Clarendon.

Austen, J. (1992). *Mansfield park*. Hertfordshire, UK: Wordsworth.

Bakhtin, M. (1981). *The dialogic imagination*. Austin, TX: University of Texas Press.

Bakhtin, M. (1986). *Speech genres and other late essays*. Austin: University of Texas Press.

Bal, M. (1985). *Narratology: Introduction to the theory of narrative*. Toronto, ON: University of Toronto Press.

Bamberg, M. (2005). Agency. In D. Herman, M. Jahn, & M.-L. Ryan (Eds). *The Routledge encyclopedia of narrative theory* (pp. 9–10). London: Routledge.

Bamberg, M. (2007). Stories: Big or small? In M. Bamberg (Ed.), *Narrative—State of the art* (pp. 165–174). Amsterdam, Netherlands & Philadelphia, PA: John Benjamins.

Bamberg, M. (2010). Who am I? Big or small—shallow or deep? *Theory & Psychology, 21*(1), 1–8.

Bamberg, M. (2012). Narrative practice and identity navigation. In J. A. Holstein & J. F. Gubrium (Eds.), *Varieties of narrative analysis* (pp. 99–124). London: Sage.

Bamberg, M., & Georgakopoulou, A. (2008). Small stories as a new perspective in narrative and identity analysis. *Text & Talk, 28*(3), 377–396.

Banfield, A. (2003). Time passes: Virginia Woolf, post-Impressionism, and Cambridge time. *Poetics Today, 24*(3), 471–516.

Bar, M. (Ed.) (2011a). *Predictions in the brain: Using our past to generate a future*. Oxford & New York: Oxford University Press.

Bar, M. (2011b). Predictions: A universal principle in the operations of the human brain. In M. Bar (Ed.), *Predictions in the brain: Using our past to generate a future* (pp. v–vii). Oxford & New York: Oxford University Press.

Barnes, J. (2011). *The sense of an ending*. London: Jonathan Cape.

Barnes, J. (2013). *Levels of life*. Toronto, ON: Random House.

Barnier, A. J., Hung, L., & Conway, M. A. (2004). Retrieval-induced forgetting of emotional and unemotional autobiographical memories. *Cognition and Emotion, 18* (4), 457–477.

Bartlett, F. C. (1932). *Remembering*. Cambridge, UK: Cambridge University Press.

Bauer, P. J. (2007). *Remembering the times of our lives: Memory in infancy and beyond*. Mahwah, NJ: Erlbaum.

Bauman, R. (1986). *Story, performance, and event: Contextual studies of oral narrative*. Cambridge, UK: Cambridge University Press.

Bauman, Z. (2000). *Liquid modernity*. Oxford: Polity Press.

Beckett, S. (1957). *Proust*. New York: Grove Press.

Beiner, G. (2008). In anticipation of a post-memory boom syndrome. *Cultural Analysis, 7*, 107 112.

Beike, D. R., Lampinen, J. M., & Behrend, D. A. (Eds.) (2004). *The self and memory*. New York: Psychology Press.

Bender, J., & Wellbery, D. (1991). Introduction. In J. Bender & D. Wellbery (Eds.), *Chronotypes: The construction of time* (pp. 1–15). Stanford, CA: Stanford University Press.

Benjamin, W. (1917/1996). On perception. In W. Benjamin, *Selected Writings, Vol. 1: 1913–1926* (pp. 93–96). Cambridge, MA: Harvard University Press.

Benjamin W. (1918/1991). Über das Programm der kommenden Philosophie (pp. 157–171). *In Gesammelte Schriften, Vol. 2 (1)*. Frankfurt am Main: Suhrkamp.

Benjamin, W. (1918/1996). On the program of the coming philosophy. In W. Benjamin, *Selected Writings, Vol. 1: 1913–1926* (pp. 100–110). Cambridge, MA: Harvard University Press.

Benjamin, W. (1968). The image of Proust. In H. Arendt (Ed.), *Illuminations*. New York: Schocken.

Benjamin, W. (1974). Über den Begriff der Geschichte [On the concept of history]. In *Gesammelte Werke, Vol. 2(2)*. Frankfurt am Main: Suhrkamp.

Benjamin, W. (2006). *Berlin childhood around 1900*. Cambridge, MA: Harvard University Press.

Benjamin, W. (2008). *The work of art in the age of mechanical reproduction*. London: Penguin.

Benjamin, W. (1999). *The Arcades project*. Cambridge, MA: The Belknap Press of Harvard University.

Bergstein, M. (2010). *Mirrors of memory: Freud, photography, and the history of art*. Ithaca, NY: Cornell University Press.

Bergson, H. (1946). *The creative mind: An introduction to metaphysics*. New York: Citatel Press. (Original work published 1934.)

Bergson, H. (1990). *Matter and memory*. New York: Zone Books. (Original work published 1896.)

Berntsen, D., & Rubin, D. C. (2004). Cultural life scripts structure recall from autobiographical memory. *Memory & Cognition, 32*, 427–442.

Berntsen, D., & Rubin, D. C. (Eds.) (2012a). *Understanding autobiographical memory: Theories and approaches*. Cambridge, UK & New York: Cambridge University Press.

Berntsen, D., & Rubin, D. C. (2012b). Introduction. In D. Berntsen & D. C. Rubin (Eds.), *Understanding autobiographical memory: Theories and approaches* (pp. 1–8). Cambridge, UK & New York: Cambridge University Press.

Biebuyck, B., & Martens, G. (2011). Literary metaphor between cognition and narration. In M. Fludernik (Ed.), *Beyond cognitive metaphor theory: Perspectives on literary metaphor* (pp. 58–75). New York: Routledge.

Bietti, L. M. (2011). Joint remembering: Cognition, communication and interaction in processes of memory-making. *Memory Studies, 5*(2), 182–205.

Bietti, L. M. (2014). *Discursive remembering: Individual and collective remembering as a discursive, cognitive and historical process.* Berlin, Germany & New York: De Gruyter.

Bietti, L. M., Stone, C. B., & Hirst, W. (Eds.) (2014). Contextualizing human memory. *Memory Studies, 7*(3), 267–271.

Birchall, D. (2001). *Onoto Watanna: The story of Winnifred Eaton.* Urbana, IL: University of Illinois Press.

Black, M. (1962). *Models and metaphors: Studies in language and philosophy.* Ithaca, NY: Cornell University Press.

Blight, D. W. (2009). The memory boom: Why and why now? In P. Boyer & J.V. Wertsch (Eds.), *Memory in mind and culture* (pp. 238–251). New York: Cambridge University Press.

Bloch, D. (2007). *Aristotle on memory and recollection: Text, translation, interpretation, and reception in Western Scholasticism.* Leiden, Netherlands: Brill.

Brown, G. D. A., & Chater, N. (2001). The chronological organization of memory: Common psychological foundations for remembering and timing. In C. Hoerl & T. McCormack (Eds.), *Time and memory: Issues in philosophy and psychology* (pp. 77–110). Oxford: Oxford University Press.

Block, R. A., & Zakay, D. (2001). Retrospective and prospective timing: Memory, attention, and consciousness. In C. Hoerl & T. McCormack (Eds.), *Time and memory: Issues in philosophy and psychology* (pp. 59–76). Oxford: Oxford University Press.

Bontempi, B., & Frankland, P. W. (2009). Memory consolidation: Cerebral cortex. In L. R. Squire (Ed.), *Encyclopedia of neuroscience* (Vol. 5, pp. 733–749). Amsterdam, Netherlands: Elsevier.

Borges, J. L. (2000). Funes the memorios. In J. L. Borges, *Labyrinths: Selected stories and other writings* (pp. 91–99). London: Penguin.

Bowie, M. (1998). *Proust among the stars.* New York: Columbia University Press.

Bowles, H. (2010). *Storytelling and drama: Exploring narrative episodes in plays.* Amsterdam, Netherlands & Philadelphia, PA: John Benjamins.

Boyer, M. C. (1996). *The city of collective memory.* Cambridge, MA: MIT Press.

Brewer, W. F. (1980). Literary theory, rhetoric, stylistics: Implications for psychology. In R. J. Spiro, B. C. Bruce, & W. F. Brewer (Eds.), *Theoretical issues in reading comprehension* (pp. 221–239). Hillsdale, NJ: Erlbaum.

Brockmeier, J. (1995/2001). The language of human temporality: Narrative schemes and cultural meanings of time. *Mind, Culture, and Activity 2,* 102–118. Revised version ((2001). Retrieved from http://www.colbud.hu/main_old/PubArchive/DP/DP04-Brockmeier.pdf

Brockmeier, J. (1996). Anthropomorphic operators of time: Chronology, activity, language and space. In J. T. Fraser & M. P. Soulsby (Eds.). *Dimensions of time and life: The study of time* (Vol. VIII, pp. 239–251). Madison, CT: International Universities Press.

Brockmeier, J. (1997). Autobiography, narrative, and the Freudian conception of life history. *Philosophy, Psychiatry, & Psychology, 4,* 175–200.

Brockmeier, J. (1998). *Literales Bewusstsein. Schriftlichkeit und das Verhältnis von Sprache und Kultur [The literate mind: Literacy and the relationship between language and culture].* Munich, Germany: Fink.

Brockmeier, J. (1999). Erinnerung, Identität und autobiographischer Prozess [Remembering, identity, and autobiographical process]. *Journal für Psychologie*, 7, 22–42.

Brockmeier, J. (2000a). Literacy as symbolic space. In J. W. Astington (Ed.), *Minds in the making* (pp. 43–61). Oxford: Blackwell.

Brockmeier, J. (2000b). Autobiographical time. *Narrative Inquiry*, 10(1), 51–73.

Brockmeier, J. (2001a). Texts and other symbolic spaces. *Mind, Culture, and Activity*, 8, 215–231.

Brockmeier, J. (2001b). From the beginning to the end: Retrospective teleology in autobiography. In J. Brockmeier & D. Carbaugh (Eds.), *Narrative and identity: Studies in autobiography, self, and* culture (pp. 246–280). Amsterdam, Netherlands & Philadelphia, PA: John Benjamins.

Brockmeier, J. (2001c). Identity. In M. Jolly (Ed.), *Encyclopedia of life writing: Autobiographical and biographical forms* (Vol. 1, pp. 455 457). London & Chicago, IL: Fitzroy Dearborn.

Brockmeier, J. (2001d). Time. In M. Jolly (Ed.), *Encyclopedia of life writing: Autobiographical and biographical forms* (Vol. 1, pp. 455–457). London & Chicago, IL: Fitzroy Dearborn.

Brockmeier, J. (2002a). Remembering and forgetting: Narrative as cultural memory. *Culture & Psychology*, 8(1), 15–43.

Brockmeier, J. (2002b). Searching for cultural memory: Introduction [to the Special Issue: "Narrative and Cultural Memory"]. *Culture and Psychology*, 8(1) 5–14.

Brockmeier, J. (2002c) (Ed.). Special volume on "Narrative and Cultural Memory." *Culture and Psychology*, 8(1), 5–152.

Brockmeier, J. (2002d). Ineffable experience. *The Journal for Consciousness Studies*, 9 (9–10), 79–95.

Brockmeier, J. (2002e). Possible lives. *Narrative Inquiry*, 12(2), 455–466. Also in M. Bamberg & M. Andrews (Eds.) (2004). *Considering counter-narratives: Narrating, resisting, making sense* (pp. 323–333). Amsterdam, Netherlands & Philadelphia, PA: John Benjamins.

Brockmeier, J. (2005). The text of the mind. In C. Erneling & D. M. Johnson (Eds.), *The mind as a scientific object: Between brain and culture* (pp. 432–452). New York: Oxford University Press.

Brockmeier, J. (2007). Über narratives Bewusstsein [On narrative consciousness]. In P. H. Breitenstein, V. Steenblock, and J. Siebert (Eds.), *Geschichte, Kultur, Bildung. Philosophische Denkrichtungen* [History, culture, Bildung: Philosophical perspectives] (pp. 12–25). Hanover, Germany: Siebert.

Brockmeier, J. (2008a). Lifetime and eternity. In J. Belzen & A. Geels (Eds.), *Autobiography and the psychological study of religious lives* (pp. 19–38). Amsterdam, Netherlands & New York: Rodopi.

Brockmeier, J. (2008b). Language, experience, and the "traumatic gap": How to talk about 9/11? In L.-C. Hydén & J. Brockmeier (Eds.), *Health, illness and culture: Broken narrative* (pp. 16–35). New York: Routledge.

Brockmeier, J. (2009). Reaching for meaning: Human agency and the narrative imagination. *Theory and Psychology*, 19(2), 213–233.

Brockmeier, J. (2010). After the archive: Remapping memory. *Culture and Psychology*, 16(1), 5 35.

Brockmeier, J. (2011). Socializing the narrative mind. *Style*, 45(2), 259–264.

Brockmeier, J. (2012a). Narrative scenarios: Toward a culturally thick notion of narrative. In J. Valsiner (Ed.), *Oxford handbook of culture and psychology* (pp. 439–467). Oxford & New York: Oxford University Press.

Brockmeier, J. (2012b). Historicizing memory. Review article on Kurt Danziger's "Marking the mind: A history of memory." *Theory and Psychology 22*(3), 370–373.

Brockmeier, J. (2012c). Écriture et mémoire [Writing and memory]. In E. Guichard (Ed.), *Écritures: sur les traces de Jack Goody. Actes du Colloque de l'École National Supérieure de l'Information e des Bibliothèques* (pp. 140–155). Villeurbanne, France: Presses de l'ENSSIB.

Brockmeier, J. (2013a). Fact and fiction: Exploring the interpretive mind. In M. Hyvärinen, M. Hatavara, & L.-C. Hydén (Eds.), *The travelling metaphor of narrative* (pp. 121–140). Amsterdam, Netherlands & Philadelphia, PA: John Benjamins.

Brockmeier, J. (2013b). Afterword: The monkey wrenches of narrative. In M. Andrews, C. Squire, & M. Tamboukou (Eds.), *Doing narrative research* (2nd ed.) (pp. 261–270). London: Sage.

Brockmeier, J. (2014). Questions of meaning: Memory, dementia, and the post-autobiographical perspective. In L.-C. Hydén, H. Lindemann, & J. Brockmeier (Eds.), *Beyond loss: Dementia, identity, personhood* (pp. 69–90). Oxford & New York: Oxford University Press.

Brockmeier, J., & Carbaugh, D. (2001a). Introduction. In J. Brockmeier & D. Carbaugh (Eds.), *Narrative and identity: Studies in autobiography, self and culture* (pp. 1–22). Amsterdam, Netherlands & Philadelphia, PA: John Benjamins.

Brockmeier, J., & Carbaugh, D. (Eds.) (2001b). *Narrative and identity: Studies in autobiography, self and culture.* Amsterdam, Netherlands & Philadelphia, PA: John Benjamins.

Brockmeier, J., & Harré, R. (2001). Narrative: Problems and promises of an alternative paradigm In J. Brockmeier & D. Carbaugh (Eds.), *Narrative and identity: Studies in autobiography, self and culture* (pp. 39–58). Amsterdam, The Netherlands & Philadelphia, PA: John Benjamins.

Brockmeier, J., & Homer, B. (2014). Exploring symbolic spaces: Writing, narrative, and art. In A. Antonietti, E. Confalonieri, & A. Marchetti (Eds.). *Metarepresentation and narrative in educational settings: Where cognitive and social development meet* (pp. 308–320). Cambridge, UK: Cambridge University Press.

Brockmeier, J., & Meretoja, H. (2014). Understanding narrative hermeneutics. *Storyworlds: A Journal of Narrative Studies, 6*(2), 1–27.

Brockmeier, J., & Olson, D. R. (2009). The literacy episteme: From Innis to Derrida. In D. R. Olson, & N. Torrance (Eds.), *The Cambridge handbook of literacy* (pp. 3–21). Cambridge, UK & New York: Cambridge University Press.

Brooks, P. (1984). *Reading for the plot: Design and intention in narrative.* Cambridge, MA: Harvard University Press.

Brown, A. D., Kramer, M. E., Romano, T. A., & Hirst, W. (2012). Forgetting trauma: Socially shared retrieval-induced forgetting and post-traumatic stress disorder. *Applied Cognitive Psychology, 26,* 24–34.

Brown, R., & Kulik, J. (1977). Flashbulb memories. *Cognition, 5,* 73–99.

Brown, S. D., & Reavey, P. (2014). Vital memories: Movements in and between affect, ethics and self. *Memory Studies, 7*(3), 328–338.

Bruner, J. S. (1973). *Beyond the information given: Studies in the psychology of knowing.* Cambridge, MA: Harvard University Press.

Bruner, J. S. (1986). *Actual minds, possible worlds.* Cambridge, MA: Harvard University Press.

Bruner, J. S. (1987a). Prologue to the English edition. In R. W. Rieber & A. S. Carton (Eds.), *The collected works of L. S. Vygotsky* (Vol. 1, pp. 1–16). New York: Plenum Press.

Bruner, J. S. (1987b). Foreword. In Luria, A. R, *The mind of a mnemonist* (pp. ix–xix). Cambridge, MA: Harvard University Press.

Bruner, J. S. (1987c). Life as narrative. *Social Research, 54*(1), 11–32.

Bruner, J. S. (1990a). *Acts of meaning.* Cambridge, MA: Harvard University Press.

Bruner, J. S. (1990b). Culture and human development: A new look. *Human Development, 43*(33), 344–355.

Bruner, J. S. (1991). The narrative construction of reality, *Critical Inquiry, 17*(Autumn), 1–21.

Bruner, J. S. (1993). The autobiographical process. In R. Folkenflik (Ed.), *The culture of autobiography* (pp. 38–56). Stanford, CA: Stanford University Press.

Bruner, J. S. (1994). The 'remembered' self. In U. Neisser & R. Fivush (Eds.), *The remembering self* (pp. 41–54). Cambridge, UK: Cambridge University Press.

Bruner, J. S. (1996). *The culture of education.* Cambridge, MA: Harvard University Press.

Bruner, J. S. (2001). Self-making and world-making. In J. Brockmeier & D. Carbaugh (Eds.), *Narrative and identity: Studies in autobiography, self and culture* (pp. 25–37). Amsterdam, Netherlands & Philadelphia, PA: John Benjamins.

Bruner, J. S. (2002). Narrative distancing: A foundation of literacy. In J. Brockmeier, M. Wang, & D. R. Olson (Eds.), *Literacy, narrative and culture* (pp. 86–93). Richmond, UK: Curzon Press.

Buckner, R. L., & Carroll, D. C. (2006). Self-projection and the brain. *Trends in Cognitive Sciences, 11*(2), 49–57.

Buckner, R. L., Andrews-Hanna, J. R., & Schacter, D. L. (2008). The brain's default network: Anatomy, function, and relevance to disease. *The Year in Cognitive Neuroscience. Annals of the New York Academy of Sciences, 1124*, 1–3.

Bühler, K. (1934). *Sprachtheorie. Die Darstellungsfunktion der Sprache* [Theory of language: The representational function of language] Jena, Germany: Gustav Fischer.

Butler, J. (1990). *Gender trouble.* New York & Abington, UK: Routledge.

Butler, J. (2005). *Giving an account of oneself.* New York: Fordham University Press.

Byrne, J. H. (Ed.). (2008). *Learning and memory: A comprehensive reference* (Vol. 4). Oxford, UK, & San Diego, CA: Elsevier.

Carr, D. (1986). *Time, narrative, and history.* Bloomington, IN: Indiana University Press.

Carr, D. (1997). Narrative and the real world: An argument for continuity. In L. P. Hinchman & S. K. Hinchman (Eds.), *Memory, identity, community: The idea of narrative in the human sciences* (pp. 7–25). Albany, NY: State University of New York Press.

Carretero, M., & Solcoff, K. (2012). Commentary on Brockmeier's remapping memory: The relation between past, present and future as a metaphor of memory. *Culture Psychology, 18*(1) 14–22.

Carruthers, M. J. (1990). *The book of memory: A study of memory in medieval culture.* Cambridge, UK: Cambridge University Press.

Carruthers, M. J. (2010). How to make a composition? Memory-craft in Antiquity and in the Middle Ages. In S. Radstone & B. Schwarz (Eds.), *Memory: Histories, theories, debates* (pp. 15–29). New York: Fordham University Press.

Carter, W. C. (2000). *Marcel Proust: A life.* New Haven, CT: Yale University Press.

Caruth, C. (1996). *Unclaimed experience: Trauma, narrative, and history.* Baltimore, MD: Johns Hopkins University Press.

Caruth, C. (Ed.) (1995). *Trauma: Explorations in memory*. Baltimore, MD: Johns Hopkins University Press.

Cassam, Q. (Ed.) (1994). *Self-knowledge*. Oxford: Oxford University Press.

Caygill, H. (1998). *Walter Benjamin: The colour of experience*. London: Routledge.

Charon, R. (2006). *Narrative medicine: Honoring the stories of illness*. New York: Oxford University Press.

Charon, R. (2012). At the membranes of care: Stories in narrative medicine. *Academic Medicine, 87* (3), 342–347.

Chatman, S. B. (1978). *Story and discourse: Narrative structure in fiction and film*. Ithaca, NY: Cornell University Press.

Chekhov, A. (2007). *The cherry orchard*. London: Oberon Books.

Chen, S.-C. (2000). To report a crime: *The Woman Warrior* as a live/life testimony. *Intergrams: Studies in Languages and Literatures, 2*(1). Retrieved from http://benz.nchu.edu.tw/~intergrams/intergrams/002/002-chen.htm

Cheung, K.-K. (1988). Don't tell": Imposed silences in *The Color Purple* and *The Woman Warrior*. *PMLA, 103*(2): 162–174.

Christensen, A. (2011, November 11). Brains like glaciers. *ScienceNordic*. Retrieved from http://sciencenordic.com/brains-glaciers

Choi, J. (2006). The metropolis and mental life in the novel. *New Literary History 37*(4), 707–724.

Clark, A. (2011). Supersizing the mind: Embodiment, action, and cognitive extension. Oxford & New York: Oxford University Press.

Coetzee, J. M. (2002, October 24). Heir of a dark history. *New York Review of Books, 49*, 24–27.

Cole, M. (1996). *Cultural psychology: A once and future discipline*. Cambridge, MA: Harvard University Press.

Connerton, P. (1989). *How societies remember*. Cambridge, UK: Cambridge University Press.

Conway, M. A., & Jobson, L. (2012). On the nature of autobiographical memory. In D. Berntsen & D. C. Rubin (Eds.), *Understanding autobiographical memory: Theories and approaches* (pp. 54–69). Cambridge, UK & New York: Cambridge University Press.

Conway, M. A. (2005). Memory and the self. *Journal of Memory and Language, 53*(4), 594–628.

Conway, M. A., & Loveday, C. (2010). Accessing autobiographical memories. In J. H. Mace (Ed.), *The act of remembering: Toward an understanding of how we recall the past* (pp. 56–70). Malden, MA: Wiley-Blackwell.

Conway, M. A., & Pleydell-Pearce, C. W. (2000). The construction of autobiographical memories in the self-memory system. *Psychological Review, 107* (2), 261–288.

Coope, U. (2005). *Time for Aristotle*. Oxford & New York: Oxford University Press.

Crownshaw, R. (2004). Reconsidering postmemory: Photography, the archive, and post-Holocaust memory in W. G. Sebald's *Austerlitz*. *Mosaic: A Journal for the Interdisciplinary Study of Literature, 37*, 215–237.

Currie, G., & Ravenscroft, I. (2002). *Recreative minds: Imagination in philosophy and psychology*. Oxford & New York: Oxford University Press.

Currie, G. (2010). *Narratives and narrators: A philosophy of stories*. Oxford: Oxford University Press.

Currie, M. (2006). *About time: Narrative, fiction and the philosophy of time*. Edinburgh, UK: Edinburgh University Press.

Donald, M. (1991). *Origins of the modern mind: Three stages in the evolution of culture and cognition*. Cambridge, MA: Harvard University Press.

Danziger, K. (1990a). *Constructing the subject: Historical origins of psychological research*. Cambridge, UK: Cambridge University Press.

Danziger, K. (1990b). Generative metaphor and the history of psychological discourse. In D. E. Leary (Ed.), *Metaphors in the history of psychology* (pp. 331–356). New York: Cambridge University Press.

Danziger, K. (1997). *Naming the mind: How psychology found its language*. Thousand Oaks, CA: Sage.

Danziger, K. (2008). *Marking the mind: A history of memory*. Cambridge, UK & New York: Cambridge University Press.

Davidson, D. (1978). What metaphors mean. In S. Sacks (Ed.), *On Metaphor* (pp. 29–45). Chicago, IL: Chicago University Press.

Davis, R. G. (2005). The self in the text versus the self as text: Asian American autobiographical strategies. In G. Huang (Ed.), *Asian American literary studies* (pp. 41–63). Edinburgh, UK: Edinburgh University Press.

Davis, R. G. (2007). *Begin here: Reading Asian North American autobiographies of childhood*. Honolulu: University of Hawai'i Press.

Davis, R. G. (2011). *Relative histories: Mediating history in Asian American family memoirs*. Honolulu: University of Hawai'i Press.

Deacon, T. W. (1997). *The symbolic species: The co-evolution of language and the brain*. New York: Norton.

De Fina, A., &. Georgakopouloplou, A. (2012). *Analyzing narrative: Discourse and sociolinguistic perspectives*. Cambridge, UK: Cambridge University Press.

De Fina, A., Schiffrin, D., & Bamberg, M. (Eds.) (2006). *Discourse and identity*. Cambridge, UK & New York: Cambridge University Press.

Dennett, D. (1992). The self as a center of narrative gravity. In F. S. Kessel, P. M. Cole, & D. L. Johnson (Eds.), *Self and consciousness: Multiple perspectives* (pp. 103–115). Hillsdale, NJ: Erlbaum.

Dennett, D. (1997). Quining qualia. In N. Block, O. Flanagan, & G. Güzeldere (Eds.), *The nature of consciousness: Philosophical debates* (pp. 619–642). Cambridge, MA: MIT Press.

Derrida, J. (1978). Freud and the scene of writing. In J. Derrida, *Writing and Difference* (pp. 246–291). Chicago, IL: University of Chicago Press.

Derrida, J. (1995). Archive fever: A Freudian impression. *Diacritics, 25*(2), 9–63.

Dijck, J. van (2007). *Mediated memories in the digital age*. Stanford, CA: Stanford University Press.

Dijck, J. van (2011). Flickr and the culture of connectivity: Sharing views, experiences, memories. *Memory Studies, 4*, 401–415.

Dijck, J. van (2013). *The culture of connectivity: A critical history of social media*. Oxford & New York: Oxford University Press.

Dongfang, S. (2001a). China: 1949 to the present. In *Encyclopedia of life writing: Autobiographical and biographical forms* (Vol. 1, pp. 210–211). London & Chicago, IL: Fitzroy Dearborn.

Dongfang, S. (2001b). China: 19th century to 1949. In *Encyclopedia of life writing: Autobiographical and biographical forms* (Vol. 1, pp. 208–210). London & Chicago: Fitzroy Dearborn.

Donley, C., & Buckley, S. (Eds.) (2000). *What's normal? Narratives of mental and emotional disorders*. Kent, OH: Kent State University Press.

Douglas, M. (1992). The person in an enterprise culture. In S. H. Heap & A. Ross (Eds.), *Understanding the enterprise culture: Themes in the work of Mary Douglas* (pp. 41–62). Edinburgh, UK: Edinburgh University Press.

Draaisma, D. (2000). *Metaphors of memory: A history of ideas about the mind*. Cambridge, UK: Cambridge University Press.

Draguhn, A. (2012, December). Is the brain made for information processing? "Rational reconstructions" in neuroscience and the "organic brain." Talk given at the University Heidelberg, Marsilius-Kolleg.

Draguhn, A., & Both, M. (2009). Dancing neurons, complex beats. *Journal for Physiology, 587*(22), 5297.

Dreyfus, J.-M., & Wolff, J. (Eds.) (2012). Memory, traces and the Holocaust in the writings of W. G. Sebald. *Melilah: Manchester Journal of Jewish Studies. Supplementary Vol. 2*, 1–88.

Dudai, Y. (2006). Reconsolidation: The advantage of being refocused. *Current Opinion in Neurobiology, 16*, 174–178.

Dudai, Y. (2011). The engram revisited: On the elusive permanence of memory. In S. Nalbantian, P. M. Matthews, & J. L. McClelland (Eds.), *The memory process: Neuroscientific and humanistic perspectives* (pp. 29–40). Cambridge, MA: MIT Press.

Eakin, P. J. (1999). *How our lives become stories: Making selves*. Ithaca, NY: Cornell University Press.

Eakin, P. J. (2004). Introduction: Mapping the ethics of life writing. In P. J. Eakin (Ed.), *The ethics of life writing* (pp. 1–16). Ithaca, NY: Cornell University Press.

Eakin, P. J. (2006). Narrative identity and narrative imperialism: A response to Galen Strawson and James Phelan. *Narrative, 14*(2), 180–187.

Eakin, P. J. (2008). *Living autobiographically: How we create identity in narrative*. Ithaca, NY: Cornell University Press.

Eakin, P. J. (Eds.). (2004). *The ethics of life writing*. Ithaca, NY: Cornell University Press.

Eakin, P. J. (2014). Autobiography as cosmogram. *Storyword: A Journal of Narrative Studies, 6*(2), 21–43.

Ebbinghaus, H. (1913). *Memory: A contribution to experimental psychology*. New York: Teachers College Columbia University. (Original work published 1885.)

Echterhoff, G. (2011). The pervasiveness of memory. *Culture and Psychology, 17*(1), 3–9.

Edelman, G., & Tononi, G. (2000). *The universe of consciousness: How matter becomes imagination*. New York: Basic.

Edelman, G. (2005). *Wider than the sky: The phenomenal gift of consciousness*. New Haven, CT: Yale.

Edelman, G. (2006). *Second nature: Brain science and human knowledge*. New Haven, CT: Yale University Press.

Edwards, D. (2005). Discursive psychology. In K. L. Fitch & R. E. Sanders (Eds.), *Handbook of language and social interaction* (pp. 257–273). Mahwah, NJ: Erlbaum.

Edwards, D. (2006). Narrative analysis. In A. Jaworski & N. Coupland (Eds.), *The discourse reader* (2nd ed.) (pp. 227–238). London: Routledge.

Edwards, J. (2009). *Language and identity*. Cambridge, UK: Cambridge University Press.

Eichenbaum, H. (Ed.) (2008). Memory systems: Introduction and overview. In J. H. Byrne (Ed.), *Memory systems (Learning and memory)* (Vol. 3, pp. 1–8). Amsterdam, Netherlands & London: Elsevier.

Einstein, A., & Infeld, L. (1966). *The evolution of physics: From early concepts to relativity and quanta*. New York: Simon and Schuster.

Elgin, C. Z. (2007). The laboratory of the mind. In W. Huemer, J. Gibson, & L. Pocci (Eds.), *A sense of the world: Essays on fiction, narrative and knowledge* (pp. 43–54). London: Routledge.

Elias, N. (1992). *Time*. Oxford: Blackwell. (Original work published 1984.)

Ender, E. (2005). *Architects of memory: Literature, science, and autobiography*. Ann Arbor, MI: The University of Michigan Press.

Erll, A., & Nünning, A. (Eds.) (2008). *Cultural memory studies: An international and interdisciplinary handbook*. Berlin, Germany & New York: de Gruyter.

Erll, A. (2008). Cultural memory studies: An introduction. In A. Erll & A. Nünning (Eds.), *Cultural memory studies: An international and interdisciplinary handbook* (pp. 1–15). Berlin, Germany & New York: de Gruyter.

Ernst, W. (2013). *Digital memory and the archive*. Minneapolis, MN: University of Minnesota Press.

Eshel, A. (2003). Against the power of time: The poetics of suspension in W. G. Sebald's "Austerlitz." *New German Critique, 88* (Winter), 71–96.

Etkind, A. (2013). *Warped mourning: Stories of the undead in the land of the unburied*. Stanford, CA: Stanford University Press.

Fanon, F. (1967). *The wretched of the earth*. Harmondsworth, UK: Penguin 1967.

Farr, I. (Ed.). (2012). *Memory*. Cambridge, MA: MIT Press.

Fasulo, A., & Zucchermaglio, C. (2002). My selves and I: Identity markers in work meeting talk. *Journal of Pragmatics, 34*, 1119–1144.

Fasulo, A. (Ed.) (2004). Special volume on "Superfici del Sé: narrazioni, scritture e identità" [Surfaces of self: Narrative, writing, and identity]. *Rassegna di Psicologia, 21*(1), 5–166.

Felman, S., & Laub, D. (1992). *Testimony: Crisis in witnessing in literature, psychoanalysis, and history*. New York: Routledge.

Fernyhough, C. (2012). *Pieces of light: The new science of memory*. London: Profile Books.

Fish, S. (1980). *Is there a text in this class: The authority of interpretive communities*. Cambridge, MA: Harvard University Press.

Fiske, K. E., & Pillemer, D. B. (2006). Adult recollections of earliest childhood dreams: A cross-cultural study. *Memory, 14*, 57–67.

Fitzgerald, J. M., & Broadbridge, C. L. (2012). Theory and research in autobiographical memory: A life-span developmental perspective. In D. Berntsen & D. C. Rubin (Eds.), *Understanding autobiographical memory: Theories and approaches* (pp. 246–266). Cambridge, UK & New York: Cambridge University Press.

Fivush, R., & Haden, C. (Eds.) (2003). *Autobiographical memory and the construction of a narrative self: Developmental and cultural perspectives*. Mahwah, NJ: Erlbaum

Fivush, R. (2009). Sociocultural perspectives on autobiographical memory. In M. Courage & N. Cowan (Eds.). *The development of memory in infancy and childhood* (pp. 283–301). New York: Psychology Press.

Fivush, R. (2011). The development of autobiographical memory. *Annual Review of Psychology, 62*, 559–582.

Fleck, L. (1979). *The genesis and development of a scientific fact*. Chicago, IL: University of Chicago Press. (Original work published 1935.)

Fludernik, M. (1996). *Towards a "natural" narratology*. London: Routledge.

Fludernik, M. (2003). Natural narratology and cognitive parameters. In D. Herman (Ed.), *Narrative theory and the cognitive sciences* (pp. 243–267). Stanford, CA: Center for the Study of Language and Information.

Fludernik, M. (2009). *An introduction to narratology*. London & New York: Routledge.

Folkenflik, R. (1993). Introduction: The institution of autobiography. In R. Folkenflik (Ed.), *The culture of autobiography* (pp. 1–20). Stanford, CA.: Stanford University Press.

Folkenflik, R. (Ed.) (1993). *The culture of autobiography*. Stanford, CA.: Stanford University Press.

Foster, J. B. (1993). *Nabokov's art of memory and European Modernism*. Princeton, NJ: Princeton University Press.

Foster, J. K., & Jelicic, M. (1999). *Memory: Systems, process, or function?* Oxford & New York: Oxford University Press.

Foster, J. K. (2009). *Memory: A very short introduction*. Oxford & New York: Oxford University Press.

Foucault, M. (1970). *The order of things: An archeology of the human sciences*. London: Tavistock. (Original work published 1966.)

Foucault, M. (1977). *Discipline and punish: The birth of the prison*. New York: Pantheon Books. (Original work published 1975.)

Foucault, M. (1980). *Power/knowledge: Selected interviews and other writings 1972–1977*. Hassocks, Sussex, UK: Harvester Press.

Foucault, M. (1988). Technologies of the self. In L. H. Martin, H. Gutman, & P. H. Hutton (Eds.), *Technologies of the self: A seminar with Michel Foucault* (pp. 16–49). Amherst, MA: University of Massachusetts Press.

Foucault, M. (1990). *The history of sexuality, Vol. 3: The care of self*. London: Penguin. (Original work published 1984.)

Frank, A. (1995). *The wounded storyteller: Body, illness, and ethics*. Chicago, IL: University of Chicago Press.

Fraser, J. T. (1987). *Time, the familiar stranger*. Amherst, MA: University of Massachusetts Press.

Fraser, J. T. (1992). Human temporality in a nowless universe. *Time & Society, 2*(2): 159–173.

Freeman, M. (1993). *Rewriting the self: History, memory, narrative*. London: Routledge.

Freeman, M. (2007). Life "on holiday." In M. Bamberg (Ed.), *Narrative—State of the art* (pp. 155–163). Amsterdam, Netherlands & Philadelphia, PA: John Benjamins.

Freeman, M. (2010a). *Hindsight: The promise and peril of looking backward*. Oxford & New York: Oxford University Press.

Freeman, M. (2010b). Telling stories: Memory and narrative. In S. Radstone & B. Schwarz (Eds.), *Memory: Histories, theories, debates* (pp. 263–277). New York: Fordham University Press.

Freeman, M. (2010c). Stories, big and small: Toward a synthesis. *Theory & Psychology, 21*(1), 1–8.

Freeman, M., & Brockmeier, J. (2001). Narrative integrity: Autobiographical identity and the meaning of the "good life." In J. Brockmeier and D. Carbaugh (Eds.), *Narrative and identity: Studies in autobiography, self and culture* (pp. 75–101). Amsterdam, Netherlands & Philadelphia, PA: John Benjamins.

Freud, S. (1968). Notiz über den „Wunderblock" [A note upon the "mystic writing pad"]. In S. Freud, *Gesammelte Werke* (Vol. 14, pp. 1–8). Frankfurt am Main: S. Fischer.

Friedman, W. J. (2001). Memory processes underlying humans' chronological sense of the past. In C. Hoerl & T. McCormack (Eds.), *Time and memory: Issues in philosophy and psychology* (pp. 139–167). Oxford: Oxford University Press.

Friedman, W. J. (2004). Time in memory. *Social Cognition, 22*, 591–605.

Fuchs, A. (2004). *Die Schmerzensspuren der Geschichte. Zur Poetik der Erinnerung in W. S. Sebalds Prosa*. Cologne, Germany: Böhlau.

Gabrieli, J. D. E. (1995). A systematic view of human memory processes. *Journal of the International Neuropsychological Society, 1*, 115–118.

Gadamer, H.-G. (1989). *Truth and method* (2nd rev. ed.). New York: Crossroad Press. (Original work published 1960.)

Garloff, K. (2006). The talk of the narrator: Moments of symbolic investiture in W. G. Sebald's *Austerlitz*. In S. Denham & M. McCulloh (Eds.), *W. G. Sebald: History, memory, trauma* (pp. 157–169). Berlin, Germany & New York: de Gruyter.

Gazzaniga, M. S. (1998). *The mind's past*. Berkeley and Los Angeles, LA: University of California Press.

Gazzaniga, M. S. (2008). *Human: The science behind what makes us unique*. New York: Ecco.

Gazzaniga, M., Ivry, R. B., & Mangum, G. R. (2013) (Eds.). *Cognitive neuroscience: The biology of the mind* (4th ed.). New York & London: Norton.

Geertz, C. (1983a). "From the native's point of view": On the nature of anthropological understanding. In C. Geertz, *Local knowledge: Further essays in interpretive anthropology* (pp. 55–70). New York: Basic Books.

Geertz, C. (1983b). Common sense as a cultural system. In G. Geertz, *Local knowledge: Further essays in interpretive anthropology* (pp. 73–93). New York: Basic Books.

Geertz, C. (1983c). *Local knowledge: Further essays in interpretive anthropology*. New York: Basic Books.

Geertz, C. (2000). *Available light: Anthropological reflections on philosophical topics*. Princeton, NJ: Princeton University Press.

Genette, G. (1980). *Narrative discourse: An essay in method*. Ithaca, NY: Cornell University Press. (Original work published 1972.)

Genette, G. (1988). Time and narrative in *À la recherche du temps perdu*. In M. Hoffman & P. Murphy (Eds.), Essentials of the theory of fiction (pp. 277–298). Durham, NC: Duke University Press.

Geok-lin Lim, S., & Hong, C. K. (2007). The postmodern dilemma for life writing: Hybridizing hyphens. *Life Writing* 4(1), 3–9.

Georgakopoulou, A. (2007). *Small stories, interaction and identities*. Amsterdam, Netherlands & Philadelphia, PA: John Benjamins.

Gerber, D. A. (2006). *Authors of their lives: The personal correspondence of British immigrants to North America in the nineteenth century*. New York: New York University Press.

Gibbs, R. W. (1994). *The poetics of mind: Figurative thought, language, and understanding*. Cambridge, UK: Cambridge University Press.

Gibson, J. J. (1979). *The ecological approach to visual perception*. Boston, MA: Houghton Mifflin.

Giddens, A. (1991). *Modernity and self-identity: Self and society in the late modern age*. Stanford, CA: Stanford University Press.

Gilbert, D. T., & Wilson, T. D. (2011). Previews, premotions, and predictions. In M. Bar (Ed.), *Predictions in the brain: Using our past to generate a future* (pp. 159–169). Oxford & New York: Oxford University Press.

Gleick, J. (2011). *The information: A history, a theory, a flood*. New York: Pantheon.

Görner, R. (Ed.) (2003). *The anatomist of melancholy: Essays in memory of W. G. Sebald*. Munich, Germany: Iudicum.

Goethe, J. W. (1891). *The autobiography of Goethe. Truth and poetry: From my life*. London: Bell and Sons. (Original work published 1811–1814.)

Goffman, E. (1969). *The presentation of self in everyday life*. London: Penguin (first publication 1959).

Goffman, E. (1974). *Frame analysis*. New York: Harper & Row.

Goffman, E. (1981). *Forms of talk*. Philadelphia: University of Pennsylvania Press.

Goodman, N. (1978). *Ways of worldmaking*. Indianapolis, IN: Hackett.

Goldie, P. (2012). *The mess inside: Narrative, emotion, and the mind.* Oxford & New York: Oxford University Press.

Gordon, M. M. (1964). *Assimilation in American life: The role of race, religion and national origins.* New York: Oxford University Press.

Gould, S. J. (2003). *The hedgehog, the fox, and the magister's pox: Mending the gap between science and the humanities.* New York: Random House.

Grafton, A., Most, G. W., & Settis, S. (2010). *The classical tradition.* Cambridge, MA: Harvard University Press.

Greimas, A. (1987). *On meaning: Selected writings in semiotic theory.* Minneapolis, MN: University of Minnesota Press.

Grice, H. (2002). *Negotiating identities: An introduction to Asian American women's writing.* Manchester, UK: Manchester University Press.

Grishakova, M., & Ryan, M.-L. (Eds.) (2010). *Intermediality and storytelling.* Berlin, Germany & New York: De Gruyter.

Gross, D. (2000). *Lost time: On remembering and forgetting in late modern culture.* Amherst, MA: University of Massachusetts.

Gubrium, J. F., & Holstein, J. A. (2008). Narrative ethnography. In S. Hesse-Biber & P. Leavy (Eds.), *Handbook of emergent methods* (pp. 241–264.). New York: Guilford Publications.

Gubrium, J. F., & Holstein, J. A. (2009). *Analyzing narrative reality.* Los Angeles: Sage.

Gunaratnam, Y., & Oliviere, D. (Eds.) (2009). *Narrative and stories in health care: Illness, dying and bereavement.* Oxford & New York: Oxford University Press.

Gusdorf, G. (1980). Conditions and limits of autobiography. In Olney, J. (Ed.). *Autobiography: Essays theoretical and critical* (pp. 28–48). Princeton, NJ: Princeton University Press.

Habermas, J. (1987). *The philosophical discourse of modernity.* Cambridge, MA: MIT (originally published 1985).

Habermas, T. (Ed.) (2011). The development of autobiographical reasoning in adolescence and beyond: New directions for child and adolescent development. *New Directions in Child Development, 131.*

Habermas, T. (2012). Identity, emotion, and the social matrix of autobiographical memory: A psychoanalytic narrative view. In D. Berntsen & D. C. Rubin (Eds.), *Understanding autobiographical memory: Theories and approaches* (pp. 33–53). Cambridge, UK: Cambridge University Press.

Hacking, I. (1995). *Rewriting the soul: Multiple personality and the sciences of memory.* Princeton, NJ: Princeton University Press.

Hacking, I. (1996a). Memory science, memory politics. In P. Antze & M. Lambek (Eds.), *Tense past: Cultural essays in trauma and memory* (pp. 76–88). New York: Routledge.

Hacking, I. (1996b). Normal people. In D. R. Olson & N. Torrance (Eds.). *Modes of thought: Explorations in culture and cognition* (pp. 59–71). Cambridge, UK: Cambridge University Press.

Hacking, I. (2002). *Historical ontology.* Cambridge, MA: Harvard University Press.

Hacking, I. (2006, August 17). Making up people. *London Review of Books, 28*(16), 23–26.

Halbwachs, M. (1992). *On collective memory.* Chicago, IL: University of Chicago Press. (Original work published 1925; 1941.)

Hamacher, W. (2002). "Now": Walter Benjamin on historical time." In H. Friese (Ed.), *The moment: Time and rupture in modern thought* (pp. 161–196). Liverpool, UK: Liverpool University Press.

Harré, R. (1996). There is no time like the present. In B. J. Copeland (Ed.), *Logic and reality: Essays on the legacy of Arthur Prior* (pp. 389–409). Oxford: Clarendon Press.

Harré, R. (1998). *The singular self: An introduction to the psychology of personhood.* London: Sage.

Harré, R. (2012). Positioning theory: Moral dimensions of social-cultural psychology. In J. Valsiner (Ed.), *The Oxford handbook of culture and psychology* (pp. 191–206). Oxford & New York: Oxford University Press.

Harré, R., & Gillett, G. (1994). *The discursive mind.* Thousand Oaks, CA: Sage.

Harris, P. (2000). *The work of imagination.* Oxford: Blackwell.

Harris, R. (2000). *Rethinking writing.* Bloomington, IN: Indiana University Press.

Harris, R. (2002). Literacy and the future of writing. In J. Brockmeier, M. Wang, & D. R. Olson (Eds.), *Literacy, narrative and culture* (pp. 35–51). Richmond, UK: CurzonRoutledge.

Harris, S. (2001). The return of the dead: Memory and photography in W. G. Sebald's "Die Ausgewanderten." *The German Quarterly, 74*(4), 379–391.

Hassabis, D., & Maguire, E. A. (2007). Deconstructing episodic memory with construction. *Trends in Cognitive Sciences, 11,* 299–306.

Hassabis, D., Kumaran, D., Vann, S. D., & Maguire, E. A. (2007). Patients with hippocampal amnesia cannot imagine new experiences. *Proceedings of the National Academy of Sciences, USA, 104,* 1726–1731.

Havelock, E. A. (1963). *Preface to Plato.* Cambridge, MA: Harvard University Press.

Hayles, N. K. (2012). *How we think: Digital media and contemporary technogenesis.* Chicago, IL: University of Chicago Press.

Haynes, J. D., Sakai, K., Rees, G., Gilbert, S., Frith, C., & Passingham, D. (2007). Reading hidden intentions in the human brain. *Current Biology 17,* 323–328.

Head, D. (2007). *Ian McEwan.* Manchester, UK: Manchester University Press.

Hedstrom, M. (2002). Archives, memory, and interfaces with the past. *Archival Science, 2,* 21–43.

Hegel, G. W. F. (1977). *Phenomenology of spirit.* Oxford: Clarendon Press.

Hegel, R. E., & Hessney, R. C. (Eds.) (1985). *Expressions of self in Chinese literature.* New York: Columbia University Press.

Heidegger, M. (1962). *Being and time.* New York: Harper and Row.

Heise, U. (1997). *Chronoschism: Time, narrative, and postmodernism.* Cambridge, UK: Cambridge University Press.

Herman, D. (1995). *Universal grammar and narrative form.* Durham, NC: Duke University Press.

Herman, D. (1999a). Towards a socionarratology: New ways of analyzing natural language narratives. In D. Herman (Ed.), *Narratologies: New perspectives on narrative analysis* (pp. 218–246). Columbus, OH: Ohio State University Press.

Herman, D. (1999b). Introduction. In D. Herman (Ed.), *Narratologies: New perspectives on narrative analysis* (pp. 1–30). Columbus, OH: Ohio State University Press.

Herman, D. (2000). Narrative theory and the intentional stance. *Partial Answers 0*(2), 233–260.

Herman, D. (2009a). *Basic elements of narrative.* Oxford: Wiley-Blackwell.

Herman, D. (2009b). Narrative ways of worldmaking. In S. Heinen & R. Sommer (Eds.), *Narratology in the age of cross-disciplinary narrative research* (pp. 71–87). Berlin, Germany & New York: Walter de Gruyter.

Herman, D. (2011a). Introduction. In D. Herman (Ed.), *The emergence of mind: Representations of consciousness in narrative discourse in English* (pp. 1–40). Lincoln, NE: University of Nebraska Press.

Herman, D. (Ed.) (2011b). *The emergence of mind: Representations of consciousness in narrative discourse in English.* Lincoln, NE: University of Nebraska Press.

Herman, D. (2011c). 1880–1945: Re-minding Modernism. In D. Herman (Ed.), *The emergence of mind: Representations of consciousness in narrative discourse in English.* Lincoln, NE: University of Nebraska Press.

Herman, D. (2011d). Post-Cartesian approaches to narrative and mind. *Style, 45* (2), 265–271.

Herman, D. (2012). Exploring the nexus of narrative and mind. In D. Herman, J. Phelan, P. Rabinowitz, B. Richardson, & R. Warhol, *Narrative theory: Core concepts and critical debates* (pp. 14–19). Columbus, OH: Ohio State University Press.

Herman, D. (2013). *Storytelling and the sciences of mind.* Cambridge, MA: MIT Press.

Hermans, H. (2000). Meaning as movement: The relativity of the mind. In G. T. Reker & K. Chamberlain (Eds.), *Exploring existential meaning* (pp. 23–38). Thousand Oaks, CA: Sage.

Hermans, H. (2002). The dialogical self as a society of mind: Introduction. *Theory & Psychology 12*(2), 147–160.

Herrnstein Smith, B. (1981). Narrative versions, narrative theories. In W. J. T. Michell (Ed.), *On narrative* (pp. 209–232). Chicago, IL: The University of Chicago Press.

Hinchman, L. P., & Hinchman, S. K. (Eds.) (1997). *Memory, identity, community: The idea of narrative in the human sciences.* Albany, NY: State University of New York Press.

Hirsch, M. (2001). Surviving images: Holocaust photography and the work of postmemory. *Yale Journal of Criticism 12*(1), 5–37.

Hirst, W., Cuc, A., & Wohl, D. (2012). Of sins and virtues: Memory and collective identity. In D. Berntsen & D. C. Rubin (Eds.), *Understanding autobiographical memory: Theories and approaches* (pp. 141–159). Cambridge, UK & New York: Cambridge University Press.

Hirst, W., & Echterhoff, G. (2008). Creating shared memories in conversations: Towards a psychology of collective memory. *Social Research, 75,* 1071–1108.

Hirst, W., & Echterhoff, G. (2012). Remembering in conversations: The social sharing and reshaping of memories. *Annual Review of Psychology, 63,* 55–79.

Hoffmann, C. R. (2010). *Narrative revisited: Telling a new story in the age of new media.* Philadelphia, PA & Amsterdam, Netherlands: John Benjamins.

Holstein, J. A., & Gubrium, J. F. (2000). *The self we live by: Narrative identity in a postmodern world.* New York: Oxford University Press.

Holstein, J. A., & Gubrium, J. F. (2011). The constructionist analytics of interpretive practice. In N. Denzin & Y. Lincoln (Eds.), *The Sage handbook of qualitative research* (4th ed.). Thousand Oaks, CA: Sage.

Holzkamp, K. (1973). *Sinnliche Erkenntnis. Historischer Ursprung und gesellschaftliche Funktion der Wahrnehmung* [Sense knowledge: Historical origin and societal function of perception] (2nd ed. 2006). Frankfurt am Main: Athenäum Fischer.

Holzkamp, K. (1983). *Grundlegung der Psychologie* [Groundwork of psychology]. Frankfurt am Main: Campus.

Holzkamp, K. (2013). *Psychology from the standpoint of the subject: Selected writings of Klaus Holzkamp*. Basingstoke, UK: Palgrave Macmillan.

Hong Kingston, M. (1989). *The woman warrior: Memoirs of a girlhood among ghosts*. New York: Random House (First publication 1976).

Hong Kingston, M. (1982). Cultural misreadings by American reviewers. In G. Amirthanayagam (Ed.), *Asian and Western writers in dialogue: New cultural identities* (pp. 55–65). London: Macmillan.

Hoskins, A. (2009a). The mediatization of memory. In J. Garde-Hansen, A. Hoskins, & A. Reading (Eds.), *Save as ... digital memories* (pp. 27–43). Basingstoke, UK: Palgrave Macmillan.

Hoskins, A. (2009b). Digital network memory. In A. Erll & A. Rigney (Eds.), *Mediation, remediation and the dynamics of cultural memory* (pp. 91–108). Berlin, Germany: de Gruyter.

Hoskins, A. (2013a). Media, memory, metaphor. Remembering and the connective turn. In R. Crownshaw (Ed.), *Transcultural memory* (pp. 24–36). London: Routledge.

Hoskins, A. (2013b). The end of decay time. *Memory Studies*, 6(4) 387–389.

Humphrey, N. (2002). *The mind made flesh: Essays from the frontiers of evolution and psychology*. Oxford: Oxford University Press.

Humphrey, R. (1968). *Stream of consciousness in the modern novel*. Berkeley & Los Angeles, LA: University of California Press.

Hunt, N. C. (2010). *Memory, trauma and war*. Cambridge, UK & New York: Cambridge University Press.

Hurwitz, B. (2006). Form and representation in clinical case reports. *Literature and Medicine*, 25(2), 216–240.

Hurwitz, B. (2011). Clinical cases and case reports: Boundaries and porosities. In A. Calanchi, G. Castgellani, G. Morisco, & G. Turchetti (Eds.), *The case and the canon: Anomalies, discontinuities, metaphors between science and literature* (pp. 45–57). Göttingen, Germany: V & R Unipress.

Hutchins, E. (1995). *Cognition in the wild*. Cambridge, MA: MIT Press.

Huyssen, A. (1995). *Twilight memories: Marking time in a culture of amnesia*. New York: Routledge.

Huyssen, A. (2003). *Present pasts: Urban palimpsests and the politics of memory*. Stanford, CA: Stanford University Press.

Hydén, L.-C. (2011). Narrative collaboration and scaffolding in dementia. *Journal of Aging Studies*, 25, 339–347.

Hydén, L.-C. (2013). Towards an embodied theory of narrative and storytelling. In M. Hatavara, L.-C. Hydén, & M. Hyvärinen, (Eds.), *The travelling metaphor of narrative* (pp. 121–140). Amsterdam, Netherlands & Philadelphia, PA: John Benjamins.

Hydén, L.-C. (2014). How to do things with others: Joint activities involving persons with Alzheimer's Disease. In L.-C. Hydén, H. Lindemann, & J. Brockmeier (Eds.), *Beyond loss: Dementia, identity, personhood* (pp. 137–154). Oxford & New York: Oxford University Press.

Hydén, L.-H., & Brockmeier, J. (2008). From the retold to the performed story: Introduction. In L.-H. Hydén & J. Brockmeier (Eds.), *Health, illness and culture. Broken narratives* (pp. 1–15). New York: Routledge.

Hydén, L.-C., & Öruluv, L. (2010). Interaction and narrative in dementia. In D. Schiffrin, A. De Fina, & A. Nylund (Eds.). *Telling stories: Language, narrative, and social life* (pp. 149–160). Washington, DC: Georgetown University Press.

Hydén, L.-C., Lindemann, H., & Brockmeier, J. (Eds.) (2014). *Beyond loss: Dementia, identity, personhood.* Oxford & New York: Oxford University Press.

Hyvärinen, M. (2008). "Life as narrative" revisited. *Partial Answers, 6*(2), 261–277.

Hyvärinen, M. (2010). Revisiting the narrative turns. *Life Writing, 7*(1), 69–82.

Hyvärinen, M. (2013). Travelling metaphors, transforming concepts. In M. Hatavara, L.-C. Hydén, & M. Hyvärinen (Eds.), *The travelling concepts of narrative* (pp. 13–41). Amsterdam, Netherlands & Philadelphia, PA: John Benjamins

Hyvärinen, M., Hydén, L.-H., Saarenheimo, M., & Tamboukou, M. (Eds.) (2010). *Beyond narrative coherence.* Amsterdam, Netherlands & Philadelphia, PA: John Benjamins.

Ingvar, D. H. (1984). Memory of the future: An essay on the temporal organization of conscious awareness. *Human Neurobiology, 4,* 127–136.

Iser, W. (1993). *The fictive and the imaginary: Charting literary anthropology.* Baltimore, MD: Johns Hopkins University Press.

Jahn, M. (2007). Focalization. In D. Herman (Ed.), *The Cambridge companion to narrative* (pp. 94–108). Cambridge, UK & New York.

Jakobson, R. (1981). *Linguistics and poetics.* In R. Jakobson, *Selected writings, Vol. III: Poetry of Grammar and Grammar of Poetry* (pp. 18–51). The Hague, Paris, New York: Mouton.

James, H. (1985). The art of fiction. In P. D. Murphy & M. J. Hoffman (Eds.), *Essentials of the theory of fiction* (pp. 14–23). Durham, NC: Duke University Press.

James, W. (1981). *The principles of psychology, Vol. 1.* Cambridge, MA: Harvard University Press. (Original work published 1890.)

James, W. (1982). *The varieties of religious experience: A study in human nature.* New York & London: Penguin. (Original work published 1902.)

Jauss, H. R. (1986). *Zeit und Erinnerung in Marcel Prousts* À la recherche du temps perdu [*Time and remembering in Marcel Prousts* À la recherche du temps perdu]. Frankfurt am Main: Suhrkamp.

Jobst, S., & Lüdke, A. (Eds.) (2010). *Unsettling history: Archiving and narrating in historiography.* Frankfurt am Main: Campus.

Johnson, M. K., Raye, C. L., Mitchell, K. J., & Ankudowich, E. (2012). The cognitive neuroscience of true and false memories. In Belli, R. F. (Ed.), *True and false recovered memories: Toward a reconciliation of the debate. Vol. 58: Nebraska Symposium on Motivation* (pp. 15–52). New York: Springer.

Jolly, M. (Ed.) (2001). *Encyclopedia of life writing: Autobiographical and biographical forms, 2 Vols.* London & Chicago, IL: Fitzroy Dearborn.

Joyce, M. (2011). Seeing through the blue nowhere: On narrative transparency and new media. In R. Page & B. Thomas (Eds.), *New narratives: Stories and storytelling in the digital age* (pp. 83–100). Lincoln, NE & London: University of Nebraska Press.

Judt, T. (1998, December 3). À la recherche du temps perdu: On Pierre Nora's "Realms of memory: The construction of the French past." *The New York Review of Books, 45,* 51–58.

Junker, M.-O. (2007). The language of memory in East Cree. In M. Amberber (Ed.), *The language of memory in a cross linguistic perspective* (pp. 235–261). Amsterdam, Netherlands: John Benjamins.

Kandel, E. R., Schwartz, J. H., Jessell, T. M., Siegelbaum, S. A., & Hudspeth, A. J. (Eds.) (2013). *Principles of neural science* (5th ed.). New York: McGraw-Hill.

Kandel, E. R., & Siegelbaum, S. A. (2013). Cellular mechanisms of implicit memory storage and the biological basis of individuality. In E. R. Kandel, J. H. Schwartz,

T. M. Jessell, S. A. Siegelbaum, & A. J. Hudspeth (Eds.), *Principles of neural science* (5th ed.) (pp. 1461–1486). New York: McGraw-Hill.

Kansteiner, W. (2010) Memory, media and *Menschen*: Where is the individual in collective memory studies? *Memory Studies* 3(1), 3–4.

Kakutani, M. (2001, October 26). In a no man's land of memories and loss. *New York Times Book Review*. Retrieved from http://query.nytimes.com/gst/fullpage.html?res=9F07E2DE1331F935A15753C1A9679C8B63

Keen, S. (2007). *Empathy and the novel*. Oxford & New York: Oxford University Press.

Kermode, F. (1983). *The art of telling: Essays on fiction*. Cambridge, MA: Harvard University Press.

Kern, S. (1983). *The culture of time and space 1880–1918*. Cambridge, MA: Harvard University Press.

Kilbourn, R. J. A. (2004). Architecture and cinema: The representation of memory in W. G. Sebald's *Austerlitz*. In J. J. Long & A. Whitehead (Eds.), *W. G. Sebald: A critical companion* (pp. 140–154). Edinburgh, UK: Edinburgh University Press.

Kirschner, S. R., & Martin, J. (Eds.) (2010). *The sociocultural turn in psychology: The contextual emergence of mind and self*. New York: Columbia University Press.

Kittler, F. (1999). *Film, gramophone, typewriter*. Stanford, CA: Stanford University Press.

Klepper, M. (2013). Introduction: Rethinking narrative identity: Persona and perspective. In C. Holler & M. Klepper (Eds.), *Rethinking narrative identity: Persona and perspective* (pp. 1–31). Amsterdam, Netherlands & Philadelphia, PA: John Benjamins.

Klein, S. B., Loftus, J., & Kihlstrom, J. F. (2002). Memory and temporal experience: The effects of episodic memory loss on an amnesic patient's ability to remember the past and imagine the future. *Social Cognition, 20*, 353–379.

Kohler Riessman, C. (2008). *Narrative methods for the human sciences*. Thousand Oaks, CA: Sage.

Kopelman, M. D., Wilson, B., & Baddeley, A. D. (1989). The Autobiographical Memory Interview: A new assessment of autobiographical and personal semantic memory in amnesic patients. *Journal of Clinical and Experimental Neuropsychology, 11*, 724–744.

Kopelman, M. D., Wilson, B.A., & Baddeley, A. D. (1990). *The Autobiographical Memory Interview*. Bury St Edmunds, UK: Thames Valley Test Company.

Korsgaard, C. M. (1996). Personal identity and the unity of agency: A Kantian response to Parfit. In C. M. Korsgaard, *Creating the kingdom of ends* (pp. 363–397). Cambridge, UK & New York: Cambridge University Press.

Koselleck, R. (2004). *Futures past: On the semantics of historical time*. New York: Columbia University Press.

Krog, A. (2005). "I, me, me, mine!": Autobiographical fiction and the "I." *English Academy Review, 22*(1), 100–107.

Lacan, J. (1994). *The seminar, Book XI: The four fundamental concepts of psychoanalysis*. London: Penguin.

LaCapra, D. (1994). *Representing the holocaust: History, theory, trauma*. Ithaca, NY: Cornell University Press.

Lachmann, R. (2008). Mnemotic and intertextual aspects of literature. In A. Erll & A. Nünning (Eds.), *Cultural memory studies* (pp. 301–310). Berlin, Germany & New York: Walter de Gruyter.

Lachmann, R. (1997). *Memory and literature*. Minneapolis, MN: University of Minneapolis Press.

Lakoff, G., & Turner, M. (1989). *More than cool reason: A field guide to poetic metaphor.* Chicago, IL: University of Chicago Press.

Lambeck, M., & Antze, P. (Eds.) (1996a). *Tense past: Cultural essays in trauma and memory.* London: Routledge.

Lambeck, M., & Antze, P. (1996b). Introduction: Forecasting memory. In P. Antze & M. Lambeck (Eds.), *Tense past: Cultural essays in trauma and memory* (pp. xi–xxxviii). London: Routledge.

Landy, J. (2004). *Philosophy as fiction: Self, deception and knowledge in Proust.* Oxford: Oxford University Press.

Larrain, A., & Haye, A. (2012). The discursive nature of inner speech. *Theory and Psychology, 22*(1), 3–22.

Lévinas, E. (1987). *Collected philosophical papers.* Dordrecht, Netherlands & Boston, MA: Nijhoff.

Lewis, B. (2011). *Narrative psychiatry: How stories can shape clinical practice.* Baltimore, MD: Johns Hopkins University Press.

Linde, C. (1993). *Life stories: The creation of coherence.* New York & Oxford: Oxford University Press.

Lindemann Nelson, H. (2001). *Damaged identities, narrative repair.* Ithaca, NY & London: Cornell University Press.

Ling, A. (2009). Chinese American women writers: The tradition behind Maxine Hong Kingston. In H. Bloom (Ed.), *Asian-American writers* (pp. 63–85). New York: Chelsea House.

Ling, A., & Chu, P. P. (1998). Maxine Hong Kingston. In G. J. Leonard (Ed.), *The Asian Pacific American heritage: A companion to literature and arts* (pp. 439–446). New Yoir: Taylor & Francis.

Lloyd, G. (1993). *Being in time: Selves and narrators in philosophy and literature.* London: Routledge.

Locke, J. (2008). *An essay concerning human understanding.* Oxford & New York: Oxford University Press. (Original work published 1690.)

Lodge, D. (2002). Consciousness and the novel. In D. Lodge, *Consciousness and the novel: Connected essays* (pp. 1–99). Cambridge, MA: Harvard University Press.

Loftus, E. F. (1979). The malleability of human memory. *American Scientist, 67,* 312–320.

Loftus, E. F. (1980). *Memory: Surprising new insights into how we remember and why we forget.* Reading, MA: Addison-Wesley.

Loftus, E. F. (1994). *The myth of repressed memory: False memories and allegations of sexual abuse.* New York: St. Martin's Press.

Loftus, E. F., & Loftus, G. R. (1980). On the permanence of storied information in the human brain. *American Psychologist, 35,* 409–420.

Lotman, Yu. M. (1990). *Universe of the mind: A semiotic theory of culture.* Bloomington, IN: Indiana University Press.

Luria, A. R. (1987). *The mind of a mnemonist.* With a foreword by J. S. Bruner. Cambridge, MA: Harvard University Press.

Luria, A. R. (1979). *The making of mind.* M. Cole & S. Cole (Eds.). Cambridge, MA: Harvard University.

MacIntyre, A. C. (2007). *After virtue: A study in moral theory.* Notre Dame, IN: University of Notre Dame Press. (Original work published 1981.)

Mackenzie, C., & Atkins, K. (2008). *Practical identity and narrative agency.* New York & London: Routledge.

Mullally, S. L., & Maguire, E. A. (2014). Memory, imagination, and predicting the future: A common brain mechanism? *The Neuroscientist, 20*(3), 220–234.

Mandler, J. M. (1984). *Stories, scripts, and scenes: Aspects of schema theory*. Hillsdale, NJ: Erlbaum.

Manier, D. (2004). Is memory in the brain? Remembering as social behavior. *Mind, Culture, and Activity, 11*(4), 251–266.

Marsella, A. J., DeVos, G. & Hsu, F. L. K. (Eds.) (1985). *Culture and self: Asian and Western perspectives*. New York: Tavistock.

Martens, L. (2011). *The promise of memory: Childhood recollection and its objects in literary modernism*. Cambridge, MA: Harvard University Press.

Martin, J., & Sugerman, J. (2009). Does interpretation in psychology differ from interpretation in natural science? *Journal for the Theory of Social Behaviour, 39*(1), 19–37.

Mascuch, M. (1996). *Origins of the individualist self: Autobiography and self-identity in England, 1591–1791*. Stanford, CA: Stanford University Press.

Matsuda, M. K. (1990). *The memory of the modern*. New York & Oxford: Oxford University Press.

Matthews, E. (2006). Dementia and the identity of the person. In J. C. Hughes, S. J. Louw, & S. R. Sabat (Eds.), *Dementia: Mind, Meaning, and the Person* (pp. 163–177). Oxford & New York: Oxford University Press.

Matz, J. (2011). The art of time, theory to practice. *Narrative, 19*(3), 273–294.

McAdams, D. (1993). *The stories we live by: Personal myths and the making of the self*. New York: Guilford Press.

McAdams, D. P. (2008). Personal narratives and the life story. In O. John, R. Robins, & L. A. Pervin (Eds.), *Handbook of personality: Theory and research* (pp. 241–261). New York: Guilford Press.

McCrone, J. (2004, February 8). Reasons to forget. *The Times Literary Supplement, 5290*, 3–4.

McDermott, K. B., Szpunar, K. K., & Arnold, K. M. (2011). Similarities in episodic future thought and remembering: The importance of contextual setting. In M. Bar (Ed.), *Predictions in the brain: Using our past to generate a future* (pp. 83–94). Oxford & New York: Oxford University Press.

McEwan, I. (2005). *Saturday*. London: Jonathan Cape.

McEwan, I. (2012, March 23). The originality of the species. *The Guardian*, Books (Online edition). Retrieved from http://www.theguardian.com/books/2012/mar/23/originality-of-species-ian-mcewan.

McGinn, C. (2004). *Mindsight: Image, dream, meaning*. Cambridge, MA: Harvard University Press.

McLean, K. C. (2008). The emergence of narrative identity. *Social and Personality Psychology Compass, 2*, 1685–1702.

McLean, K. C., & Pasupathi, M. (Eds.) (2010). *Narrative development in adolescence: Creating the storied self*. New York: Springer.

McLean, K. C., & Pasupathi, M. (2011). Old, new, borrowed, and blue? The emergence and retention of meaning in autobiographical storytelling. *Journal of Personality, 79*(1), 135–163.

McQuire, S. (1998). *Visions of modernity: Representation, memory, time and space in the age of the camera*. London: Sage.

McTaggart, J. M. E. (1908). The unreality of time. *Mind, 17*, 457–473.

Mead, G. H. (1934). *Mind, self, and society from the standpoint of a social behaviorist*. Chicago, IL: The University of Chicago Press.

Medved, M. I., & Brockmeier, J. (2004). Making sense of traumatic experiences: Telling your life with Fragile X syndrome. *Qualitative Health Research*, *14*(6), 741–759.

Medved, M. I., & Brockmeier, J. (2008). Continuity amid chaos: Neurotrauma, loss of memory, and sense of self. *Qualitative Health Research*, *18*(4), 469–479.

Medved, M. I., & Brockmeier, J. (2010). Weird stories: Brain, mind, and self. In M. Hyvärinen, L.-H. Hydén, M. Saarenheimo, & M. Tamboukou (Eds.), *Beyond narrative coherence* (pp. 17–32). Amsterdam, Netherlands & Philadelphia, PA: John Benjamins.

Medved, M. I., & Brockmeier, J. (2015). When memory goes awry. In A. L. Tota & T. Hagen (Eds.), *The Routledge international handbook of memory studies* (pp. 268–284). London: Routledge.

Menary, R. (Ed.) (2010). *The extended mind*. Cambridge, MA: MIT Press.

Meretoja, H. (2013). Philosophical underpinnings of the narrative turn in theory and fiction. In M. Hatavara, L.-C. Hydén, & M. Hyvärinen (Eds.), *The traveling concepts of narrative* (pp. 93–118). Amsterdam, Netherlands & Philadelphia, PA: John Benjamins.

Meretoja, H. (2014a). Narrative and human existence: Ontology, epistemology and ethics. *New Literary History*, *45*(1), 89–109.

Meretoja, H. (2014b). *The narrative turn in fiction and theory: The crisis and return of storytelling from Robbe-Grillet to Tournier*. Basingstoke, UK: Palgrave Macmillan.

Michaelian, K. (2010). Is memory a natural kind? *Memory Studies*, *4*(2), 170–189.

Middleton, D., & Brown, S. D. (2005). *The social psychology of experience: Studies in remembering and forgetting*. London: Sage.

Middleton, D., & Edwards, D. (Eds.) (1990a). *Collective remembering*. London: Sage.

Middleton, D., & Edwards, D. (1990b). Introduction. In D. Middleton & E. Edwards (Eds.), *Collective remembering* (pp. 1–21). London: Sage.

Middleton, D., & Edwards, D. (1990c). Conversational remembering. In D. Middleton & E. Edwards (Eds.) *Collective remembering* (pp. 22–45). London: Sage.

Mildorf, J. (2010). Narratology and the social sciences. In J. Alber & M. Fludernik (Eds.), *Postclassical narratology: Approaches and analyses* (pp. 234–251). Columbus, OH: Ohio State University Press.

Mildorf, J. (2012). Second-person narration in literary and conversational storytelling. *Storyworlds: A Journal of Narrative Studies*, *4*, 75–98.

Minami, M. (2000). The relationship between narrative identity and culture: Commentary on Jens Brockmeier's "Autobiographical time." *Narrative Inquiry*, *10*(1), 75–80.

Misch, G. (1950). *A history of autobiography in Antiquity, 2 vols*. London: Routledge & Paul.

Misch, G. (1985). *Geschichte der Autobiographie, 4 vols. in 8 books* (2nd ed.). Frankfurt am Main: Klostermann.

Mitchell, W. J. T. (1994). *Picture theory: Essays on verbal and visual representation*. Chicago, IL: University of Chicago Press.

Montaigne, M. de (1993). *The complete essays*. London: Penguin. (Original work published 1580.)

Moore, C., & Lemmon, K. (Eds.) (2001). *The self in time: Developmental perspectives*. Mahwah, NJ: Erlbaum.

Moulin, C. J. A. (Ed.) (2011). *Models of memory and memory systems (Human memory, Vol. 2)*. Los Angeles, LA: Sage.

Mühlhäusler, P., & Harré, R. (1990). *Pronouns and people: The linguistic construction of social and personal identity*. Oxford: Blackwell.

Müller, G. (1968). *Morphologische Poetik: Gesammelte Aufsätze*. Darmstadt, Germany: Wissenschaftliche Buchgesellschaft.

Munn, N. (1992). The cultural anthropology of time: A critical essay. *Annual Review of Anthropology, 21*, 93–123.

Munn, N. (1995). An essay in the symbolic construction of memory in the Katuli "Gisalo." In D. de Coppet & A. Iteanu (Eds.), *Cosmos and society in Oceania* (pp. 83–104). Oxford: Berg.

Murakami, K. (2012). Time for memory: Beyond spatial metaphors. *Culture and Psychology, 18*(3), 3–13.

Murakami, K. (2014). Commemoration reconsidered: Second World War veterans' reunion as pilgrimage. *Memory Studies, 7*(3), 339–353.

Muscuch, M. (1996). *Origins of the individual self: Autobiography and self-identity in England, 1591–1791*. Stanford, CA: Stanford University Press.

Nahin, P. J. (2001). *Time machines. Time travel in physics, metaphysics, and science fiction*. New York: Springer.

Nalbantian, S. (2003). *Memory in literature: From Rousseau to neuroscience*. Basingstoke, UK: Palgrave Macmillan.

Nalbantian, S., Matthews, P. M., & McClelland, J. L. (Eds.) (2011). *The memory process: Neuroscientific and humanistic perspectives*. Cambridge, MA: MIT Press.

Namer, G. (2000). *Halbwachs e la mémoire sociale*. Paris: L'Harmattan.

Nehamas, A. (1985). *Nietzsche: Life as literature*. Cambridge, MA: Harvard University Press.

Neisser, U. (1967). *Cognitive psychology*. New York: Appleton Century Crofts.

Neisser, U., & Winograd, E. (Eds.) (1988). *Remembering reconsidered: Ecological and traditional approaches to the study of memory*. New York: Cambridge University Press.

Nelson, K. (1996). *Language in cognitive development: The emergence of the mediated mind*. New York: Cambridge University Press.

Nelson, K. (2006). Development of representation in childhood. In E. Blaystock & F. I. M. Craik (Eds.), *Lifespan cognition* (pp. 178–192). Oxford & New York: Oxford University Press.

Nelson, K. (2007a). *Young minds in social worlds: Experience, meaning, and memory*. Cambridge, MA: Harvard University Press.

Nelson, K. (2007b). Developing past and future selves for time travel narratives. *Behavioral and Brain Sciences, 30*, 327–328.

Nelson, K. (Ed.) (1989). *Narratives from the crib*. Cambridge, MA: Harvard University Press.

Niiya, B. (1999). Asian American autobiographical tradition. In G. J. Leonard (Ed.), *The Asian American heritage: A companion to literature and the arts* (pp. 427–434). London & New York: Garland.

Nora, P. (1989). Between memory and history: Les lieux de mémoire. *Representations, 26*, 7–25.

Nora, P. (Eds.) (1996–1998). *Realms of memory: Rethinking the French past, 3 vol*. New York: Columbia University Press.

Norrick, N. R. (2000). *Conversational narrative: Storytelling in everyday talk*. Amsterdam, Netherlands & Philadelphia, PA: John Benjamins.

Norrick, N. R. (2007). Conversational storytelling. In D. Herman (Ed.), *The Cambridge companion to narrative* (pp. 127–141). Cambridge, UK & New York: Cambridge University Press.

Nowotny, H. (1994). *Time: The modern and the postmodern experience*. Cambridge, UK: Polity Press.

Nünning, A., Gymnich, M., & Sommer, R. (Eds.). *Literature and memory: Theoretical paradigms, genres, functions*. Tübingen, Germany: Narr.

Nyberg, L., Kim, A. S. N., Habib, R., Levine, B., & Tulving, E. (2010). Consciousness of subjective time in the brain. *Proceedings of the National Academy of Sciences of the United States of America, 107*(51), 22356–22359.

Oatley, K. (2007). Narrative modes of consciousness and selfhood. In P. D. Zelazo, M. Moscovitch & E. Thompson (Eds.), *The Cambridge handbook of consciousness* (pp. 375–402). New York: Cambridge University Press.

Oatley, K. (2008). The mind's flight simulator. *The Psychologist, 21*, 1030–1032.

Oatley, K. (2011). *Such stuff as dreams: The psychology of fiction*. Malden, MA & Oxford, UK: Wiley-Blackwell.

Oatley, K. (2012). *The passionate muse: Exploring emotion in stories*. Oxford & New York: Oxford University Press.

Oatley, K., & Djikic, M. (2008). Writing as thinking. *Review of General Psychology, 12*(1), 9–27.

Ochs, E., & Capps, L. (2001). *Living narrative: Creating lives in everyday storytelling*. Cambridge, MA: Harvard University Press.

Olick, J. K. (2003). *States of memory: Continuities, conflicts, and transformations in national retrospection*. Durham, NC: Duke University Press.

Olick, J. K. (2008a). Collective memories: A memoire and prospect. *Memory Studies, 1*, 23–29.

Olick, J. K. (2008b). From collective memory to the sociology of mnemotic practices and products. In A. Erll & A. Nünning (Eds.), *Cultural Memory Studies: An International and Interdisciplinary Handbook* (pp. 151–161). Berlin & New York: de Gruyter.

Olick, J. K. (2011). Collective memory: The two cultures. In J. K. Olick, V. Vinitzky-Seroussi, & D. Levy (Eds.), *The collective memory reader* (pp. 225–228). Oxford: Oxford University Press.

Olick, J. K., Vinitzky-Seroussi, V., & Levy, D. (Eds.) (2011). *The collective memory reader*. Oxford: Oxford University Press.

Olick, J. K., Vinitzky-Seroussi, V., & Levy, D. (2014). Response to our critics. *Memory Studies, 7*(1), 131–138.

Olney, J. (1998). *Memory and narrative: The weave of life-writing*. Chicago, IL: University of Chicago Press.

Olson, D. R. (1994). *The world on paper*. Cambridge, UK: Cambridge University Press.

Olson, D. R. (2001). What writing is. *Pragmatics and Cognition, 9*, 239–258.

Olson, D. R. (2006). The documentary tradition in mind and society. In D. R. Olson & M. Cole (Eds.), Technology, literacy, and the evolution of society: Implications of the work of Jack Goody (pp. 289–303). Mahwah, NJ: Erlbaum.

Ondaatje, M. (2007). *Devisadero*. Toronto, ON: McClelland & Steward.

Page, R. (2013). Seriality and storytelling in social media. *Storyworlds: A Journal of Narrative Studies, 5*, 31–54.

Page, R., & Thomas, B. (Eds.) (2011). *New narratives: Stories and storytelling in the digital age*. Lincoln & London: University of Nebraska Press.

Painter, G. D. (1977). *Marcel Proust: A biography*. Harmondsworth, UK: Penguin.

Palmer, A. (2004). *Fictional minds*. Lincoln, NE: University of Nebraska Press.

Palmer, A. (2010). Social minds in the novel. Columbus, OH: Ohio State University Press.

Palmer, A. (2011). Social minds in fiction and criticism. *Style, 45*(2), 196–240.

Pane, S. (2005). Trauma obscura: Photographic media in W. G. Sebald's *Austerlitz*. *Mosaic: A Journal for the Interdisciplinary Study of Literature, 38*(1), 37–55.

Parfit, D. (1984). *Reasons and persons*. Oxford: Clarendon Press.

Peirce, C. S. (1992). *The essential Peirce. Selected philosophical writings. Vol. 2*. Bloomington, IN: Indiana University Press.

Pentzold, C. (2009). Fixing the floating gap: The online encyclopedia Wikipedia as a global memory place. *Memory Studies, 2*, 255–272.

Petrelli, D., Whittaker, S., & Brockmeier, J. (2008). AutoTopography: What can physical mementos tells us about digital memories? In *The balance between art and science: Human computer interaction 2008: Stories and memories* (pp. 53–62): Proceeding of the twenty-sixth annual SIGCHI conference on human factors in computing systems. doi: acm.org/10.1145/1357054.1357065

Phelan, J. (2005). *Living to tell about it: A rhetoric and ethics of character narration*. Ithaca, NY: Cornell University Press.

Phelan, J., & Booth, W. G. (2005). Narrator. In D. Herman, M. Jahn, & M.-L. Ryan (Eds.), *Routledge encyclopedia of narrative theory* (pp. 388–392). London & New York: Routledge.

Piaget, J. (1969). *The child's conception of time*. New York: Basic Books.

Pillemer, D. B. (1998). *Momentous events, vivid memories: How unforgettable moments help us understand the meaning of our lives*. Cambridge, MA: Harvard University Press.

Pillemer, D. B., & White, S. H. (1989). Childhood events recalled by children and adults. *Advances in Child Development and Behavior, 21*, 297–340.

Pipa, G. (2010, February 24). Our brain plays jazz. Talk given at the Redwood Center for Theoretical Neuroscience at the University of California, Berkeley.

Plato. (1921). *Theaetetus. Sophist* (Loeb Classical Library Vol. 7). Cambridge, MA: Harvard University Press.

Polkinghorne, D. E. (1988). *Narrative knowing and the human sciences*. Albany, NY: State University of New York Press.

Polkinghorne, D. (2004). Ricoeur, narrative and personal identity. In C. Lightfoot, C. Lalonde, & M. Chandler (Eds.), *Changing conceptions of psychological life* (pp. 27–48). Mahwah, NJ: Erlbaum.

Prebble, S. C., Addis, D. R., & Tippett, L. J. (2013). Autobiographical memory and sense of self. *Psychological Bulletin, 139*(4), 815–840.

Prentice, C., Devadas, V., & Johnson, H. (Eds.) (2010). *Cultural transformations: Perspectives on translocations in a global age*. Amsterdam, Netherlands: Rodopi.

Proust, M. (1983). *Remembrance of things past*. 3 vols. Harmondsworth, UK: Penguin. (Original work published 1913–1927.)

Radstone, S., & Schwarz, B. (Eds.) (2010). *Memory: Histories, theories, debates*. New York: Fordham University Press.

Randall, W. L. (2007). From computer to compost: Rethinking our metaphors for memory. *Theory and Psychology, 17*(5), 611–633.

Randall, W. L. (2010). The narrative complexity of our past: In praise of memory's sins. *Theory & Psychology, 20*(2), 147–169.

Randall, W. L. (2011). Memory, metaphor, and meaning: Reading for wisdom in the stories of our lives. In G. Kenyon, E. Bohlmeijer, & W. L. Randall (Eds.), *Storying later life. Issues, investigations, and interventions in narrative gerontology* (pp. 20–38). Oxford & New York: Oxford University Press.

Randall, W. L., & McKim, E. (2008). *Reading our lives: The poetics of growing old*. Oxford & New York: Oxford University Press.

Rasmussen, S. J. (2012). Cultural anthropology. In J. Valsiner (Ed.), *Oxford hand-book of culture and psychology* (pp. 96–115). Oxford & New York: Oxford University Press.

Richardson, B. (1987). Time is out of joint: Narrative models and the temporality of the drama. *Poetics Today*, *8*, 299–309.

Richardson, B. (2006). *Unnatural voices: Extreme narration in modern and postmodern contemporary fiction*. Columbus, OH: Ohio State University Press.

Ricoeur, P. (1980). Narrative time. [Special issue: "On narrative"] *Critical Inquiry*, 7(1), 169–190.

Ricoeur, P. (1981). The narrative function. In P. Ricoeur, *Hermeneutics and the human sciences* (pp. 274–296). Cambridge, UK: Cambridge University Press.

Ricoeur, P. (1984, 1985, 1988). *Time and narrative, Vols. 1-3*. Chicago, IL: University of Chicago Press.

Ricoeur, P. (1991a). Life in quest of narrative. In D. Wood (Ed.), On *Paul Ricoeur: Narrative and interpretation* (pp. 20–33). London: Routledge.

Ricoeur, P. (1991b). Narrative identity (D. Wood, Trans). In D. Wood (Ed.), *On Paul Ricoeur: Narrative and interpretation* (pp. 188–199). London: Routledge.

Ricoeur, P. (1991c). Narrative identity (M. S. Muldoon, Trans.). *Philosophy Today*, 35(1), 73–81.

Ricoeur, P. (1992). *Oneself as another*. Chicago, IL: University of Chicago Press.

Ricoeur, P. (2003). *The rule of metaphor*. London: Routledge. (First English edition, 1977).

Ritivoi, A. D. (2002). *Yesterday's self: Nostalgia and the immigrant identity*. Lanham, MD: Rowman and Littlefield.

Ritivoi, A. D. (2006). *Paul Ricoeur: Tradition and innovation in rhetorical theory*. Albany, NY: State University of New York Press.

Ritivoi, A. D. (2009). Explaining people: Narrative and the study of identity. *Storyworlds: A Journal of Narrative Studies*, *1*, 25–41.

Roberts, G. (Ed.) (2001). *The history and narrative reader*. London & New York: Routledge.

Roberts, R. (2010). *Conversations with Ian McEwan*. Jackson, MS: University Press of Mississippi.

Roediger, H. L., Dudai, Y., & Fitzpatrick, S. M. (Eds.) (2007). *Science of memory: Concepts*. Oxford: Oxford University Press.

Roediger, H. L., & DeSoto, K. A. (2015). The psychology of reconstructive memory. In J. Wright (Ed.), *The international encyclopedia of the social and behavioral sciences* (2nd ed.). Oxford: Elsevier. Retrieved from http://psych.wustl.edu/memory/Roddy%20article%20PDF's/BC_Roediger %20&%20DeSoto%20(in%20press).pdf

Rorty, R. (1979). *Philosophy and the mirror of nature*. Princeton, NJ: Princeton University Press.

Rorty, R. (1989). *Contingency, irony, and solidarity*. Cambridge, UK: Cambridge University Press.

Rorty, R. (1990). Pragmatism as anti-representationalism. In J. P. Murphy (Ed.), *Pragmatism: From Peirce to Davidson* (pp. 1–6). Boulder, CO: Westview Press.

Rorty, R. (2004). Being that can be understood is language. In B. Krajewski (Ed.), *Gadamer's repercussions* (pp. 21–29). Los Angeles, LA: University of California Press.

Rorty, R. (2005). A queasy agnosticism. Review of McEwan's "Saturday," *Dissent*, Fall. Retrieved from http://www.dissentmagazine.org/article/?article=191

Rose, D. (2014). *Enchanted objects: Design, human desire, and the internet of things.* New York: Scribner.

Rose, S. (2006). *The 21st-century brain: Explaining, mending and manipulating the mind.* London: Vintage.

Rose, S. (2010). Memories are made of this. In S. Radstone & B. Schwarz (Eds.), *Memory: Histories, theories, debates* (pp. 198–208). New York: Fordham University Press.

Rosner, J. (2007). (Ed.). *The messy self.* Boulder, CO & London: Paradigm.

Rossi, P. (1991). *Il passato, la memoria, l'oblio* [Past, memory, and forgetting] Bologna, Italy: Molino.

Rossington, M., & Whitehead, A. (Eds.) (2007). *Theories of memory.* Baltimore, MD: Johns Hopkins University Press.

Rubin, D. C. (1996). *Remembering our past: Studies in autobiographical memory.* Cambridge, UK: Cambridge University Press.

Rubin, D. C. (1998). Beginnings of a theory of autobiographical remembering. In C. P. Thompson, D. J. Herrmann, D. Bruce, J. D. Reed, D. G. Payne, & M. P. Toglia (Eds.), *Autobiographical memory: Theoretical and applied perspectives* (pp. 47–67). Mahwah, NJ: Erlbaum.

Rubin, D. C. (2005). A basic-systems approach to autobiographical memory. *Current Directions in Psychological Science, 14*(2), 79–83.

Rubin, D. C. (2006). The basic-systems model of episodic memory. *Perspectives on Psychological Science, 1*(4), 277–311.

Rubin, D. C. (Ed.) (1986). *Autobiographical memory.* Cambridge, UK & New York: University Press.

Rubin, D. C. (Ed.) (1996). *Remembering our Past: Studies in Autobiographical Memory.* Cambridge & New York: University Press.

Rubin, D. C. (2012). The basic system model of autobiographical memory. In D. Berntsen & D. C. Rubin (Eds.), *Understanding autobiographical memory: Theories and approaches* (pp. 11–31). Cambridge, UK: Cambridge University Press.

Rubin, D. C., & Greenberg, D. L. (2003). The role of narrative in recollection: A view from cognitive and neuropsychology. In G. Fireman, T. McVay, & O. Flanagan (Eds.), *Narrative and consciousness: Literature, psychology, and the brain* (pp. 53–85). Oxford & New York: Oxford University Press.

Rudd, A. (2009). In defense of narrative. *European Journal of Philosophy, 17*(1), 60–75.

Rumelhart, D. E. (1975). Notes on a schema for stories. In D. G. Bobrow & A. Collins (Eds.), Representation and understanding: Studies in cognitive science (pp. 211–236). New York: Academic Press.

Ryan, M.-L. (2007). Toward a definition of narrative. In D. Herman (Ed.), *The Cambridge companion to narrative* (pp. 22–35). Cambridge, UK: Cambridge University Press.

Ryan, M.-L. (2009). From narrative games to playable stories: Toward a poetic of interactive narrative. *Storyworlds: A Journal of Narrative Studies, 1,* 43–59.

Sacks, H. (1992). *Lectures on conversation.* Oxford: Basil Blackwell.

Sacks, O. (2013, February 21). Speak, memory. *The New York Review of Books, 60*(3), 19–21.

Salutin, R. (1995, March 21). Reservations about a worthy project. *The Globe and Mail,* p. 12.

Sarbin, T. R. (1986). The narrative as root metaphor for psychology. In T. R. Sarbin (Ed.), *Narrative psychology: The storied nature of human conduct* (pp. 3–21). New York: Praeger.

Sarbin, T. R. (1998). Believed-in imaginings: A narrative approach. In J. de Riviera & T. R. Sarbin (Eds.), *Believed-in imaginings: The narrative construction of reality* (pp. 15–30). Washington, DC: American Psychological Association.

Sarbin, T. R. (2000). Worldmaking, self and identity. *Culture & Psychology, 6*, 253–258.

Sartwell, C. (2000). *End of story: Toward an annihilation of language and history*. Albany, NY: State University of New York Press.

Sample, I. (2007, February 7). The brain scan that can read people's intentions: Call for ethical debate over possible use of new technology in interrogation. *The Guardian*, pp. 1–2.

Sato, G. K. (2005). Asian American history: War, memory, and representation. In G. Huang (Ed.), *Asian American literary studies* (pp. 15–40). Edinburgh, UK: Edinburgh University Press.

Saunders, M. (2008). Life-writing, cultural memory, and literary studies. In A. Erll & A. Nünning (Eds.), *Cultural memory studies: An international and interdisciplinary handbook* (pp. 321–331). Berlin, Germany & New York: de Gruyter.

Saunders, M. (2010). *Self-impression: Life-writing, autobiographiction and the forms of modern literature*. Oxford & New York: Oxford University Press.

Schacter, D. L. (1990). Perceptual representation systems and implicit memory: Toward a resolution of the multiple memory systems debate. *Annals of the New York Academy of Sciences, 608 (The development and neural bases of higher cognitive functions)*, 543–571.

Schacter, D. L. (1995). Memory distortion: History and present status. In D. L. Schacter, J. T. Coyle, G. D. Fischbach, M. M. Mesulam, & L. E. Sullivan (Eds.), *Memory distortion: How minds, brains and societies reconstruct the past* (pp. 1–43). Cambridge, MA: Harvard University Press.

Schacter, D. L. (1996). *Searching for memory: The brain, the mind, and the past*. New York: Basic Books.

Schacter, D. L. (2001). *The seven sins of memory: How the mind forgets and remembers*. Boston, MA: Houghton Mifflin.

Schacter, D. L., & Addis, D. R. (2007). The cognitive neuroscience of constructive memory: Remembering the past and imagining the future. *Philosophical Transactions of the Royal Society (B), 362*, 773–786.

Schacter, D. L, Addis, D. R., & Buckner, R. L. (2008). Episodic simulation of future events: Concepts, data, and applications. *The Year in Cognitive Neuroscience, Annals of the New York Academy of Sciences, 1124*, 39–60.

Schacter, D. L., Addis, D. R., Hassabis, D., Martin, V. C., Spreng, R. N., & Szpunar, K. K. (2012). The future of memory: Remembering, imagining, and the brain. *Neuron, 76*, 677–694.

Schacter, D. L., Benoit, R. G., De Brigard, F., & Szpunar, K. K. (2015). Episodic future thinking and episodic counterfactual thinking: Intersections between memory and decisions. *Neurobiology of Learning and Memory, 117*, 14–21.

Schacter, D. L., Guerin, S. A., & St. Jacques, P. L. (2011). Memory distortion: An adaptive perspective. *Trends in Cognitive Sciences, 15*, 467–474.

Schacter, D. L., & Tulving, E. (1994). What are the memory systems of 1994? In D. L. Schacter & E. Tulving (Eds.), *Memory systems* (pp. 1–38). Cambridge, MA: MIT Press.

Schacter, D. L., & Wagner, D. (2013). Learning and memory. In E. R. Kandel, J. H. Schwartz, T. M. Jessell, S. A. Siegelbaum, & A. J. Hudspeth (Eds.), *Principles of neural science* (5th ed.) (pp. 1441–1460). New York: McGraw-Hill.

Schapp, W. (1954). *In Geschichten verstrickt: Zum Sein von Mensch und Ding* [Entangled in stories: On the being of Man and thing] (4th ed., 2004). Frankfurt am Main: Klostermann.

Schiff, B. (2012). The function of narrative: Toward a narrative psychology of meaning. *Narrative Works, 2*(1), 33–47. Retrieved from http://journals.hil.unb.ca/index.php/NW/article/view/19497/21063

Schiff, B. (2013). Fractured narratives: Psychology's fragmented narrative psychology. In M. Hatavara, L.-C. Hydén, & M. Hyvärinen, (Eds.), *The travelling metaphor of narrative* (pp. 245–264). Amsterdam, Netherlands & Philadelphia, PA: John Benjamins.

Schraube, E. (2013). First-person perspective and sociomaterial decentering: Studying technology from the standpoint of the subject. *Subjectivity, 6*(1), pp. 12–32.

Sebald, W. G. (1990). Jean Améry und Primo Levi. In I. Heidelberger-Leonard (Ed.), *Über Jean Améry* (pp. 24–35). Heidelberg, Germany: Winter.

Sebald, W. G. (1993, April 19). Wildes Denken. Interview with Siegrid Löffler. *Profil*, 48–52.

Sebald, W. G. (1998). *The rings of Saturn*. London: The Harvill Press. (Original work published 1995.)

Sebald, W. G. (2001a). *Austerlitz*. New York: Random House. (Original work published 2001.)

Sebald, W. G. (2001b, December 3). Ich fürchte das Melodramatische. An Interview. *Der Spiegel, 11*, 228–34.

Sell, R. D. (2000). *Literature as communication*. Amsterdam, Netherlands & Philadelphia, PA: John Benjamins.

Shattuck, R. (1962). *Proust's binoculars: A study of memory, time and imagination in À la recherche du temps perdu*. New York: Random House.

Shen, D. (2002). Defence and challenge: Reflections on the relation between story and discourse. *Narrative, 10*(3), 222–234.

Sider, G. M., & Smith, G. A. (1997). *Between history and histories: The making of silences and commemorations*. Toronto, ON: University of Toronto Press.

Silverman, M. (2013). *Palimpsestic memory: The Holocaust and colonialism in French and Francophone fiction and film*. New York & Oxford: Berghahn.

Simmel, G. (1903). Die Großstädte und das Geistesleben [The metropolis and mental life]. In T. Petermann (Ed.), *Die Großstadt*. Jahrbuch der Gehe-Stiftung, Bd. 9 (pp. 185–206). Dresden, Germany: v. Zahn & Jaensch [English translation in K. Wolff (Ed.), *The Sociology of Georg Simmel*. New York: Free Press, 1964].

Simmel, G. (1971). The metropolis and mental life. In D. N. Levine (Ed.), *On individuality and social forms*. Chicago, IL: University of Chicago Press, 1971.

Singer, J. A., & Salovey, P. (1993). *The remembered self: Emotions and memory in personality*. New York: The Free Press.

Singer, W. (2005). The brain—An orchestra without a conductor. *MaxPlanckResearch, 3*, pp. 14–18.

Singer, W. (2007). Understanding the brain. *European Molecular Biology Organization Reports, 8*, 16–19.

Singer, W. (2009). The brain, a complex self-organizing system. *European Review 17*(2), 321–329.

Sklar, H. (2012). Narrative empowerment through comics storytelling: Facilitating the life stories of the intellectually disabled. *Storyworlds: A Journal of Narrative Studies 4*, 123–149.

Skowronski, J. J., Walker, R. W., & Betz, A. L. (2004). Who was I when that happened? The timekeeping self in autobiographical memory (pp. 183–206). In D. R. Beike, J. M. Lampinen, & D. A. Behrend (Eds.), *The self and memory*. New York: Psychology Press.

Smith, B., & Sparkes, A. C. (2008). Changing bodies, changing narratives and the consequences of tellability: A case study of becoming disabled through sport. *Sociology of Health & Illness, 30*(2), 217–236.

Smith, S., & Watson, J. (2010). *Reading autobiography: A guide for interpreting life narratives.* Minneapolis, MN: University of Minnesota Press.

Smith, S. (1991). Maxine Hong Kingston's Woman Warrior: Filiality and woman's autobiographical storytelling. In R. R. Warhol and D. Price Herndl (Eds.), *Feminisms: An anthology of literary theory and criticism* (pp. 1058–1078). New Brunswick, NJ: Rutgers University Press.

Snell, B. (1982). *The discovery of the mind: The Greek origins of European thought.* New York: Dover.

Sontag, S. (2000, February 25). A mind in mourning. W. G. Sebald's travels in search of some remnant of the past. *The Times Literary Supplement, 5056,* 3–5.

Sparkes, A. C., & Smith, B. (2008). Men, spinal cord injury, memories, and the narrative performance of pain. *Disability & Society, 23*(7), 679–690.

Sparkes, A. C., & Smith, B. (2012). Narrative analysis as an embodied engagement with the lives of others. In J. A. Holstein & J. F. Gubrium (Eds.), *Varieties of narrative analysis* (pp. 53–73). London: Sage.

Spreng, R. N., Mar, R. A., & Kim, A. S. (2009). The common neural basis of autobiographical memory, prospection, navigation, theory of mind and the default mode: A quantitative meta-analysis. *Journal of Cognitive Neuroscience, 21,* 489–510.

Squire, L. R. (2004). Memory systems of the brain: A brief history and current perspective. *Neurobiology of Learning and Memory, 82,* 171–177.

Stam, H. (Ed.) (2010). Self and dialogue [Special issue]. *Theory and Psychology, 20*(3), 299–463.

Staley, W. (2013, October 20). The incredible factory of frites. *The New York Times Magazine,* pp. 42–48.

Steedman, C. (2009). Literacy, reading, and concepts of the self. In D. R. Olson & N. Torrance (Eds.), *The Cambridge handbook of literacy* (pp. 221–241). Cambridge, UK: Cambridge University Press.

Stone, C. B., Coman, A., Brown, A. D., Koppel, J., & Hirst, W. (2012). Toward a science of silence: The consequences of leaving a memory unsaid. *Perspectives on Psychological Science, 7*(1), 39–53.

Straub, J. (2005). Telling stories, making history. In J. Straub (Ed.), *Narration, identity, and historical consciousness* (pp. 44–98). New York: Gerghan.

Straub, J. (2008). Psychology, narrative, and cultural memory: Past and present. In A. Erll & A. Nünning (Eds.), *Cultural memory studies: An international and interdisciplinary handbook* (pp. 215–228). Berlin & New York: de Gruyter.

Strawson, G. (2004). Against narrativity. *Ratio, 17*(4), 428–452.

Strawson, G. (2011). *Locke on personal identity: Consciousness and concernment.* Princeton, NJ: Princeton University Press.

Suddendorf, T., & Corballis, M. C. (2007). The evolution of foresight: What is mental time travel, and is it unique to humans? *Behavioral and Brain Sciences, 30,* 299–351.

Suddendorf, T., Addis, D. R., & Corballis, M. C. (2011). Mental time travel and the shaping of the human mind. In M. Bar (Ed.), *Predictions in the brain: Using our past to generate a future* (pp. 344–354). Oxford & New York: Oxford University Press.

Summit, J. (2008). *Memory's Library: Medieval books in early modern England.* Chicago, IL: University of Chicago Press.

Sutton, J. (2009). Looking beyond memory studies: Comparisons and integrations. *Memory Studies, 2*(3), 299.

Sutton, J., Harris, C. B., Keil, P. G., & Barnier, A. J. (2010). The psychology of memory, extended cognition, and socially distributed remembering. *Phenomenology and the Cognitive Sciences, 9*(4), 521–560.

Svoboda, E., McKinnon, M. C., Levine, B. (2006). The functional neuroanatomy of autobiographical memory: A meta-analysis. *Neuropsychologica, 44*, 2189–2208.

Szondi, P. (2006). Hope in the past. In W. Benjamin, *Berliner childhood around 1900* (pp. 1–33). Cambridge, MA: Harvard University Press. (Original work published 1961.)

Szpunar, K. K. (2010). Episodic future thought: An emerging concept. *Perspectives on Psychological Science, 5*, 142–162.

Szpunar, K. K., Addis, D. R., McLelland, V. C., & Schacter, D. L. (2013). Memories of the future. New insights into the adaptive value of episodic memory. *Frontiers in Behavioral Neuroscience, 7*, Article 47.

Szpunar, K. K., Chan, J. C. K., & McDermott, K. B. (2009). Contextual processing in episodic future thought. *Cerebral Cortex, 19*, 1539–1548.

Szpunar, K. K., & Tulving, E. (2011). Varieties of future experience. In M. Bar (Ed.), *Predictions in the brain: Using our past to generate a future* (pp. 3–12). Oxford & New York: Oxford University Press.

Szymborska, W. (1998). *Poems, new and collected, 1957–1997.* New York: Harcourt Brace.

Tadié, J.-Y. (2000). *Marcel Proust.* New York: Viking. (Original work published 1996.)

Taylor, C. (1985a). *Philosophy and the human sciences: Philosophical papers 2.* Cambridge, UK: Cambridge University Press.

Taylor, C. (1985b). Self-interpreting animals. In C. Taylor, *Human agency and language: Philosophical papers 1* (pp. 45–76). Cambridge, UK: Cambridge University Press.

Taylor, C. (1985c). *Human agency and language: Philosophical papers 1.* Cambridge, UK: Cambridge University Press.

Taylor, C. (1989). *Sources of the self: The making of the modern identity.* Cambridge, UK: Cambridge University Press

Taylor, C. (2003). *Modern social imaginaries.* Durham, NC & London: Duke University.

Taylor, S. (2010). *Narratives of identity and place.* London & New York: Routledge.

Terdiman, R. (1993). *Present past: Modernity and the memory crisis.* Ithaca, NY: Cornell University Press

Terdiman, R. (2010). Memory in Freud. In S. Radstone & B. Schwarz (Eds.), *Memory: Histories, theories, debates* (pp. 93–108). New York: Fordham University Press.

Thomas, K. (2009). *The ends of life: Roads to fulfillment in early modern England.* Oxford: Oxford University Press.

Thomas, R. (1992). *Literacy and orality in Ancient Greece.* Cambridge, UK: Cambridge University Press.

Thomas, R. (2009). The origins of Western literacy: Literacy in Ancient Greece and Rome. In D. R. Olson, & N. Torrance (Eds.), *The Cambridge handbook of literacy* (pp. 346–361). Cambridge, UK & New York: Cambridge University Press.

Thorne, A., & McLean, K. C. (2003). Telling traumatic events in adolescence: A study of master narrative positioning. In R. Fivush & C. Haden (Eds.), *Autobiographical memory and the construction of a narrative self: Developmental and cultural perspectives* (pp. 169–185). Mahwah, NJ: Erlbaum.

Tóibín, C. (2006, November 30). A thousand prayers. *New York Review of Books, 53*(19), 50–53.

Tomasello, M. (1999). *The cultural origins of human cognition*. Cambridge, MA: Harvard University Press.

Tomasello, M. (2005). *Constructing a language: A usage-based theory of language acquisition*. Cambridge, MA: Harvard University Press.

Tomasello, M. (2008). *Origins of human communication*. Cambridge, MA: MIT Press.

Tomasello, M. (2014). *A natural history of human thinking*. Cambridge, MA: Harvard University Press.

Tulving, E. (1972). Episodic and semantic memory. In E. Tulving & W. Donaldson (Eds.), *Organization of memory* (pp. 382–403). New York: Academic Press.

Tulving, E. (1983). *Elements of episodic memory*. New York: Oxford University Press.

Tulving, E. (1985a). How many memory systems are there? *American Psychologist, 40*, 385–398.

Tulving, E. (1985b). Memory and consciousness. *Canadian Psychology, 26*, 1–12.

Tulving, E. (2002a). Milestones in cognitive neuroscience. An interview. In M. Gazzaniga, R. B. Ivry, & G. R. Mangum (Eds.), *Cognitive neuroscience: The biology of the mind* (2nd ed.) (pp. 322–323). New York & London: Norton.

Tulving, E. (2002b). Episodic memory: From mind to brain. *Annual Review of Psychology, 53*, 1–25.

Tulving, E. (2005). Episodic memory and autonoesis: Uniquely human? In H. S. Terrace & J. Metcalfe (Eds.), *The missing link in cognition* (pp. 4–56). New York & Oxford: Oxford University Press.

Tulving, E. (2007). Are there 256 different kinds of memory? In J. S. Nairne (Ed.), *The foundations of remembering* (pp. 39–52). New York: Psychology Press.

Tulving, E., & Kim, A. S. N. (2009). Autonoetic consciousness. In T. Bayne, A. Cleeremans, & P. Wilken (Eds.), *The Oxford companion to consciousness* (pp. 96–98). Oxford & New York: Oxford University Press.

Turkle, S. (2011). *Alone together: Why we expect more from technology and less from each other*. New York: Basic Books.

Ungerer, F. (2007). Iconic text strategies: Path, sorting and weighting, kaleidoscope. In E. Tabakowska, C. Ljungberg, & O. Fischer (Eds.), *Insistent images: Iconicity in language and literature* (pp. 229–245). Amsterdam, Netherlands & Philadelphia, PA: John Benjamins.

Valsiner, J. (2012). *A guided science: History of psychology in the mirror of its making*. New Brunswig, NJ: Transaction Publishers.

Valsiner, J. V. (2007). *Culture in minds and societies*. Los Angeles, CA: Sage.

van Fraassen, B. (1991). Time in physical and in narrative structure. In J. Bender & D. E. Wellbery (Eds.), *Chronotypes: The construction of time* (pp. 19–37). Stanford, CA: Stanford University Press.

Veale, K. (2004). Online memorialisation: The web as a collective memorial landscape for remembering the dead. *Fibreculture, 3*. Retrieved from http://journal.fibreculture.org/issue3/issue3_veale.html

Vernant, J.-P. (2006). *Myth and thought among the Greeks*. New York: Zone Books. (Original work published 1965.)

Vu, N., & Brockmeier, J. (2003). Human experience and narrative intelligibility. In N. Stephenson, H. L. Radtke, R. Jorna, & H. J. Stam (Eds.), *Theoretical psychology: Critical contributions* (pp. 455–466). Toronto, ON: Captus University Publications.

Vygotsky, L. S. (1978). *Mind in society: The development of higher psychological processes*. Cambridge, MA: Harvard University.

Wagoner, B. (2012). Culture in constructive remembering. In J. Valsiner (Ed.), *Oxford handbook of culture and psychology* (pp. 1034–1055). Oxford & New York: Oxford University Press.

Walsh, D. (1969). *Literature and knowledge*. Middletown, CT: Wesleyan University Press.

Walsh, R. (2011). The common basis of narrative and music: Somatic, social, and affective foundations. *Storywords: A Journal of Narrative Studies, 3*, 49–72.

Wang, J. M. (2008). *When "I" was born: Women's autobiography in modern China*. Madison, WI: University of Wisconsin Press.

Wang, Q. (2013). *The autobiographical self in time and culture*. Oxford & New York: Oxford University Press.

Wang, Q., & Brockmeier, J. (2002). Autobiographical remembering as cultural practice: Understanding the interplay between memory, self, and culture. *Culture & Psychology, 8*(1), 45–64.

Watson, J. (1993). Toward an anti-metaphysics of autobiography. In R. Folkenflik (Ed.), *The culture of autobiography* (pp. 57–79). Stanford, CA.: Stanford University Press.

Watt, I. (1996). *Myth of modern individualism: Faust, Don Quixote, Don Juan, Robinson Crusoe*. Cambridge, UK: Cambridge University Press.

Weber, R. (2003). Die fantastische befragt die pedantische Genauigkeit. Zu den Abbildungen in W. G. Sebalds Werken. *Text + Kritik, 158* [Special issue on W. G. Sebald], 63–75.

Weinrich, H. (2004). *Lethe: The art and critique of forgetting*. Ithaca, NY: Cornell University Press.

Weinstein, D., & Weinstein, M. A. (1993). *Postmodern(ized) Simmel*. London: Routledge.

Weintraub, K. J. (1978). *The value of the individual: Self and circumstance in autobiography*. Chicago, IL: University of Chicago Press.

Weiten, T., & Wolf, B. (Eds.) (2012). *Gewalt der Archive: Studien zur Kulturgeschichte der Wissensspeicherung* [The violence of the archives: Studies in the cultural history of knowledge repository]. Konstanz, Germany: Konstanz University Press.

Wertsch, J. V. (1998). *Mind as action*. New York: Oxford University Press.

Wertsch, J. V. (2007). Mediation. In H. Daniels, M. Cole, & J. V. Wertsch (Eds.), *The Cambridge companion to Vygotsky* (pp. 178–192). New York: Cambridge University Press.

Wertsch, J. V. (2009). Collective memories. In P. Boyer & J.V. Wertsch (Eds.), *Memory in mind and culture* (pp. 117–137). New York: Cambridge University Press.

Wertsch, J. V. (2011). Beyond the archival model of memory and the affordances and constraints of narratives. *Culture Psychology 17*(1), 21–29.

Whittaker, S., Kalnikaite, V., Petrelli, D., Bergman, O., Clough, P., & Brockmeier, J. (2012). Socio-technical lifelogging: Deriving design principles for a future proof digital past. *Human Computer Interaction 27*(1–2) [Special issue on "Designing for personal memories: Past, present, and future"], 37–52.

Williams, B. (2009). Life as narrative. *European Journal of Philosophy, 17*(2), 305–314.

Wilson, A., & Ross, M. (2003). The identity function of autobiographical memory: Time is on our side. *Memory, 11*(2), 137–149.

Wilson, R. A. (1995). *Cartesian psychology and physical minds: Individualism and the sciences of the mind*. Cambridge, UK: Cambridge University Press.

Winter, J. (2000). The generation of memory: Reflections on the memory boom in contemporary historical studies. *Bulletin of the German Historical Institute, 27*, 69–92.

Winter, J. (2006). *Remembering war: The Great War between memory and history in the twentieth century.* New Haven, CT: Yale University Press.

Winter, J. (2008). Sites of memory and the shadow of war. In A. Erll & A. Nünning (Eds.), *Cultural memory studies: An international and interdisciplinary handbook* (pp. 61–74). Berlin & New York: de Gruyter.

Wittgenstein, L. (1984). *Vermischte Bemerkungen. Werkausgabe Vol. 8.* Frankfurt am Main: Suhrkamp.

Wittgenstein, L. (2009). *Philosophical investigations* (4th rev. ed.). Chichester, UK: Wiley-Blackwell. (Original work published 1953.)

Wixted, J. T. (2004). The psychology and neuroscience of forgetting. *Annual Review of Psychology, 55,* 235–269.

Wood, J. (2008). *How fiction works.* New York: Farrar, Straus & Giroux

Wood, M. (2005). *Literature and the taste of knowledge.* Cambridge, UK & New York: Cambridge University Press.

Woolf, V. (1954). *A writer's diary.* New York: Harcourt, Brace and Company.

Wu, Pei-Yi (1990). *The Confucian's progress: Autobiographical writings in traditional China.* Princeton, NJ: Princeton University Press.

Wu, T. (2010). *The master switch: The rise and fall of information empires.* New York: Knopf.

Wundt, W. (1900–1920). *Völkerpsychologie: Eine Untersuchung der Entwicklungsgesetze von Sprache, Mythos und Sitte, 10 vols.* [Cultural psychology: An investigation into the laws of development of language, myth, and custom.]. Leipzig, Germany: Engelmann.

Yamada, Y., & Kato, Y. (2006a). Directionality of development and the Ryoko model. *Culture and Psychology, 12,* 260–272.

Yamada, Y., & Kato, Y. (2006b). Images of circular time and spiral repetition: The generative life cycle model. *Culture & Psychology, 12,* 143–160.

Yates, F. (1966). *The art of memory.* London: Routledge and Kegan Paul.

Young, J. E. (1993). *The texture of memory: Holocaust memorials and meaning.* New Haven, CT: Yale University Press.

Young, J. E. (2008). The texture of memory: Holocaust memorials in history. In A. Erll & A. Nünning (Eds.), *Cultural memory studies: An international and interdisciplinary handbook* (pp. 357–365). Berlin & New York: de Gruyter.

Young, M. (1988). *The metronomic society: Natural rhythms and human time-tables.* London: Thames and Hudson.

Zahavi, D. (2007). Self and other: The limits of narrative understanding. *Royal Institute of Philosophy Supplement, 60* [Thematic issue on "Narrative and understanding persons"], 179–202.

Zalewski, D. (2009, February 23). The background hum: Ian McEwan's art of unease. *The New Yorker, 23,* 46–61.

Zemon Davis, N. (1995). *Women on the margins: Three seventeenth-century lives.* Cambridge, MA: Harvard University Press.

Zerubavel, E. (2003). *Time maps: Collective memory and the social shape of the past.* Chicago, IL: University of Chicago Press.

Zunshine, L. (2006). *Why we read fiction: Theory of the mind and the novel.* Columbus, OH: Ohio State University Press.

INDEX

"n" indicates material in endnotes.

"distributed memory," 60
Djikic, M., 145
Douglas, Mary, 222–23
Draaisma, Douwe, 66, 73, 79, 80, 86
Draguhn, Andreas, 57, 332n.10
Dudai, Yadin, 55, 92, 332n.10
durée, 264
dynamic nominalism, 318, 320

Eakin, Paul John, 103, 143, 177,
 190–91, 252, 333n.10
East Cree language, 1
Eaton, Winnifred, 240
Ebbinghaus, Hermann, 5, 11, 73,
 78–79, 81, 94
écriture, 94
Edelman, G., 56, 93
Edwards, Derek, 122, 198–200
Edwards, John, 173
Einstein, Albert, 51, 260, 261, 264, 272–74
Elgin, Catherine, 42
Elias, Norbert, 229
Emigrants, The (Sebald), 289
emotional function of language, 211–12
emotions, 49, 266
encoding. *See also* inscription
 brain imaging of, 329n.3
 challenging, 330–31n.1
 and compost heap metaphor, 92
 computer disk drive analogy for,
  9, 56–58
 consensus on process of, 6–7
 vs. consolidation/reconsolidation of
  memories, 328n.10
 in episodic memory, 154
 historical perspective on, 71, 74
 neurophysiological activities
  associated with, 47, 55, 58
 and "retrieval-induced"
  forgetting, 136
 in semantic memory, 154
 in systems model, 154
Ender, E., 277
England, 34, 227, 293, 313
engrams, 55–57, 92, 332n.10, 334n.15.
 See also long-term memory
Enlightenment, European, 77,
 221, 223
enterprise cultures, 222–23
episodic memory

and Augustine's memories, 162
and autobiographical memory,
 150, 162
based on information processing
 paradigm, 163
classification of, 149
and consciousness, 188
encoding, storing, and retrieval
 in, 154
and future thought, 327–28n.9
imagistic content of, 162, 166
interviews on, 334n.13
morphing and transformative nature
 of, 40–41
neurophysiological activities
 associated with, 48, 327n.8
in *Saturday*, 152
vs. semantic, 6, 148
sensory information stored in,
 334n.15
time travel with, 260
episteme framework, 74–78, 176,
 219–20, 224–25, 316
Erll, Astrid, 30
Eshel, Amir, 289, 300, 304
ethnographic studies of memory,
 197–202
evolutionary framework, 65–66,
 72, 74, 76
experiencing/experience
 actual events, and invented
  memories, 52
 Benjamin on, 329n.4
 in brain, site of, 333n.11
 color of our, 104, 109
 complex, 105–18
 in consciousness, 166
 creation/re-creation in, 109
 feelings associated with events, 49
 and identity construction, 173–74
 vs. imagining, 49, 55
 interpretability of complex,
  106, 114–17
 James (Henry) on, 166
 James (William) on, 140
 language and complex,
  105–9, 329n.8
 meaning-making in, 105
 and narrative, 103–18, 195, 248,
  329n.6, 333n.12

forgetting (*Cont.*)
  as creative ongoing open
    processes, viii
  cultural approach to, 61, 316
  darkness in, 89
  digital media impact on, 39
  Freud's approach to, 142, 330n.1
  global practices of, 95
  historical frameworks for, 66–70,
    72–73, 75–78
  on Lethe river, 98, 259
  in literature and art, 42–43
  Loftus & Loftus on theories of, 7–8
  mnemonic silence in, 135–36
  narrative in, 275–78
  neurophysiological activities
    associated with, 47
  Nietzsche on, 331n.6
  nonsubstantialist conceptions of, 64
  palimpsestic quality of, 69
  power and, in "structural
    amnesia," 249
  Proust on, 269
  and remembering in autobiographical
    process, 137
  resistance to and subversion of
    forced, 250
  "retrieval-induced," 136
  in Sebald's *Austerlitz*, 290
  as sins, 10, 55, 94, 115, 137
  as social activity, 308
  social and political changes
    impacting, 31, 35
  temporality of, 139
  unconscious, link to, 142
Foster, J. K., 9
Foucault, Michel, 34, 74, 76–77, 220,
  223–25, 228, 317–21, 338n.1
Frank, Arthur, 104
Frankland, P. W., 328n.10
free direct thought, 160, 264
free indirect speech, 135, 137, 159
free indirect thought, 160
Freeman, Mark, 104, 106,
  146, 253–54
Freud, Sigmund, 69, 98, 138, 142, 193,
  330n.1, 331n.10, 335n.3
Fuchs, Anne, 300
functional magnetic resonance imaging
  (fMRI), 6, 146, 329n.3

Gadamer, Hans-Georg, 109, 116–17,
  176, 329n.8
Gazzaniga, M. S., 333n.11
Geertz, Clifford, 59–60, 202,
  223, 231–32
Genette, G., 268, 297–98, 304, 336n.6
Georgakopoulou, Alexandra, 178,
  182–83, 198
Gerber, David, 235
Germany, 31, 32, 227
Geschichte der Autobiographie
  (Misch), 186
Gibson, James, 164
Giddens, Anthony, 190
glacier metaphor, 93
Gleick, James, 326n.2
God, remembered by, 226–27
Goethe, Johann Wolfgang, 331n.10
Goffman, Erving, 182
Goldie, Peter, 164
Goodman, Nelson, 123
Gordon, Milton, 241
Göttingen School, 73
Gould, Stephen Jay, 318
Greece, culture of literacy in, 67
Greimas, Algirdas, 130
The Guardian, 87–88, 131
Guatemala, 31
Gubrium, J. F., 198
Gulf War, 15
Gusdorf, Georges, 186
gwei, 251

Habermas, Jürgen, 19
habitual memory, 152–53
Hacking, Ian, 3–4, 5, 27, 42,
  221–23, 316–22
Halbwachs, Maurice, 16, 30–31, 39, 94,
  230, 265, 326n.1
Hardy, Thomas, 262
Harré, Rom, 121, 122, 137–38, 252
Harris, Roy, 40
Hart, Francis, 333n.9
Harvey, William, 80–81, 86, 328–29n.3
Havel, Václav, 31
Havelock, Eric, 67
Hayles, N. Katherine, 36
Haynes, John-Dylan, 88
Head, Dominic, 130
Hebb, Donald, 332n.10

identity construction/formation (*Cont.*)
  narrative hermeneutics of, 14,
    180–81, 191–92
  narrator in, 102
  with neurotrauma, 203–4
  postautobiographical perspective on,
    217–18, 308
  poststructuralist arguments
    on, 34–35
  pragmatism on, 200
  reading in, 174–75
  self-exploration in, 43
  self-interpretations in, 138
  sense of self in, 129, 337n.10
  and social and political power, 178
  temporality in, 190, 205, 277, 305
  transcendent model of Western, 333n.9
  Tulving on, 188–89
illness narratives, 111–12, 172, 205
imagery, 161–67
imaginary, narrative theory of, 120–21
imagining, 48–55, 165, 266, 301,
  327nn.7–9
imperatives, 211
implicit memory, 149, 152–54. *See also*
  nondeclarative memory
"In a no man's land of memories and
  loss" (Kakutani), 286–87
individualism, 224–25, 229, 236, 237,
  334n.17
individualist cultures, 225
individualist identity, 181, 188, 309
individualist memory, 57, 221,
  225, 229–33
individualist mind, 126, 189, 230
individualist time, 52
individuality, 25, 186–87, 228, 237–38,
  241, 335n.3
individual memory
  appreciation of, 227
  brain as location of, 2, 7
  and collective memory, 39, 200–201,
    229–33, 254–55, 334n.18, 335n.3
  confounding of, with digital
    media, 36
  construction of, 16
  and cultural memory, 160–61,
    200–201, 229–33, 238,
    334n.18, 335n.2
  experimental study of, 115

in Sebald's *Austerlitz*, 291
and social memory, 200–201,
  229–33, 334n.18, 335nn.2–3
social networks and making
  of, 38–39
of traumatic pasts, 15–16, 32
individual time, 52, 261–62
information processing model
  archive metaphor in, 9
  for autobiographical memory, 11, 148
  and biological universalism, 6
  computational, 11, 57, 148
  shift from, 5–6, 325n.3
  and systems model, 6,
    148–50, 331n.9
  Tulving's model based on, 163
inner discourses, 142, 200–201
Inouye, Daniel K., 335n.5, 335n.7
inscription, 68–71, 74, 82, 91, 93. *See
  also* encoding
installations
  Census, 27, 311–16
  at London's Homerton University
    Hospital, 4–5, 325n.1
  storehouse metaphor in creation of, 5
intentionality, 61, 110, 173, 279–80,
  283, 334n.17
intentions, 9, 37, 57, 87–88, 122, 279
internalized life story, 138
Internet, 38–40, 94–96, 227, 266,
  326nn.2–3
interpretation
  of artworks, 315
  of autobiographical memory, 38,
    114–15, 323
  in autobiographical process, 137
  vs. autonoetic consciousness, 48
  changing frameworks for, 168
  of complex experiences, 106,
    114–17, 175
  in connective memory, 39
  independence of memories
    from, 98–99
  narrative framework for, 173, 197
  neurophysiological activities
    associated with, 48, 327n.8
  in perception, 48
  vs. pure memory, 23
  during recall, 98, 193
  by self (*see* self-interpretation)

temporalization of, 50–51, 110, 261
for understanding events, 120
of what it's all about, 141
interpretive communities, 116
intertextualism, 34
invented memories, 52, 54
invention, 68
involuntary memory, 258–59,
269–71, 282
Iser, Wolfgang, 120–21
Islam, 226

Jakobson, Roman, 210–14, 334n.20
James, Henry, 166, 172
James, William, 24, 139–41, 163,
331n.5, 331–32n.10
Japan, 52
Japanese Nightingale, A (Eaton), 240
jazz performance metaphor, 92
Johnson, Marcia, 327n.8
Joyce, James, 43, 103, 131, 262, 286
Judaism, 226
Judt, Tony, 31–32

Kafka, Franz, 262, 286, 287, 331n.4
Kakutani, Michiko, 286–87
Kandel, Eric R., 81, 325n.3
Kantian philosophy, 104, 274
Kermode, F., 117
Kern, Stephen, 263–65, 336n.3
Kiefer, Anselm, 27, 309, 311–16
Kilbourn, R. J. A., 292–93
knowledge
archeology of, 317
and autobiographical identity, 224
and autobiographical memory, 162
in Benjamin's concept of the
now, 338n.4
in epistemological nominalism, 60
and experiential memory, 109, 149
in experimental psychology, 78
Foucault's unity of power and, 77,
220, 224–25, 317
through literature, 112
"memory cue" for activation of, 196
as mirror, 202–3
in semantic memory, 148, 334n.15
stories intertwined with, 165
storing (*see* storehouse metaphor)
temporal, 260

Korsgaard, Christine, 173
Koselleck, R., 338n.1
Krebs, Hans, 9
Krog, Antjie, 252
Kronos, 313

Lacan, Jacques, 138
Lambeck, Michael, 20, 35
Landy, J., 270
language
action orientation of, 122–23, 125
autobiographical meanings and
resources of, 45, 205
in autobiographical memory, 194
Bakhtin's conception of, 201
Bühler's psychology of, 212
and complex experiences,
105–9, 329n.8
computer-based digital literacy and
understanding, 42
and contextualist vs. individualist
approaches to time, 52
creation of realities through,
99, 122–23
in cultural semiosphere, 61
and culture, 321
with dementia, 205
development of, 197
as epiphenomenon, 195
evolutionary framework for, 65–66
formalist philosophy of, 338n.2
functions of, 202–3, 209–16, 337n.2
and identity construction, 173,
205, 332n.1
and images, 161–67
independence of memories
from, 98–99
inherent polyphony of, 159
intersubjective nature of, 209–16
mind and, 197, 230
philosophy of Wittgenstein, 62
Plato on, 212
as psychological tool, 106
realist view of, 202
reality effect of, 166
and recall, 98, 162, 194
representational view of,
202–3, 209–12
and self-understanding, 173
sound dimension of, 213

language (*Cont.*)
  structuralist philosophy of, 102, 338n.2
  and thoughts, 330n.1
  as transparent, 166
  Wittgenstein's philosophy of, 62
  writing framework for, 66–72
Lashley, Karl, 332n.10
lead, 311–15
learning, 11, 77–78, 230
Leibniz, Gottfried Wilhelm, 274, 337n.8
Les Lieux de Mémoire (Nora), 16, 325n.6
Lethe (river of forgetfulness), 98, 259
Lévinas, Emanuel, 329n.8
Li, Yiyun, 246–47
library metaphor, 68–71
lieux de mémoire, 33–34
Life as narrative (Bruner), 173, 322
lifeblogs, 39
lifelogging, 95–96
life stories, 173–75, 180, 195
life writing. *See also* autobiographical narratives
  of Asian Americans, 242
  autobiographical self-resolution in, 76, 144
  and cultural constructions of memory, 275
  diversity of forms in, 224
  identity construction in, 44, 143
  illness narratives, 111–12, 172, 205
  of immigrants, 234–35
  of modernists and postmodernists, 43
  narrative in, 103, 143
  to negotiate group membership, 228
  self-defining memories in, 138
  self in, 44, 143
  on storehouse metaphor, 44
  temporal self-localization in, 275, 278–79
  themes in, 44
  on what-it-is-like, 106, 110–14, 116, 119, 122, 145
Linde, Charlotte, 228
Lindemann Nelson, Hilde, 174, 177, 179
Ling, Amy, 240–41, 251
linguistic mode, 14, 160, 168
literacy, 67–69, 144, 145

literary and artistic domain, 42–46
literary modernism. *See* modernist literature
literary narratives, 46, 100, 120, 125–26
literary pragmatism, 160
literary theory, 100–101, 139
literature
  and autobiographical process, 99–101, 143
  Chinese, 237–38, 243
  forgetting and remembering in, 42–44
  as "form of lived experience," 112
  imagery in, 161–67
  knowledge through, 112
  landscape of consciousness in, 130, 157, 279
  McEwan on science and, 130
  modernist (*see* modernist literature)
  postmodernist, 43, 103, 125, 174–75, 253–54, 268
  realist, 102, 166, 262, 337n.2
  in self-interpretation, 120
  structuralists on, 100
  substantialization of memory in, 63
Lloyd, Genevieve, 270
Locke, John, 187–91, 193, 202, 216–18, 220–24, 253
Lodge, David, 42
Loftus, E. F. and G. R., 7–8
long-term memory. *See also* engrams
  "activation" of, 196
  borderline between short-term and, 149
  declarative (*see* declarative memory)
  episodic (*see* episodic memory)
  explicit, 149, 152–54, 163
  measurability of, 163
  models of (*see* information processing model; systems model)
  neurophysiological activities associated with, 328n.10
  phoenix metaphor for, 92
  retention time of, 148–49
  semantic (*see* semantic memory)
  storehouse metaphor for, 55, 58, 92
Lotman, Iuri, 52
Lowe, Pardee, 335n.6
Luria, Alexander R., 141, 147–48, 151

MacIntyre, Alasdair, 173, 175, 176
magnetoencephalography
    (MEG), 329n.3
Mandler, J. M., 334n.15
Mann, Thomas, 43, 103, 166, 262
Mansfield Park (Austen), 63
Marking the mind (Danziger), 64–66
martyrs, 226
Matsuda, Matt, 330n.12
Matz, Jesse, 268
McAdams, Dan, 195
McCrone, John, 10
McDermott, K. B., 328n.9
McEwan, Ian
    narrative strategies of, 130
    psychology of protagonists in works
        of, 130
    on real world details in
        Saturday, 331n.3
    Saturday, 24, 129–68, 248–49,
        264, 338n.3
    work-shadowing
        neurosurgeon, 331n.2
McGinn, Colin, 53
McKim, Elizabeth, 174–76
McTaggart, John, 50–51, 261
Mead, George Herbert, 200, 326n.1
Medved, Maria, 178, 203
memorialization, 16, 31
"memories of the future," 49, 327n.9
memory. *See also* remembering
    absence of, 89
    "activation" of, 196
    as an arbiter of truth and
        authenticity, 16
    archetype of, 71, 72
    as associative, 93
    autobiographical (*see*
        autobiographical memory)
    as biological entity (*see*
        substantialization of memory)
    categorizing/classification of, 21
    coherence of, 15
    collective (*see* collective memory)
    communicative, 335n.2
    connective, 39, 95
    conceptions of content of, 6, 207
    consolidation/reconsolidation of,
        328n.10
    contextualist, 57

continuity of, 15, 54
conversions of, 115–16
cultural (*see* cultural memory)
declarative (*see* declarative memory)
distorted, 10, 36, 54
"distributed," 60
ecological, 95
elusiveness of, 1–5
episodic memory (*see* episodic
    memory)
epistemology of, 154
ethical status of, 15–16
experiential, 109, 149
"extended," 60
false, 54
formation of, 318
frameworks for, 65–78, 316–17
habitual, 152–53
Hacking's historical epistemology of,
    3–4, 27
historical, 16, 33
"iconic," 149
implicit, 149, 152–54
individual (*see* individual memory)
individualist, 57, 221, 225, 229–33
in information theory, 326n.2
intergenerational, 294
intertextualist arguments on, 34–35
invented, 52, 54
involuntary, 258–59, 269–71, 282
and learning, 11, 77–78
long-term (*see* long-term memory)
malleability of, 4, 17, 36, 54
as meaning constructions, 34–35, 45,
    50, 136
mechanical theory of, 57, 136
mixed, of immigrants, 234–42
models of, 147–48
modernist literature vs. traditional
    view of, 43–45
of "momentous events," 138, 197
moral weight of, 15–16
"morphing" of, 95
mutability of, 36, 41
as a natural kind, 3, 6, 8, 23, 60,
    80, 84, 90
nonconscious, 152–53
nondeclarative, 149, 152–53, 155
ontology of, 3–4, 15, 26–27,
    154, 316–17

social, 153, 308
mnemonic silence, 135–36, 142
mnemonic values, 74, 77
Mnemosyne, 68–69, 85, 313
mnemosyne, 67, 69
model, 14, 147, 328n.1
modernism. *See also* modernity
   in autobiographical time's
     development, 267–68
   and culture of autobiography, 267
   literature (*see* modernist literature)
   melancholia of, 291
   memory research and, 231, 261
   myths of, 236
   and narrative practices, 103
   as a social and cultural
     movement, 336n.3
   time in, 261–66
modernist literature. *See also*
    postmodernist literature
   on autobiographical identity, 45
   on individualist memory, 231
   lived practices as, 174–75, 268
   narrative techniques in, 44, 103, 125
   self-examination in, 43–45
   simultaneity in, 266–67, 270,
     276, 280–83
   strategies and techniques of, 131
   time in, 261–84
   on urbanization, 336n.2
modernity. *See also* postmodernity
   autobiographical self-exploration in,
     43, 227–28
   discourse of, on problems and
     crises of, 19
   dissolving of traditions and
     certainties in, 18
   identity construction with, 228–29
   "liquid," from globalization, 234–35
   mnemonic continuity of, 16
   myths of, 236
   organization of continuity in, 19
   personal identity, challenge to, 235
   simultaneity in, 266–67
   Western vs. Occidental rationalism
     in, 18–19
Montaigne, Michel de, 43, 331n.10
Moore, Gordon, 326n.2
Mrs Dalloway (Woolf), 131
Mühlhäusler, P., 252

Müller, Günter, 299
multiple personality disorder, 221
Munn, Nancy, 64
Murakami, Kyoko, 156
musical performance metaphor, 92–93
music and narrative, 213
Musil, Robert, 43
MySpace, 38–39
myths
   American, during WWII, 240–41
   in ancient Greek society, 67–69
   vs. autobiographical narratives, 248
   Census and, 313
   Chinese, in *The Woman Warrior*, 244,
     248–49, 251
   cultural creation of, 2
   of individuality, 236
   of Lethe, 98
   meaning-making with, 273
   of modernity, 236
   personal, self-narratives as, 195

Nabokov, Vladimir, 43, 44, 103
Nalbantian, Suzanne, 43, 275
narrated time, 110, 299–300
narrative. *See also* stories
   in academic memory research,
     334n.13
   action orientation of, 125–26, 178
   affective mode, 14, 160, 168
   affective potential of, 213
   agency, 176–80, 191, 217
   as alternative metaphor for
     memory, 91
   anachronies, 157, 297–98
   anthropological argument for, 121
   Aristotelian idea of, 102, 125
   and artworks, 315
   autobiographical (*see*
     autobiographical narratives)
   in autobiographical process, 20,
     99–102, 156–61, 168, 200, 308
   Bruner's narrative psychology, 196,
     279, 330n.1
   cognitive mode, 14, 160, 168
   in cognitive psychology, 195, 199,
     334n.15
   collaboration on, 206–9, 334n.19
   consciousness, 139
   "consciousness factor" in, 112

narrative (*Cont.*)
for contextualizing, 40
as culturally-mediated psychological
activity, 106
cultural models of, 322–23
digital media impact on, 40
embodied engagement with,
208–9, 213
emotions in, 211
enactment model, 148, 153–56, 331n.8
as epiphenomenon, 195, 199
experience (*see* narrative experience)
fictional (*see* fictional narratives)
fine-tuning, 211–12
first-person (*see* first-person
narrative)
functions of, 85
"grammar," 337n.2
hermeneutics (*see* narrative
hermeneutics)
hindsight in, 146, 185
historical traditions of, 330n.15
identity (*see* narrative identity)
illness, 111–12, 172, 205
imagination, 119–21, 123, 166, 177
"intelligibility," 236
"interior monologue," 264
as interpretive framework, 173
intersubjective nature of, 113
investigative framework for, 179
Labov's structural analysis of, 198
as language form, 13–14, 51
light/dark in, 87–89
linear sequences of action in, 268
linguistic mode, 14, 160, 168
literary, 46, 100, 120, 125–26
meaning-making in, 105, 160
and metaphor, 85–89, 101
as method, 101–2
mimetic function of, 337n.2
mind-creating and mind-representing
forms of, 43–44, 126
as model, 14, 147
in neurocognitive psychology, 195
nonfictional, 26, 41, 125, 248,
289–90, 333n.10
nonlinear, 268
options for, 177
perspectives in, 158–60
polychronic, 267–68, 304

postclassical understanding of,
124–27, 160
realist conventions for, 102
realist view of, 202
representational view of, 202–3
rhetorical devices in, 161
Ricoeur on, 85
second-person, 159–60, 212
sequentiality in, 40, 287, 298
seriality in, 40
social development through, 196
strong (*see* strong narrative thesis)
synthesis, 168
in systems model, 194–95
third-person, 135, 159, 191
thought presentation in, 160
time, 271–79, 298–300, 304
tonal and rhythmic aspects of, 213
"transparency," 166
worldmaking by, 123, 126–27
and writing, 145–47
Narrative and Identity (Brockmeier &
Carbaugh), 332–33n.3
narrative enactment model, 148,
153–56, 331n.8
narrative experience
Carr on, 329n.6
core qualities of, 103–18
Herman on, 330n.9
personality psychology on, 195
primordial level of, 333n.12
in stream of consciousness, 139–40
narrative hermeneutics
of autobiographical
remembering, 20
of autobiographical
self-understanding, 14
of experiencing, 51–52, 105, 107
of fiction, 125
of historical stories, 330n.12
of identity construction, 14,
180–81, 191–92
temporalization of, 51–52, 261
narrative identity
agency in, 176–80
with Alzheimer's disease, 205–18
and autobiographical memory, 323
in autobiographical process, 180–81,
183–84, 199–200, 203–4,
209–10, 218

Swedish Center for Dementia Research
(CEDER), 206, 334n.19
synecdoche, 161
systems model
for autobiographical memory, 11–12,
148–54, 194
for autobiographical process
examination, 148–55
brain imaging support for, 6, 7, 148
and information processing model, 6,
148–50, 331n.9
interconnections in, 8, 150
vs. narrative enactment model,
148, 153–54
narrative in, 194–95
quantitative measurability of, 155, 163
storehouse metaphor in, 7–9
Szondi, Peter, 281–83
Szpunar, K. K., 328n.9
Szymborska, Wislawa, 110

Taoist literary traditions, 238
Taylor, Charles, 43, 117–18, 173, 190,
229, 254, 338n.1
Taylor, Stephanie, 236–37
technological and media domain, 35–42
television, 166
temporality. *See also* time
in autobiographical process, 26, 123,
139, 261, 267–84, 304
biological vs. human, 337n.7
in consciousness, 190
contextualist vs. individualist, 52
derivative and phenomenological
forms of, 336n.1
of experiences, 50–51, 106, 109–10
"fuzzy," 304
human, 273, 337n.7
in identity construction, 190, 205,
277, 305
in narrative, levels of analysis
of, 297–98
in Proust's *Recherche*, 262,
270, 282–83
of remembering, 139, 257–61, 264
and urbanization, 266
temporalization
of autobiographical remembering, 52
individual and historical processes
of, 308

of interpretation, 50–51, 110, 261
material and symbolic aids for, 273
McTaggart's forms of, 50–51, 261
meaning-making process in, 268–69,
273–74, 277–79
narrative hermeneutics of, 51–52, 261
in Proust's *Recherche*, 268–69, 280
in Sebald's *Austerlitz*, 287
Terdiman, Richard, 18
testimony, 32–33
Theaetetus (Plato), 69, 85
theory of mind, 49, 327n.9
Theresienstadt, 293–303
third person narrative, 135, 159, 191
Thomas, Keith, 34
thought report, 160
Thousand Years of Good Prayers, A (Yiyun
Li), 247
time. *See also* temporality *and*
temporalization
absolutist account of, 262–64, 274
Aristotle on, 259
autobiographical (*see*
autobiographical time)
in autobiographical identity, 190
in autobiographical memory, 52
autobiographical self in, 305
Benjamin's concept of the now,
301–2, 338n.4
cognitive psychology on, 259
and collective memory, 265
contextualist, 52
as cultural and historical
constructions, 52, 263, 272
derivative and phenomenological
forms of, 336n.1
discourse (*see* discourse time)
economics and, 263
Einsteinian model of, 51, 264, 272–74
existential root of our sense of, 51
in fairy tales and folktales, 268
flux of (*see* durée)
individual, 52, 261–62
localizing experiences in, 50
McTaggert's "unreality of time,"
51, 261
in modernist literature, 261–84
narrated, 110, 299–300
narrative, 271–79, 298–300, 304
Newtonian (*see* Newtonian time)

Vertigo (Sebald), 289
Vietnamese fables and tales, 236
Vietnam War, 15
visual memory, 12, 48, 66, 164
"vital" memories, 138
vocatives, 211
Vu, Nhi, 236, 248
Vygotsky, Lev, 36, 65, 106–08, 142,
     196–97, 209–11, 216, 326n.1,
     329n.7, 330n.1

Wagner, D., 325n.3
Wagoner, B., 91
Walsh, Dorothy, 112
Walsh, Richard, 213
Wang, Qi, 238, 323
Watson, Julia, 186–87
Watt, Ian, 236
Weber, Max, 18–19
Weinrich, Harald, 70, 89, 98
Weintraub, Karl Joachim, 333n.9
Wellbery, David, 274
what-it-is-like quality of stories, 106,
     110–14, 116, 119, 122, 145
White, S. H., 196
Whitehead, A., 32
Wikipedia, 38–39, 40
Wilde, Oscar, 322
Winter, Jay, 18, 34
witnessing, 16
Wittgenstein, Ludwig, 62, 86, 125,
     164, 178, 209–11, 216, 230, 254,
     321, 338n.2
Woman Warrior, The (Kingston),
     242–55, 335n.8
Wong, Jade Snow, 240, 335n.6
Wood, J., 165
Wood, Michael, 112
Woolf, Virginia, 43, 131, 166, 262, 264,
     278, 286

World War I (WWI), 18
World War II (WWII), 15–16, 32,
     240–41, 291
writing
     in autobiographical
          process, 144–47
     communication framework
          from, 144
     computer-based digital literacy and
          understanding, 42
     consciousness in, 130, 190–91
     Danziger on, 67, 70, 73
     in discursive metaphors for
          remembering, 93–94
     Freud on memory as
          unconscious, 69
     life (see life writing)
     metaphor usage in, 82–83
     and mind, 130, 144, 146
     and narrative, 145–47
     Olson on, 67, 70, 145
     vs. oral storytelling, 145, 207
     palimpsestic quality of, 69, 94
     remembering framework from,
          66–74, 76
     stream of consciousness impact from,
          144, 146
     The Woman Warrior on Chinese vs.
          American, 244–45
Wu, Tim, 326n.3
Wundt, W., 163

Yiyun Li, 246–47
Young, James, 16
YouTube, 38–39, 266

Zalewski, Daniel, 129–30
Zemon Davis, Natalie, 228
zooming, 157
Zucchermaglio, Christina, 201